AIDS, Culture, and Africa

UNIVERSITY PRESS OF FLORIDA

Florida A&M University, Tallahassee
Florida Atlantic University, Boca Raton
Florida Gulf Coast University, Ft. Myers
Florida International University, Miami
Florida State University, Tallahassee
New College of Florida, Sarasota
University of Central Florida, Orlando
University of Florida, Gainesville
University of North Florida, Jacksonville
University of South Florida, Tampa
University of West Florida, Pensacola

AIDS, Culture, and Africa

Edited by Douglas A. Feldman

University Press of Florida
Gainesville/Tallahassee/Tampa/Boca Raton
Pensacola/Orlando/Miami/Jacksonville/Ft. Myers/Sarasota

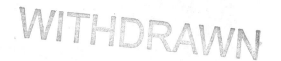

13 12 11 10 09 08   6 5 4 3 2 1

Library of Congress Cataloging-in-Publication Data
AIDS, culture, and Africa / edited by Douglas A. Feldman.
p. ; cm.
Includes bibliographical references and index.
ISBN 978-0-8130-3253-5 (alk. paper)
1. AIDS (Disease)—Social aspects—Africa. I. Feldman, Douglas A.
[DNLM: 1. Acquired Immunodeficiency Syndrome—ethnology—
Africa South of the Sahara. 2. Acquired Immunodeficiency Syn-
drome—prevention & control—Africa South of the Sahara.
3. Cultural Characteristics—Africa South of the Sahara. 4. Risk
Assessment—Africa South of the Sahara. 5. Sexual Behavior—
ethnology—Africa South of the Sahara. 6. Socioeconomic Factors—
Africa South of the Sahara. WC 503.7 A28775 2008]
RA643.86.A35A345 2008
362.196'979200968—dc22   2008020122

The author and publisher thank The College at Brockport, State
University of New York, for providing funding assistance.

The University Press of Florida is the scholarly publishing agency
for the State University System of Florida, comprising Florida A&M
University, Florida Atlantic University, Florida Gulf Coast University,
Florida International University, Florida State University, New College of Florida, University of Central Florida, University of Florida,
University of North Florida, University of South Florida, and University of West Florida.

University Press of Florida
15 Northwest 15th Street
Gainesville, FL 32611-2079
http://www.upf.com

In memory of my brother-in-law, Edward Ginsberg (1928–2005)

Contents

Tables

Preface

Kigali, Rwanda, August 1985: I was in the main hospital, Centre Hôpitalier de Kigali, in the Rwandan capital interviewing AIDS patients there to try to find out how they became HIV infected. Back in the United States, most people with AIDS were gay men; but here in Africa, I was being told that most were heterosexual. What in the world was going on? Why should the same disease behave differently in two different places? Maybe, I thought, extreme homophobia was preventing the truth to come out. Perhaps African men were secretly having lots of sex with other men, but no one wanted to talk about it. Or maybe, just maybe, male and female couples were routinely engaging in anal sex in order to prevent pregnancies. So there I was, literally sitting by their deathbeds, ready to stay as long as necessary until I learned from my informants the truth.

Nine of the ten patients were men; most were fairly wealthy men who traveled throughout central Africa on business. After gaining their informed consent, I asked them about their health history and their sex history. Were they having anal sex with their wives or mistresses? All of them insisted that they were not. Were they having sex with another male? Again, they all insisted that they were not. One had confided to me that he often had vaginal sex with female partners even when he had an outbreak of genital herpes. But absolutely no same-sex or heterosexual anal sex behavior.

On my final visit to the hospital, I was told of one last AIDS patient, a woman, on a bed in the rear of the hospital ward. When I approached her, I was startled by what I saw. All skin and bones, her eyes closed, with dozens of flies swirling around her. I thought she had already died. But then she began to stir, her eyes opened, and I introduced myself and told her about the study. With great effort, she managed to sit up, and she agreed to participate. Her face was very gaunt, and her voice was little more than a whisper. And she told me her story.

Rangira (a pseudonym) was thirty-six, Tutsi, a mother of three children. When she started developing AIDS symptoms, her husband began to blame her for becoming infected, and angrily threw her out of the house. The children stayed with the husband and his family, while Rangira had no choice but to return home to her mother. The bitter irony is that Rangira had remained faithful to her husband during their long marriage, and it was her husband who undoubtedly had an extramarital relationship and infected her, though he had not yet developed symptoms.

Over several months, her health continued to deteriorate and her weight continued to drop, until finally she was admitted to the hospital, too weak to walk on her own. She told me how she was shunned by her family, friends, and neighbors, as the word spread that she had AIDS. But as she talked, I was drawn to her quiet sense of dignity, her resolve not to let the disease conquer her spirit, even as it destroyed her body. As she attempted to sit up straight on her hospital bed, she told me how important it was to her to make sure that her health and sexual history that she was giving me was totally accurate. She had never had anal sex; she knew that her husband was seeing other women; and she was a faithful wife and devoted mother.

At the end of the interview, as I was leaving, a reporter for the British Broadcasting Corporation (BBC) was also in the hospital ward covering the then new story about AIDS in Africa. She asked if she could photograph the female patient that I just spoke with outside in the daylight. I told her that the woman was far too ill to be moved or bothered. But when Rangira heard that the reporter wanted to photograph her, she insisted that it happen. With the assistance of one of the nurses, she managed to climb into a wheelchair and was wheeled out to the daylight for her close-up. She wanted to be remembered and for the world to know about her experience, as she solemnly posed for her photo. Within days her photo was broadcast throughout the world. For a time, she became the face of the ravages of AIDS in Africa.

A few days later, as I prepared to leave Rwanda, I wanted to go back to the hospital to say good-bye to Rangira and thank her. But it was too late. I was told that she had died the day after I saw her.

Looking back today, I wonder—given that she and her husband were Tutsi, the main target of the horrific genocide that gripped Rwanda in 1994—whether she would have survived the genocide nine years after her death from AIDS. Did her husband and children survive?

＊   ＊   ＊

The cultural and biological dimensions of HIV/AIDS in sub-Saharan Africa have been analyzed by anthropologists since 1985. Today, dozens of anthropologists are conducting research in Africa, looking at cultural factors that increase the spread of the epidemic, discovering how to most effectively prevent HIV transmission through condom promotion and other safer sex practices, and understanding how African communities are affected by this devastating disease. This volume presents all original, never-before-published chapters by international anthropologists and other social/behavioral scientists who are leaders in this field. It paves the way for a deeper cultural understanding necessary to effectively reverse the catastrophic growth of HIV/AIDS on the African continent.

The volume begins (chapter 1) with a review of the literature on the anthropological contribution to our understanding of HIV/AIDS in Africa. This includes discussions on condoms, HIV prevention campaigns, government involvement, food policy, male circumcision, traditional healers, the role of poverty, AIDS orphans, social and economic consequences, gender inequality, sex workers, the epidemiology of HIV transmission, sex outside marriage, breast-feeding, indigenous AIDS-like illnesses, vaccine trials, voluntary counseling and testing, ethical issues, anthropological research, and policy concerns.

Lee and Susser, in chapter 2, then examine how HIV/AIDS has impacted a traditional foraging community in Namibia. They find that greater gender equality among the Ju/'hoansi may be a factor in the lower HIV rates within that population. Kornfield and Babalola (chapter 3) look at how HIV-positive men and women in Rwanda delay HIV testing and continue to practice unprotected sex long after their diagnoses. For example, some HIV-positive men continue to have sex with sex workers even after their diagnosis so that their friends do not suspect that they are HIV infected, and they get remarried after their wives die. Also, some HIV-positive women engage in sex work to bring in additional money when their husbands are not able to work, and after their husbands die.

Macintyre and Kendall (chapter 4) broadly look at societal-level behavioral change and the importance of social proximity to the epidemic. Brown (chapter 5) discusses the importance of the current research by anthropologists on male circumcision as a possible HIV intervention in Africa. Longfield (chapter 6) focuses on partner categories and risk perceptions in Côte d'Ivoire for future target-specific interventions.

Turning to research by anthropologists in Zambia, Simpson (chapter 7) looks at how ideas of masculinity lead to rejection of condom use and promotes sexual risk-taking. Feldman and colleagues (chapter 8) examine how the stigma of AIDS often results in negative attitudes and a lack of empathy toward persons with AIDS among Zambian high school students. In nearby Namibia, Lorway (chapter 9) looks at how homophobia has led to the neglect of HIV prevention for men who have sex with men throughout much of the continent and how fear of AIDS is allowing antigay African leadership to promote bigotry and hate.

Shifting our attention to Uganda, where the declining HIV rates there have encouraged an American conservative policy of stressing sexual abstinence and partner reduction, and diminishing the role of condoms (the "ABc" Campaign—Abstinence, Be faithful, and a small "c" for a de-emphasized use of condoms), Onjoro (chapter 10) supports the ABc approach, arguing that program failures in Africa and the success in Uganda should lead us to reject condom promotion programs. However, McCombie and Eshel (chapter 11) argue that we need to reinterpret the lower HIV rates for Uganda and examine how language is used in sexual behavior surveys. They believe that the ABc approach should not be applied throughout Africa. Swezey and Teitelbaum (chapter 12), also taking an anti-ABc approach, look at the changing family structure in Uganda and decision making for care seeking and resource use within families with AIDS. Rwabukwali (chapter 13) points out that poverty is not necessarily a risk factor for HIV, since many poor Ugandan women do not engage in multiple sexual practices.

Preston-Whyte (chapter 14) tells us that political economy issues explain HIV patterns in Africa far more than do cultural issues. The conclusion (chapter 15) discusses the political and economic factors that have been turning HIV prevention, care, and treatment in a different, and ultimately alarming, direction, and what might be done to change that.

This volume brings together anthropologists and other social/behavioral scientists to discuss their research and policy issues on HIV/AIDS in Africa. However, it is written primarily for the nonanthropologist, with any anthropological terminology clearly defined. It should be of interest to international health researchers, health policy makers, epidemiologists, health educators, political scientists, sociologists, psychologists, government and nongovernmental organization officials, health practitioners, and many others, as well as medical and applied anthropologists.

Acknowledgments

I would like to thank Jackie Deats, Ashley Heiman, and Jenna Landahl for their assistance with the index, and John Byram, Eli Bortz, and Michele Fiyak-Burkley of the University Press of Florida for their assistance with the production of this book. I would also like to thank The College at Brockport, State University of New York, for funding assistance.

1

AIDS, Culture, and Africa

The Anthropological Perspective

DOUGLAS A. FELDMAN

Since 1985, anthropologists have been making significant contributions to the study of HIV/AIDS in sub-Saharan Africa. Without a steady or consistent source of funding, especially in the earlier years, anthropological research on HIV/AIDS in Africa has informed other major fields, including epidemiology, public health, health education, biomedicine, health policy analysis, and other social and behavioral sciences, for more than two decades. A considerable body of literature has accumulated on HIV/AIDS in Africa, contributing to the overall growth of medical, applied, and public anthropology.

Some of the earlier contributions during the mid and late 1980s by anthropologists focused on the social epidemiology of HIV—the search for sociocultural practices and cofactors that would explain the much higher rate of heterosexual transmission in Africa than in North America and Europe (Bond and Vincent 1996a). That interest of the biomedical community was based less on a concern for the fate of Africa than on a potential fear that the same pattern of heterosexual HIV transmission might quickly hit the shores (and bedrooms) of North America and Europe.

But by the early 1990s, as it became clearer that heterosexual HIV transmission was not a lethal threat to most North Americans and Europeans, and as more anthropologists entered the research arena with more diverse interests, the primary perspective of anthropologists on AIDS in Africa has moved beyond social epidemiology to an understanding of the sociocultural and economic consequences of the disease; exploration of the social, cultural, and historic context of AIDS; a critique of the political economy and gender inequality in Africa; and an examination of HIV prevention, educational, and intervention programs.

It could be argued, however, that the abandonment of social epidemiologic interests by anthropologists was too hasty, and many of the key questions on the intersection of biological and cultural factors in the transmissibility of HIV can only be answered through anthropological knowledge, insight, and research. This point is not a trivial one. The degree to which the epidemic in Africa is spread through which customs and practices, and which kinds of sexual behavior, and the precise trajectory of the epidemic are critical concerns, which a biocultural anthropological perspective is uniquely situated to investigate. And, by and large, anthropology has ignored these social epidemiologic questions and, regrettably, gone in a different direction.

Other topics pursued by anthropologists studying AIDS in Africa have been highly diverse and include: male circumcision, HIV transmission, risk behavior, food policy, the role of anthropologists, "dry sex" (the fairly common activity of delubricating the vagina prior to sex), workshops, ethics, male condoms, female condoms, churches, breast-feeding, public policy, public awareness, traditional healers, research methods, household studies, global funding, the relationship between HIV and other sexually transmitted diseases (STDs), ethnomedicine, abstinence-only programs, men who have sex with men (MSM), female sex workers, poverty, the need for antiretroviral medications, women, values and beliefs, ethnography, AIDS-like indigenous diseases, the extended family, AIDS orphans, social stigma, the origin of HIV, fear, vaccine trials, and voluntary counseling and testing. This review of the literature is by no means exhaustive, representing perhaps only a third of the works on HIV/AIDS by anthropologists, but is intended to give the reader a sense of the diversity of HIV-related research on Africa conducted by anthropologists.

Several anthropologists have looked, for example, at male condoms for HIV prevention. Taylor (1990) discusses the cosmological importance in pregenocide Rwanda of having an uninterrupted flow of fluids, including semen, and suggests that this would make it even more difficult to promote condoms there. Susser and Stein (2000) describe the Ju/'hoansi of Namibia, where a woman can insist that a man use a condom, and she can withhold sex if he refuses. Among other groups throughout southern Africa, however, the use of a condom is seen as a challenge to a man's masculine authority.

Bond and Dover (1997), in a study of migrant workers in rural Zambia, find that the underlying and pervasive ideal is that sex is essentially a procreative act. An emphasis on male potency and male and female fertility often overrides anxieties about contracting HIV and other STDs. Condom use is only negotiated within some short-term relationships, and even then not consistently. While both men and women have negative attitudes toward condoms, women (because of their economic and ideological dependence on men) are in a much weaker position to negotiate condom use.

Rwabukwali and colleagues (1994), in a study of sixty-five HIV-positive and sixty-five HIV-negative Bagandan women, found that cultural norms traditionally encourage multiple sexual partners for men, and that women feel helpless in preventing HIV. They argue strongly for promoting condom use by men.

In an excellent study conducted by Kornfield and Namente (1997) in Malawi, where 40 percent of marriages end in divorce or separation, and women engage in ritual sexual "cleansing" (having intercourse) with their deceased husband's brother, most people are very religious, but do not use condoms. In a study conducted in the 1980s by Schoepf (1988) in what is now the Democratic Republic of the Congo (DRC), the church was teaching that AIDS is a divine punishment and only so-called sinners are at risk, while most secondary school students at that time did not know what a condom was and had never even seen one.

In a study of 100 female sex workers in South Africa, Varga (1997) learned that condoms are perceived as suggestive of filth, disease, infidelity, and mistrust. Sex workers never used condoms with their male lovers, and inconsistently with their male clients. She concludes that the high level of HIV/AIDS awareness had a minimal impact on condom use. Feldman and colleagues (1997) conducted a study of 276 Zambian teens during the early 1990s and found out that unprotected vaginal intercourse was common, and sometimes unprotected heterosexual anal sex was practiced (see below). Interestingly, Stewart (1999) found in a study of 600 young males and females in Uganda that they were three times more likely to accept condoms from male interviewers than from female interviewers. In another study in Ghana, focusing on methodology, McCombie and Anarfi (2002) learned that adolescent females were more likely to reveal to male interviewers than to female interviewers that they had engaged in prior sexual activity.

Female condoms have been suggested as a viable alternative to male condoms by Susser and Stein (2000). They argue that female condoms are the most socially acceptable device by both men and women in southern Africa, but cost factors and gender inequality have limited their availability.

Green, who originally supported the expansion of condom use in Africa (1988), has more recently questioned it (2003). Indeed, his new anticondom position has been used by some in the George W. Bush administration to justify an abstinence-only/partner-reduction strategy for Africa that de-emphasizes condom promotion. New epidemiologic evidence from Uganda clarifies that it was indeed primarily condom promotion that reduced the HIV rate from 15 percent to 6 percent from the early 1990s to the present. However, an artificially created condom shortage that occurred during 2005 in Uganda and a policy shift away from condoms may likely lead to a return to double-digit HIV seroprevalence in that country and in other nations in Africa where the U.S. President's Emergency Plan for AIDS Relief (PEPFAR) funding dominates. Indeed, during an artificially created condom shortage in Uganda during 2004–2005, there was a simultaneous increase in HIV rates in that country. Male and female condom use remains an important area where anthropologists need to continue doing research, and to speak out publicly in promoting an effective AIDS policy in Africa (Feldman 2003a, 2003b, 2004, 2005).

More broadly, HIV prevention and education have been a major concern of anthropologists. Early research in Rwanda showed that by the mid-1980s, the general public in Rwanda had very poor knowledge and awareness of HIV/AIDS. Even though it was at that time a highly stigmatized disease, most did not know how it was transmitted (Feldman et al. 1987). While the research in Rwanda shows no evidence of significant heterosexual anal intercourse (Feldman 1986), research among Zambian out-of-school youth shows that 35 percent of a sample of sixty adolescent females engaged in anal sex, almost always without a condom (Feldman et al. 1997). Halperin (1999) finds that women in three African countries were less aware of HIV risk through heterosexual anal intercourse than through vaginal intercourse. Yet 4 to 8 percent of three samples of females with AIDS acknowledged practicing anal sex, and 12 percent of a sample of female college students in Togo acknowledged engaging in anal penetration.

Indeed, Halperin and Williams (2001), looking at the failure of controlling HIV in South Africa and the relative success in Uganda, argue that Africa needs less of the slick Madison Avenue–type of HIV prevention campaigns found in South Africa and more of the grassroots campaigns found in Uganda. Halperin and colleagues (2004) also discuss the need to move forward in designing and implementing evidence-based prevention programs. HIV prevention workshops, particularly when they are led by peers, emphasize the cultural values of the target population, and seek to change the norms preventing safer sex practices, can be very effective in changing risk-taking behaviors (Feldman 2000).

Some anthropologists have focused on understanding the social dimensions and ethnohistorical context of HIV/AIDS. While there has been much discussion about the need for evidence-based interventions in Africa, Bond and Vincent (1996b, 2000) looked at the historical context of HIV in Uganda. Civil war and violence were endemic in Uganda until 1986. With the new government led by President Yoweri Moseveni beginning that year, there was a strong public campaign against HIV/AIDS. At first, members of high-risk groups were targeted (truck drivers, traders, and female sex workers). But, the authors point out, now the targeting is broader, including those in "poverty, the weak, and the vulnerable" (2000: 363). Van der Vliet (1994) examines the early history of AIDS in South Africa during the apartheid era, and finds that the conservative political ideology neglected the epidemic, often blaming persons with AIDS for their predicament.

Food policy and HIV is also a topic that has interested some anthropologists. Hunter and colleagues (1993) indicate that 8 percent of households in a region of Uganda had significant reductions in crops and livestock specifically due to AIDS mortality or morbidity. Barnett and Blaikie (1989) point out that AIDS is clearly impacting food policy in Africa. They suggest that research is needed to determine the types of coping mechanisms in the face of labor and food shortages, how land tenure systems and methods of labor organization are likely to respond to falling populations, and whether a possible return to hunting in some areas of declining population would be feasible.

Male circumcision and HIV have also been a strong interest of anthropologists (for example, Halperin et al. 2002). The late Priscilla Reining and Francis Conant are two anthropologists who, during the 1980s, discussed a link between male circumcision and HIV in Africa (Bongaarts et al. 1989). Halperin and Bailey (1999) point to a greater than eightfold increased risk of HIV infection for African uncircumcised men. In a cross-sectional study conducted in Uganda by Bailey and colleagues (1999), it was learned that differences in sex practices do not account for the higher risk of HIV infection found among uncircumcised men. They argue in favor of male circumcision as a prevention intervention strategy in areas where circumcision is absent in Africa.

In a study among the Luo in Kenya, Bailey and colleagues (2002) found that the Luo accepted the idea of male circumcision to reduce risk of HIV infection, but the authors acknowledge some barriers to circumcision, as well as a lack of knowledge and resources among local clinicians to perform the circumcisions. The efficacy of male circumcision in HIV prevention is an area where anthropologists need to closely follow in the near future. Recent trial studies conducted by anthropologists and others show that introducing adult male circumcision into an area where it did not occur previously was widely accepted, although some men did not follow the recommendation to abstain from sex for a month after the operation, resulting ironically in an increase of HIV transmission. The evidence is clear that in Africa, circumcision prevents HIV infection. But why doesn't this also occur in Europe, where most men are not circumcised and the HIV rates remain relatively low? Also, would men who become circumcised be more likely to engage in risky sex?

Traditional healers and HIV have remained an interest among some anthropologists (for example, Feldman 1986; Green 1992a, 1992b, 2000). Beginning in the late 1980s, Green (1988) stressed the need to work with traditional healers for effective educational, counseling, and condom distribution services. In research conducted in Mozambique, Green and colleagues (1993) point out that traditional healers regard AIDS, unlike other STDs, as a new disease for which they lack medicines. Green and colleagues (1995) also describe a South African HIV/STD prevention program in 1992 that began with 28 traditional healers and successfully grew in less than a year to over 1,500 traditional healers. Green (1997) points out that at least 80 percent of sub-Saharan Africans rely primarily or exclusively on traditional healers for their health care needs. He stresses that traditional healers in HIV prevention programs can significantly improve the effectiveness of these programs (Green 1999b).

Schoepf (1992a) also points out that traditional healers have considerable authority not just in rural Africa, but in poor urban communities as well. During 2004, Randall Tobias, the former head of PEPFAR, lamented that there are only 500 physicians available for providing antiretroviral medication treatment in the whole of Mozambique, totally oblivious to the 85,000 traditional healers in that nation who could be trained to provide HIV treatments (Green 1999a). Biomedical practitioners must work together with traditional healers to help contain the epidemic (Green 1994). Anthropologists need to work with PEPFAR administrators to integrate traditional healers into HIV prevention and treatment programs where appropriate.

Anthropologists see poverty as both a catalyst and an inhibitor to HIV transmission. Halperin (2000) suggests that poverty is not always associated with AIDS, pointing to Botswana as a fairly prosperous nation with an extraordinarily high HIV rate. Feldman (1986) observed that most of the AIDS patients who were interviewed in the hospital in Rwanda were fairly wealthy, and pointed out that in Zambia in the mid-1990s, the banking industry was particularly hit hard among top administrative personnel who died of AIDS (Feldman and Wang Miller 1998). Van der Vliet (2004) complains that South Africa has missed several opportunities to control the enormous growth of AIDS because of President Thabo Mbeki's destructive insistence that AIDS is caused by "poverty" rather than by HIV.

On the other hand, Schoepf (2004a) maintains that the conditions of poverty further accelerated the spread of HIV in the DRC. She argues that broader socioeconomic changes that reduce poverty and gender subordination are necessary to control the epidemic (Schoepf 1992b, 1993), and that AIDS is the result of social conditions, rather than a virus spread by the behavior of individuals (Schoepf 1991). Susan Hunter and colleagues (1997) cite their research in Tanzania showing that families with sufficient resources, whether headed by men or women, are coping better than those without sufficient resources. Seeley and colleagues (1994), in a study in rural Uganda, discovered that people in the poorest households were most likely to be HIV positive. More research is needed by anthropologists to examine the microeconomics of HIV/AIDS and the African family.

In a household study of families with AIDS in Uganda, only four out of twenty-four informants told everyone in the household about their AIDS diagnosis (McGrath and Ankrah 1993). Clearly, fear and stigma play a central role in decision-making patterns in AIDS households. The authors emphasize the importance in providing outside assistance for families responsible for caring for persons with AIDS. Also in Uganda, Seeley and Kajura (1993) found during a six-month study that twenty-seven of the thirty extended families studied were not able to provide adequate support for people with AIDS within their households. Hunter (1990) points out that while many of the AIDS orphans are taken in by their grandparents or other extended kin, these households are often under considerable socioeconomic stress and need urgent government assistance.

More generally, the social and economic consequences of HIV/AIDS continue to interest many anthropologists (Bond et al. 1996; Brummelhuis and Herdt 1995; Feldman, ed. 1990; Reynolds Whyte and Harwood 1998; Setel 1999; Setel and Lewis 1999; Wallman 1996). Barnett and Blaikie (1992) conducted an eighteen-month study in Uganda that focused on the social and economic consequences of the disease and learned that there is a very heavy human cost. Hunter (2003) argues that the exploitation of developing nations by the West is directly responsible for the spread of the disease in Africa. She also condemns the initial reluctance of pharmaceutical firms to lower their cost of antiretroviral medications. Feldman (1991) points out that AIDS is one of many problems facing Africa today, but it has had a devastating impact particularly on the African family.

Gender inequality and the status of women in Africa are central to the epidemic spread of HIV (Schoepf 2004b). Varga (2001b) suggests that we need to study male sexuality and reproductive health more in order to focus on male power and gender inequality.

Female sex workers have often been blamed for spreading the epidemic. However, Porter (1994) examined the data for Ghana and found that migrating men brought HIV back with them from Côte d'Ivoire and infected the local sex workers in Ghana, who in turn infected other nonmigrating men, who then infected their wives and children. Renaud (1997) conducted an ethnography of a female sex worker community in Senegal, where the women lived in makeshift huts by the side of a road. With sex work legal in Senegal, the women were given free condoms and HIV education and testing, resulting in a low HIV rate. Varga (2001a) describes her research in South Africa among a sample of 100 female sex workers, twenty-five male truck driver clients, and ten male personal partners. Condom use was inconsistent at best. When clients became personal partners, the condoms usually came off. Denial of risk, fatalism, economic pressure, and unwillingness to learn one's HIV status all played a role in creating a very high HIV rate among the sex workers, their clients, and their personal partners.

Hrdy (1988), in a very problematic work, wrongly accepts the popular notion that same-sex sexuality among men is rare and inconsequential in Africa. However, Murray and Roscoe's (1998) superb volume nearly a decade later documents the widespread existence of homosexuality in numerous traditional African societies, which has been significantly repressed today by missionary influences and governmental oppression. Niang (a Senegalese anthropologist) and colleagues (2002) describe MSM in Senegal, indicating that they have distinct identities and social roles that go beyond sexual practices. *Ibbis* are men who tend to adopt feminine mannerisms, while *yoos* are men who also have sex with men but do not consider themselves gay. Only 23 percent of Senegalese MSM who engage in insertive anal sex use a condom, while even fewer (14 percent) who engage in receptive anal sex use a condom. Niang and colleagues (2003) point out that MSM in Africa receive little attention because of the widespread denial and stigmatization of male same-sex sexual behavior. They suggest the need for nonstigmatizing sexual health information and services for African MSM. Certainly, more anthropological research will be needed for this neglected but at high risk population.

Hrdy's work (1988) did a disservice to our understanding of the sociocultural factors that may influence HIV transmissibility by effectively ending discussion in that area. Hrdy reviews the evidence for nonvaginal transmission and concludes that other factors—same-sex behavior, heterosexual anal sex, female circumcision, exposure to blood, use of shared implements, or contact with nonhuman primates—play no or a minimal role in the continuing spread of HIV in Africa. With the exception of same-sex behavior and perhaps to a lesser extent heterosexual anal sex, he may be right about these factors. But his study closed the door to our understanding of the role of other potentially important cofactors, such as the pervasive practice of dry sex in southern and other parts of Africa, the role of elongating the labia majora among some central African cultures, prior immunosuppression and intestinal parasitic infestation, the increase of urban African women who have sex during menstruation, the importance of having sex with one's brother-in-law upon the death of a husband in order to release his spirit (a practice known as the levirate), and the false and dangerous notion that sex with a virgin—often a child—would cure AIDS (Brokensha 1988; Feldman 1987, 1990). Anthropologists can have an excellent understanding of the overlay of cultural practices and HIV prevalence, which would be very useful—when combined with microbiological evidence—in delineating the possible sequence of HIV transmission patterns.

The initial research that has been conducted by anthropologists in the areas of HIV transmission and social epidemiology was important in beginning to clarify how the disease spreads in Africa. Bond (1992) maintains that dry sex causes internal abrasions, which facilitates HIV transmission, and describes, for example, how the Society for Women and AIDS has been holding workshops in Zambia informing women of this risk. Brown and colleagues (1993) conducted focus groups in central Zaire (now the DRC) to learn that both men and women like a dry, tight vagina, and women use thirty different substances—mostly leaves and powders—to achieve that goal. Brown and Brown (2000), in a literature review, report that traditional intravaginal substances and practices are found in eleven African countries. While there are no prospective studies yet to link these practices to disease transmission, research is needed to examine the effects of the vaginal pH, flora, and epithelium. Among the Kolda and Laobe of southern Senegal, 40 percent of adult women use plants and powders to dry their vaginas prior to sex (Niang 1995).

Halperin and Epstein (2004) assert that the much higher rate of heterosexually transmitted HIV in Africa than in North America and Europe can be explained by the pervasive pattern among African married men of having a mistress. However, this does not explain why the subset of white suburban married men in North America and Europe who also have a mistress do not have a similar epidemiologic pattern of high HIV seropositivity. It appears likely that the differential pattern of decreased susceptibility through vaginal intercourse between North American and Europe versus

Africa may be attributable to the nature of the subtype, since HIV-1 subtype B is prevalent in North America and Europe, while other subtypes are prevalent in Africa. Other cofactors, both biological and sociocultural, may play an important role as well.

McGrath and colleagues (1992; 1993) indicate that sex outside of marriage among Ugandan married women is permissible for several reasons: after the birth of twins, at funerals, at weddings, for revenge against an unfaithful husband, for economic reasons, and for greater sexual satisfaction. However, the Ugandan worldview allows for greater sexual freedom for men than for women, and while men are expected to be unfaithful, women generally are not.

Raphael (1990, 1994), long before the World Health Organization (WHO) and the United Nations Children's Fund (UNICEF) came to a similar conclusion, recommended that alternatives be found for HIV-positive mothers in Africa to breast-feed their children. WHO and UNICEF had originally insisted that children of HIV-positive mothers faced a greater risk from using polluted water mixed with baby formula than from breast-feeding, until a reanalysis of the epidemiologic data showed just how risky breast-feeding by HIV-positive mothers can actually be.

A household survey conducted in Rwanda in 1985 established that AIDS-like symptoms were new in that country, and were not previously endemic (Feldman 1989). Also, traditional healers had not seen the disease previously in that country (Feldman 1986), but traditional healers had seen a disease, locally named *kaliondeonde*, with similar symptoms in central and eastern Zambia for several decades before the 1980s (Feldman 1993, 1998). Kornfield and Namate (1997) describe two similar AIDS-like illnesses (*tsempho* and *kanyera*) in Malawi. Mogensen (1995) looks at the beliefs surrounding another AIDS-like illness (*kahungo*) in southern Zambia among the Tonga.

The social dimensions of HIV vaccine trials in Africa has also been of anthropological interest. In interviews conducted among nearly 1,200 Ugandan military men about HIV vaccine trials, McGrath and colleagues (McGrath, George, et al. 2001; McGrath, Mafigiri, et al. 2001) found that the men were often unclear if the trials cure or prevent disease, had a poor level of knowledge of clinical trials procedures (but this improved incrementally over follow-up), and were concerned about possible side effects, yet wanted to participate in the vaccine trials in order to be protected from HIV/AIDS.

Yoder and Matinga (2004) looked at the issue of voluntary counseling and testing. They found that in Malawi, 14.5 percent of adult men and women who visited voluntary counseling and testing sites tested positive for HIV. But during a twelve-month period, only 1 percent of the estimated 760,000 HIV-positive persons in Malawi were actually tested and counseled at these sites. The authors recommend significantly expanding these sites in Malawi, and argue that it is essential that counseling services remain included at all test sites.

Ethical questions surrounding AIDS research have also been of anthropological concern. For example, Bond (1997) discusses her fieldwork on a commercial farm in southern Zambia to design an HIV prevention program for farm workers. She learned that the older migrant male workers on the farm were coercively having sex with some of the young girls brought in from the surrounding villages to work on the farm. When she expressed her concern, the farm management "solved" the problem by firing the underage workers. While some in the local community supported this action, others were angered by it, placing the anthropologist in a "no-win" ethical situation.

Adequate funding for anthropological research on HIV/AIDS has remained a serious problem, although it has improved somewhat from the mid and late 1980s, when hardly any funds were available for ethnographic research. Even today, anthropologists make up only a very small part of the total workforce hired by major organizations that are funded by the U.S. Agency for International Development (USAID) and are based in the United States and doing research and conducting interventions on AIDS in Africa, while most of the research questions in need of investigation are essentially anthropological or ethnographic in nature. Setel (1997) adroitly points out that AIDS research and intervention projects that have allocated multiple senior staff and teams of assistants necessary for demographic surveillance and epidemiologic monitoring often operate with only a single expatriate social scientist and a junior African colleague for research assistance. Training opportunities for Africans in anthropology and ethnographic research have lagged far behind those in epidemiology, demography, and international health.

However, it is likely that anthropologists will continue in the decade or more to come to make significant contributions and advances to our understanding of AIDS in Africa. Biological anthropologists need to join with cultural anthropologists in fully comprehending the nature of the epidemic. Anthropological knowledge is the encapsulated totality of all known and knowable human experience. Anthropologists need to speak out assertively on policy issues concerning the direction of HIV prevention, as well as AIDS care and treatment. The neoconservative ideological agenda is, often successfully, using the AIDS crisis as a mechanism to change the values, beliefs, and behaviors of Africans throughout the continent, to the detriment of African cultures. And, of course, anthropologists need to continue using ethnography, short-term and long-term, to understand the social and cultural dimensions of this devastating disease.

Acknowledgments

Parts of this chapter were presented as a paper at the Society for Applied Anthropology in Santa Fe, New Mexico, in April 2005 and at the Centers for Disease Control and Prevention (CDC) in Atlanta in December 2005. I would like to thank Rachel Langer for her assistance. I would also like to thank the many anthropologists who sent me their publications and bibliographies on HIV/AIDS in preparation of this literature review. This chapter is intended to give the reader a sense of the diversity of interests of anthropologists working on AIDS in Africa. Due to the enormity in the growth of the anthropological literature on this topic, it was not possible to include most of the available publications. My apologies to those anthropologists whose works, therefore, were not included in this chapter.

References Cited

Bailey, R. C., R. Muga, R. Poulussen, and H. Abicht. 2002. "The Acceptability of Male Circumcision to Reduce HIV Infections in Nyanza Province, Kenya." *AIDS Care* 14: 27–40.

Bailey, R. C., S. Neema, and R. Othieno. 1999. "Sexual Behaviors and Other HIV Risk Factors in Circumcised and Uncircumcised Men in Uganda." *Journal of Acquired Immune Deficiency Syndromes* 22: 294–301.

Barnett, T., and P. Blaikie. 1989. "AIDS and Food Production in East and Central Africa: A Research Outline." *Food Policy* (February): 2–6.

———. 1992. *AIDS in Africa*. New York: Guilford.

Bond, G. C., J. Kreniske, I. Susser, and J. Vincent, eds. 1996. *AIDS in Africa and the Caribbean*. New York: Harper Collins.

Bond, G. C., and J. Vincent. 1996a. "AIDS in Uganda: The First Decade." In *AIDS in Africa and the Caribbean*, ed. G. C. Bond, J. Kreniske, I. Susser, and J. Vincent, 85–97. New York: Harper Collins.

———. 1996b. "Community Based Organizations in Uganda: A Youth Initiative." In *AIDS in Africa and the Caribbean*, ed. G. C. Bond, J. Kreniske, I. Susser, and J. Vincent, 99–113. New York: Harper Collins.

———. 2000. "The Moving Frontier of AIDS in Uganda: Contexts, Texts, and Concepts." In *Contested Terrains and Constructed Categories: Contemporary Africa in Focus*, ed. G. C. Bond and N. C. Gibson, 345–363. Boulder, Colo.: Westview Press.

Bond, V. 1992. "Winds of Change in Zambia." *WorldAIDS* 21 (May): 3–4.

———. 1997. "'Between a Rock and a Hard Place': Applied Anthropology and AIDS Research on a Commercial Farm in Zambia." *Health Transition Review* 7 (Supplement 3): 69–83.

Bond, V., and P. Dover. 1997. "Men, Women and the Trouble with Condoms: Problems Associated with Condom use by Migrant Workers in Rural Zambia." *Health Transition Review* 7 (Supplement 3): 377–391.

Bongaarts, J., P. Reining, P. Way, and F. Conant. 1989. "The Relationship between Male Circumcision and HIV Infection in African Populations." *AIDS* 3: 373–377.

Brokensha, D. 1988. "Overview: Social factors in the Transmission and Control of African AIDS." In *AIDS in Africa: The Social and Policy Impact*, ed. N. Miller and R. C. Rockwell, 167–173. Lewiston, N.Y.: Edwin Mellen Press.

Brown, J. E., O. Bibi Ayowa, and R. C. Brown. 1993. "Dry and Tight: Sexual Practices and Potential AIDS Risk in Zaire." *Social Science and Medicine* 37 (8): 989–994.

Brown, J. E., and R. C. Brown. 2000. "Traditional Intravaginal Practices and the Heterosexual Transmission of Disease: A Review." *Sexually Transmitted Diseases* 27 (4): 183–187.

Brummelhuis, H. T., and G. Herdt, eds. 1995. *Culture and Sexual Risk: Anthropological Perspectives on AIDS*. New York: Gordon and Breach.

Feldman, D. A. 1986. "Anthropology, AIDS, and Africa." *Medical Anthropology Quarterly* 17 (2): 38–40.

———. 1987. "Role of African Mutilations in AIDS Discounted." *New York Times*, January 7.

———. 1989. "A Household Survey for AIDS-Related Complex in Rwanda." *Medical Anthropology* 10: 143–149.

———. 1990. "Assessing the Viral, Parasitic, and Sociocultural Cofactors in AIDS Transmission in Rwanda." In *Culture and AIDS*, ed. D. A. Feldman, 45–54. Westport, Conn.: Praeger.

———. 1991. "The Sociocultural Impacts of AIDS in Central and East Africa." In *AIDS and the Social Sciences: Common Threads*, ed. R. Ulack and W. F. Skinner, 124–133. Lexington: University Press of Kentucky.

———. 1993. "Is It AIDS? Or Is It Kaliondeonde?" Paper presented at the American Anthropological Association, Washington, D.C., November.

———. 1998. "The Origin of HIV/AIDS." In *The AIDS Crisis: A Documentary History*, ed. D. A. Feldman and J. Wang Miller, 1–6. Westport, Conn.: Greenwood Press.

———. 2000. "Changing Risky Sexual Behavior in Zambia." *Anthropology Newsletter* (October): 70–71.

———. 2003a. "Problems with the Uganda Model for HIV/AIDS Prevention." *Anthropology News* (October): 6.

———. 2003b. "Reassessing AIDS Priorities and Strategies for Africa: ABC vs. ACCDG-LMT." *AIDS and Anthropology Bulletin* 15 (2): 5–8.

———. 2004. "Too Many Strings Constrict U.S. Funding for AIDS Fight." *Rochester (N.Y.) Democrat and Chronicle*, August 3.

———. 2005. "A Global AIDS Consensus?" *Anthropology News* (May): 4.

————, ed. 1990. *Culture and AIDS*. Westport, Conn.: Praeger.

Feldman, D. A., and J. Wang Miller, eds. 1998. *The AIDS Crisis: A Documentary History*. Westport, Conn.: Greenwood Press.

Feldman, D. A., S. R. Friedman, and D. C. Des Jarlais. 1987. "Public Awareness of AIDS in Rwanda." *Social Science and Medicine* 24 (2): 97–100.

Feldman, D. A., P. O'Hara, K. S. Baboo, N. W. Chitalu, and Y. Lu. 1997. "HIV Prevention among Zambian Adolescents: Developing a Value Utilization/Norm Change Model." *Social Science and Medicine* 44 (4): 455–468.

Green, E. C. 1988. "AIDS in Africa: An Agenda for Behavioral Scientists." In *AIDS in Africa: The Social and Policy Impact*, ed. N. Miller and R. C. Rockwell, 175–196. Lewiston, N.Y.: Edwin Mellen Press.

————. 1992a. "The Anthropology of Sexually Transmitted Disease in Liberia." *Social Science and Medicine* 35 (12): 1457–1468.

————. 1992b. "Sexually Transmitted Disease, Ethnomedicine and Health Policy in Africa." *Social Science and Medicine*. 35 (2): 121–130.

————. 1994. *AIDS and STDs in Africa: Bridging the Gap Between Traditional Healing and Modern Medicine*. Boulder, Colo.: Westview Press.

————. 1997. "The Participation of African Traditional Healers in AIDS/STD Prevention Programmes." *Tropical Doctor* 27 (Supplement 1): 56–59.

————. 1999a. "Engaging Indigenous African Healers in the Prevention of AIDS and STDs." In *Anthropology in Public Health: Bridging Differences in Culture and Society*, ed. R. A. Hahn and K. W. Harris, 63–83. New York: Oxford University Press.

————. 1999b. "Involving Healers." *AIDS Action* 44 (October–December): 3.

————. 2000. "Photoessay: The WHO Forum on Traditional Medicine in Health Systems, Harare, Zimbabwe, February 14–18, 2000." *Journal of Alternative and Complementary Medicine* 6 (5): 379–382.

————. 2003. *Rethinking AIDS Prevention: Learning from Successes in Developing Countries*. Westport, Conn.: Greenwood.

Green, E. C., A. Jurg, and A. Dgedge. 1993. "Sexually-Transmitted Diseases, AIDS and Traditional Healers in Mozambique." *Medical Anthropology* 15: 261–281.

Green, E. C., B. Zokwe, J. David Dupree. 1995. "The Experience of an AIDS Prevention Program Focused on South African Traditional Healers." *Social Science and Medicine* 40 (4): 503–515.

Halperin, D. T. 1999. "Heterosexual Anal Intercourse: Prevalence, Cultural Factors, and HIV Infection and Other Health Risks, Part I." *AIDS Patient Care and STDs* 13 (12): 717–730.

————. 2000. "Old Ways and New Spread AIDS in Africa." *San Francisco Chronicle*, November 30.

Halperin, D. T., and R. C. Bailey. 1999. "Male Circumcision and HIV Infection: 10 Years and Counting." *Lancet* 354 (9192): 1813–1815.

Halperin, D. T., and H. Epstein. 2004. "Concurrent Sexual Partnerships Help to Explain Africa's High HIV Prevalence: Implications for Prevention." *Lancet* 364 (9428): 4–6.

Halperin, D. T., M. J. Steiner, M. M. Cassell, E. C. Green, N. Hearst, D. Kirby, H. D.

Gayle, and W. Cates. 2004. "The Time Has Come for Common Ground on Preventing Sexual Transmission of HIV." *Lancet* 364 (November 27): 1913–1915.

Halperin, D. T., H. A. Weiss, R. Hayes, B. Auvert, R. C. Bailey, J. Caldwell, T. Coates, N. Padian, M. Potts, A. Ronald, R. Short, B. Williams, and J. Klausner. 2002. "Response to Ronald Gray et al., Male Circumcision and HIV Acquisition and Transmission: Cohort Studies in Rakai, Uganda." *AIDS* 16 (5): 810–812.

Halperin, D. T., and B. Williams. 2001. "No Way to Fight AIDS in Africa." *Washington Post*, August 26.

Hrdy, D. B. 1988. "Cultural Practices Contributing to the Transmission of HIV in Africa." In *The Heterosexual Transmission of HIV in Africa*, ed. D. Koch-Weser and H. Vanderschmidt, 255–264. Cambridge, Mass.: Abt Books.

Hunter, S. S. 1990. "Orphans as a Window on the AIDS Epidemic in Sub-Saharan Africa: Initial Results and Implications of a Study in Uganda." *Social Science and Medicine* 31 (6): 681–690.

———. 2003. *Black Death: AIDS in Africa*. New York: Palgrave Macmillan.

Hunter, S. S., E. Bulirwa, and E. Kisseka. 1993. "AIDS and Agricultural Production: Report of a Land Utilization Survey, Masaka and Rakai Districts of Uganda." *Land Use Policy* (July): 241–258.

Hunter, S. S., F. Kaijage, P. Maack, A. Kiondo, and P. Masanja. 1997. "Using Rapid Research to Develop a National Strategy to Assist Families Affected by AIDS in Tanzania." *Health Transition Review* 7 (Supplement 3): 393–420.

Kornfield, R., and D. Namate. 1997. *Cultural Practices Related to HIV/AIDS Risk Behaviour: Community Survey in Phalombe, Malawi*. STAFH Project, Report Series No. 10. Lilongwe, Malawi: Support to AIDS and Family Health Project.

McCombie, S. C., and J. K. Anarfi. 2002. "The Influence of Sex of Interviewer on the Results of an AIDS Survey in Ghana." *Human Organization* 61 (1): 51–57.

McGrath, J. W., and E. M. Ankrah. 1993. "AIDS and the Urban Family: Its Impact in Kampala, Uganda." *AIDS Care* 5 (1): 55–78.

McGrath, J. W., K. George, G. Svilar, E. Ihler, D. Mafigiri, M. Kabugo, and E. Mugisha. 2001. "Knowledge about Vaccine Trials and Willingness to Participate in an HIV/AIDS Vaccine Study in the Ugandan Military." *Journal of Acquired Immune Deficiency Syndromes* 27: 381–388.

McGrath, J. W., D. Mafigiri, M. Kamya, K. George, R. Senvewo, G. Svilar, M. Kabugo, and E. Mugisha. 2001. "Developing AIDS Vaccine Trials Educational Programs in Uganda." *Journal of Acquired Immune Deficiency Syndromes* 26: 176–181.

McGrath, J. W., C. B. Rwabukwali, D. A. Schumann, J. Pearson-Marks, S. Nakayiwa, B. Namande, L. Nakyobe, and R. Mukasa. 1993. "Anthropology and AIDS: The Cultural Context of Sexual Risk Behavior among Urban Baganda Women in Kampala, Uganda." *Social Science and Medicine* 36 (4): 429–439.

McGrath, J. W., D. A. Schumann, J. Pearson-Marks, C. B. Rwabukwali, R. Mukasa, B. Namande, S. Nakayiwa, and L. Nakyobe. 1992. "Cultural Determinants of Sexual Risk Behavior for AIDS among Baganda Women." *Medical Anthropology Quarterly* 6 (2): 153–161.

Mogensen, H. O. 1995. *AIDS Is a Kind of Kahungo That Kills: The Challenge of Using*

Local Narratives When Exploring AIDS among the Tonga of Southern Zambia. Boston: Scandinavian Press.

Murray, S. O., and W. Roscoe, eds. 1998. *Boy-Wives and Female Husbands: Studies in African Homosexualities.* New York: Palgrave.

Niang, C. I. 1995. "Traditional Women's Associations as Channels for HIV/AIDS/STD Prevention." *AIDS STD Health Promotion Exchange* 3: 4–6.

Niang, C. I., M. Diagne, Y. Niang, A. M. Moreau, D. Gomis, M. Diouf, K. Seck, A. S. Wade, P. Tapsoba, and C. Castle. 2002. *Meeting the Sexual Health Needs of Men Who Have Sex with Men in Senegal.* Horizons Program report, 1–18. New York: Population Council.

Niang, C. I., P. Tabosa, E. Weiss, M. Diagne, Y. Niang, A. M. Moreau, D. Gomis, A. S. Wade, K. Seck, and C. Castle. 2003. "'It's Raining Stones': Stigma, Violence and HIV Vulnerability among Men Who Have Sex with Men in Dakar, Senegal." *Culture, Health and Sexuality* 5 (6): 499–512.

Porter, R. W. 1994. "AIDS in Ghana: Priorities and Policies." In *Global AIDS Policy*, ed. D. A. Feldman, 90–106. Westport, Conn.: Bergin and Garvey.

Raphael, D. 1990. "HIV and Breastmilk." In *Current Directions in Anthropological Research on AIDS*, ed. D. A. Feldman, 3–5. Miami: AIDS and Anthropology Research Group, Society for Medical Anthropology.

———. 1994. "The Politics of International Health: Breastfeeding and HIV." In *Global AIDS Policy*, ed. D. A. Feldman, 129–141. Westport, Conn.: Bergin and Garvey.

Renaud, M. L. 1997. *Women at the Crossroads: A Prostitute Community's Response to AIDS in Urban Senegal.* New York: Gordon and Breach.

Reynolds Whyte, S., and A. Harwood, eds. 1998. *Questioning Misfortune: The Pragmatics of Uncertainty in Eastern Uganda.* New York: Cambridge University Press.

Rwabukwali, C. B., D. A. Schumann, J. W. McGrath, D. Carroll-Pankhurst, R. Mukasa, S. Nakayiwa, L. Nakyobe, and B. Namande. 1994. "Culture, Sexual Behavior, and Attitudes towards Condom Use among Baganda Women." In *Global AIDS Policy*, ed. D. A. Feldman, 70–89. Westport, Conn.: Bergin and Garvey.

Schoepf, B. G. 1988. "Women, AIDS, and Economic Crisis in Central Africa." *Canadian Journal of African Studies* 22 (3): 625–644.

———. 1991. "Ethical, Methodological and Political Issues of AIDS Research in Central Africa." *Social Science and Medicine* 33 (7): 749–763.

———. 1992a. "AIDS, Sex and Condoms: African Healers and the Reinvention of Tradition in Zaire." *Medical Anthropology* 14: 225–242.

———. 1992b. "Women at Risk: Case Studies from Zaire." In *The Time of AIDS: Social Analysis, Theory and Method*, ed. G. Herdt and S. Lindenbaum, 259–286. Newbury Park, Calif.: Sage.

———. 1993. "AIDS, Action-Research with Women in Kinshasa, Zaire." *Social Science and Medicine* 37 (11): 1401–1413.

———. 2004a. "AIDS, History and Struggles Over Meaning." In *HIV and AIDS in Africa: Beyond Epidemiology*, ed. E. Kalipen, S. Craddock, J. R. Oppong, and J. Ghosh, 15–28. Malden, Mass.: Blackwell.

———. 2004b. "AIDS in Africa: Structure, Agency and Risk." In *HIV and AIDS in Africa: Beyond Epidemiology*, ed. E. Kalipen, S. Craddock, J. R. Oppong, and J. Ghosh, 121–132. Malden, Mass.: Blackwell.

Seeley, J., and E. Kajura. 1993. "The Extended Family and Support for People with AIDS in a Rural Population in South West Uganda: A Safety Net with Holes?" *AIDS Care* 5 (1): 117–122.

Seeley, J., S. S. Malamba, A. J. Nunn, D. W. Mulder, J. F. Kengeya-Kayondo, and T. G. Barton. 1994. "Socioeconomic Status, Gender, and Risk of HIV-1 Infection in a Rural Community in South West Uganda." *Medical Anthropology Quarterly* 8 (1): 78–89.

Setel, P. W. 1997. "Sexual Networking, Knowledge, and Risk: Contextual Social Research for Confronting AIDS and STDs in Eastern and Southern Africa." *Health Transition Review* 7 (Supplement 3): 1–3.

———. 1999. *A Plague of Paradoxes: AIDS, Culture and Demography in Northern Tanzania.* Chicago: University of Chicago Press.

Setel, P. W., and M. Lewis, eds. 1999. *Histories of STDs and HIV/AIDS in Sub-Saharan Africa.* Westport, Conn.: Greenwood.

Stewart K. 1999. Research Report: HIV/AIDS and Adolescents in Rural Uganda. *AIDS and Anthropology Bulletin* 11 (1): 5–6.

Susser, I., and Z. Stein. 2000. "Culture, Sexuality, and Women's Agency in the Prevention of HIV/AIDS in Southern Africa." *American Journal of Public Health* 90 (7): 1042–1048.

Taylor, C. 1990. "AIDS and the Pathogenesis of Metaphor." In *Culture and AIDS*, ed. D. A. Feldman, 55–66. Westport, Conn.: Praeger.

van der Vliet, V. 1994. "Apartheid and the Politics of AIDS." In *Global AIDS Policy*, ed. D. A. Feldman, 107–128. Westport, Conn.: Bergin and Garvey.

———. 2004. "South Africa Divided against AIDS: A Crisis of Leadership." In *AIDS and South Africa: The Social Expression of a Pandemic*, ed. K. D. Kauffman and D. L. Lindauer, 48–96. New York: Palgrave MacMillan.

Varga, C. A. 1997. "The Condom Conundrum: Barriers to Condom Use among Commercial Sex Workers in Durban, South Africa." *African Journal of Reproductive Health* 1 (1): 74–88.

———. 2001a. "Coping with HIV/AIDS in Durban's Commercial Sex Industry." *AIDS Care* 13 (3): 351–365.

———. 2001b. "The Forgotten Fifty Per Cent: A Review of Sexual and Reproductive Health Research and Programs Focused on Boys and Young Men in Sub-Saharan Africa." *African Journal of Reproductive Health* 5 (3): 175–195.

Wallman, S., and G. Bantebya-Kyomuhendo. 1996. *Kampala Women Getting By: Well-being in the Time of AIDS.* Athens: Ohio University Press.

Yoder, P. S., and P. Matinga. 2004. *Voluntary Counselling and Testing (VCT) for HIV in Malawi: Public Perspectives and Recent VCT Experiences. Measure DHS+*. Calverton, Md.: ORC Macro.

2

Confounding Conventional Wisdom

The Ju/'hoansi and HIV/AIDS

RICHARD B. LEE AND IDA SUSSER

Over the last thirty years, the Ju/'hoansi have become one of the classic cases in the anthropological literature documenting the lifeways of a contemporary hunting and gathering society (Lee 1979, 2003; Lee and DeVore 1976; Marshall 1976). Less well known is the fact that the Ju/'hoansi, straddling the border between Botswana and Namibia, are located in the heart of the world region hardest hit by AIDS. The most recent UNAIDS estimates put Namibia's HIV-positive rates at 22.5 percent and Botswana's at 38.0 percent; the latter is the highest national rate in the world. How would the Ju/'hoansi, for all their renowned cultural resilience, fare in the geographical epicenter of the worst epidemic in world history?

Since 1996, the authors have been working in capacity-building projects to stem the tide of AIDS in Namibia and Botswana. We have conducted training workshops at the University of Namibia over an eight-year period involving over 200 students and health professionals, and have combined this with regular tracking of the situation regarding HIV/AIDS among the Ju'hoansi. We visited the Tjumkui/Nyae Nyae-area Ju/'hoansi in Namibia in 1996, 1997, 2000, and 2003 and the Dobe-area Ju/'hoansi of Botswana in 1999 and 2001, first under a multiyear Fogarty Foundation grant to Columbia University and then supported by our respective universities (Lee 2004).[1]

As late as 1987, when Lee did fieldwork in the Dobe area of Botswana, there were no cases of AIDS reported. In that year a South African medical team, under the direction of Trefor Jenkins of the South African Institute for Medical Research, did a rapid nutritional and health assessment of about 140 Ju/'hoansi, a twenty-year follow-up to an initial baseline survey in 1967–1968. During the research, Jeanette Peterson, a Danish doctor from the Maun Hospital, was touring the district to alert communities about a new disease, sexually transmitted and invariably fatal. The Jenkins team joined her to present the AIDS story to a mixed audience of Herero and Ju/'hoansi. Jenkins, John Hansen, and Lee decided to add HIV testing to the blood workups previously scheduled. Of the collected samples from close to 150 individuals in blind testing, not one sample returned HIV positive. However, Jenkins, working across the border in Namibia the following year, brought back two seropositive samples from Tjumkui (Hansen et al. 1994).

Within a few years, the national rates in both Botswana and newly independent Namibia had started their steep climb, approaching their record high levels by the mid-1990s. However, the situation in the Dobe and Nyae Nyae areas was still largely unknown. Interest in this topic was one of the factors that brought Lee and Susser together in 1996 to undertake capacity-building research and teaching in Namibia and Botswana.

Since that time, six field trips have given us the opportunity to gauge a sense of the way HIV/AIDS has entered the lives of the Ju/'hoansi. By 2001, estimating from very fragmentary data, about fifty cases had emerged in a total population of 2,500 on both sides of the border. This number converts to a 3.3 percent seropositive rate in persons fifteen to forty-nine years old. Compared to Botswana's and Namibia's much higher rates, remarkably, this rate is about 60 to 90 percent lower than national averages. The lower rates among the San peoples generally are confirmed by recent statements by senior Namibian government officials, including those by President Sam Nujoma. In addressing the people of Tjumkui on July 13, 2003, he said: "I am happy to report that Tjumkui District does not have much AIDS. The people here are careful. They understand the risks and we want to keep it that way. The people from outside, from Windhoek, from Walvis Bay, from Caprivi are diseased. It is they who bring it here. Watch out for them when they come here. You can tell who they are. They dress well" (Nujoma 2003).

In spite of the problematic implications of his claim that people can blame outsiders for AIDS and tell if a person will transmit AIDS simply by their clothes, this statement recognizes that—for the moment—there is less HIV/AIDS in the Tjumkui District than elsewhere in Namibia. However, our most recent field trip to the San settlements Tjumkui and Baraka, Namibia, in July 2003 indicated that the nature of the epidemic was undergoing a transition and that there is a possibility that these rates could climb rapidly, approaching the levels observed in other parts of the region.

In this chapter, we address three questions: First, how are we to explain these much lower AIDS rates among the Ju/'hoansi? Second, what accounts for the rapid growth in rates in the period 2002–2004? And third, what possibilities exist for turning the situation around so that a worst-case scenario does not materialize?

The Lower Rates: Macro and Micro Factors

In neither the Dobe nor the Nyae Nyae area has the area's clinics made any attempts to survey the incidence of HIV by means of anonymous testing or sentinel surveys. People with AIDS may die without a definitive diagnosis. In the absence of serious survey data or even correct diagnoses, how do we know anything about the incidence of AIDS?

Dobe, in Botswana, twenty kilometers west of the subdistrict capital of Qangwa and only two kilometers from the Namibia border, had a resident population of about a dozen men from outside the community (such as, border guards and livestock inspectors) and a similar number of unmarried young local women. If AIDS was present, it might not be recognized as such, but the presence of a debilitating or incapacitating illness in persons in the age range of fifteen to forty-nine years would suggest the likelihood of the presence of the disease.

We undertook a house-to-house survey of all seven villages at the Dobe waterhole in July 2001, moving from village to village and asking patiently and discreetly whether anyone in that village was incapacitated or had experienced bouts of debilitating illness. The survey revealed not a single case of any illness resembling AIDS in persons of any age in the village of Dobe, with a population of 175 people.

In interviews, we asked repeatedly if anyone knew of other Ju/'hoansi living with AIDS or who had died of AIDS, and three names kept coming up, all women across the border in Tjumkui. Yet epidemiologists would agree that a similar survey elsewhere in Botswana, in a settlement of comparable size, would have revealed dozens of examples.

In explaining the much lower rates among the Ju/'hoansi, we have to invoke both macro and micro factors. Geographic isolation must play a role. Far from the urban centers and truck routes, the Ju/'hoan areas experienced low levels of interactions with outsiders. However, since the 1990s a succession of civil servants, soldiers, tourism workers, and traders, almost all male, have found their way into the interior. Additional factors for the low rates must be sought.

Ju/'hoan Women's Autonomy

Long before the AIDS crisis, ethnographic fieldwork in the 1960s and 1970s documented women's high status and freedom of action among the Ju/'hoansi. Young women could and did veto marriage plans. Women's voices were heard in the tribal councils. Women provided 70 percent of the food, and this economic autonomy was an important source of their strength. Accounts of women's experiences of work, sex, and family in the writings of Patricia Draper (1975), Lorna Marshall (1976), Harriet Rosenberg (1997), and Marjorie Shostak (1981) provide us with a rich history on which to base our current understandings of Ju/'hoan response to the threat of HIV.

Almost every observer of the African AIDS tragedy pinpoints the lethal impact of gendered inequality as a driving force in the epidemic. In our research among the dominant non-San ethnic groups elsewhere in Namibia, such as the Owambo, we noted that men more than women maintained multiple partners and that women repeatedly voiced frustration at their powerlessness to insist on condom use with boyfriends and spouses. Today in southern Africa as a whole, women comprise 55 to 60 percent of people with AIDS (Lee 2004; Preston-Whyte et al. 2000; Stein and Susser 2000).

Based on Ju/'hoan women's history of autonomy, one would predict that Ju/'hoan women differ in their sense of empowerment from women of other ethnic groups. In fact, women and young girls among the Ju/'hoansi revealed a greater degree of confidence in sexual negotiation with men, a sense of their own empowerment, than did the Owambo women (Stein and Susser 2000).

For example, we asked a young Ju/'hoan woman at Baraka in 1996 whether she would ask her husband to use a condom. She stated emphatically, "Yes, I would ask him, and if he did not agree, I would refuse sex." While Owambo women eagerly responded to demonstrations of the female condom and asked us where they could obtain them, Ju/'hoan women saw no particular advantage to the female condom, saying that if they wanted a man to use a condom, they would simply ask him to use a male one, distributed free at the local clinic.

In a group discussion with young married women in Dobe in 2001, one of us (Susser) asked the women if they would be able to make use of a box of male condoms. "Give us some and we will teach our husbands how to use them," they said.

While this does not indicate whether actual behavior change would follow, the remarks of the Ju/'hoansi women expressed a sense of entitlement and straightforwardness with respect to sexual decisions, which was not evidenced among the Owambo women. Nor was there the atmosphere of status striving and peer pressure that we observed among Windhoek high school and university students (Lee 2001).

When we interviewed young men in Dobe in 1999, their responses corroborated the women's views. They talked as if women had the power to turn down sexual advances, and they said that if a young woman were to accept such advances, they would see that as representing the opportunity to marry her, again in sharp contrast to the attitudes of young Owambo men. The terms in which young Ju men speak, coupled with the language used by young Ju/'hoan women—for example, seeing the opportunity to "teach" their boyfriends about condoms—suggests a kind of autonomy and sense of self-confidence that could augur well for the future as Ju women encounter men from other ethnic groups.

Taken together, these lines of evidence support the idea that women's autonomy is a powerful weapon against the spread of AIDS and may account in large part for the lower rates observed. Nevertheless, we need to ask to what extent the rapid changes in recent years have affected Ju/'hoan women's ability to retain control of their sexuality and their life choices.

Forces Driving the Epidemic Come to Tjumkui

In July 2003, we arranged to spend a period of time doing fieldwork in the Namibian areas of the Ju/'hoan world. The town of Tjumkui, population about 1,000, was once a remote San village, but it is now the administrative center for the San region and is connected to the urban centers of Namibia by an all-weather road. The town site includes a clinic, police station, stores, and rows of cement houses reminiscent of South African Bantustans. There is also a coed boarding school, the Tjumkui Junior Secondary School, housing 450 students ages thirteen to nineteen years, half of them female. A safari lodge opened in 1997 to provide a base from which tourists could visit the San villages and witness healing rituals staged for their consumption. Recently, the town was connected to the national telecommunications system with satellite phones powered by solar panels.

The population is divided roughly in two halves, with residents of Ju/'hoan ethnicity equaling in number outsiders of several different Namibian ethnic groups, including Owambo, Kavango, Herero, and Damara. The Tjumkui East region includes some 1,200 other Ju/'hoansi dispersed at thirty-five settlements, located at distances from Tjumkui ranging from ten to fifty kilometers.

Founded during the apartheid era as a government station in 1960, the village of Tjumkui has been the locus of massive state intervention in the lives of the Ju, accompanied by welfare dependency, rising interpersonal violence, and alcohol abuse. It also has—however faint—an aura of cosmopolitan sophistication, offering a taste of urban pleasures in a vast area of widely dispersed settlements. John Marshall's (2003) five-part film series, *A Kalahari Family*, chronicles the turbulent history of the Nyae Nyae area, of which Tjumkui is the principal settlement.

Apart from the shops, the clinic, the Dutch Reformed Mission church, and other grassroots churches, by far the most popular attractions are the sixteen shebeens, informal enterprises for the sale of alcohol, one for every sixty residents of Tjumkui. The shebeens range in permanence from a few stools or benches in front of a woman's traditionally built *rondavel*—a one-room African dwelling of wattle-and-daub construction—to more substantial structures with pool tables and sound systems blaring the latest pop music. Shebeens offer home-brewed *tombo* for N$1.00 per pitcher (U.S.$0.14), and commercially bottled beer for N$10.00 (U.S.$1.40). Brandy and other spirits are also available.

The shebeens are the main forums of social life for the people of Tjumkui, sites for people of different social classes and ethnicities, insiders and outsiders, to mingle. They are also sites where Ju/'hoan girls and young women go to drink and make liaisons with men from the outside, where sex is the major transactional medium.

On our first trip to the area, seven years earlier, when we approached officials of the Nyae Nyae Farmers Cooperative, a grassroots nongovernmental organization (NGO), to conduct research on AIDS, the representatives (all men) were well aware of the nature of the disease, its lethality, and its mode of transmission. But instead of implicating men as the main vectors of the disease, in their view AIDS was introduced among them by Ju/'hoan women.

Given that it was the local women who had sexual relations with male outsiders from high HIV areas, the men's perceptions were accurate, if incomplete. At Tjumkui, it was common knowledge that nonlocal men—road crews, traders, civil servants—drank at shebeens, and then had liaisons with San women. Drinking was widely seen as the major problem.

Clearly, Tjumkui as the main center for the spread of HIV has had a certain history; in the 1980s South African army units were based there, later replaced by border guards and other administrative personnel, posted far from home and seeking the local nightlife. The good-quality gravel road and an airstrip further increased accessibility. On the Botswana side of the border, Qangwa, the administrative center, plays a similar role, though on a much smaller scale.

In contrast to Tjumkui and Qangwa, other, more remote San villages had fewer outside visitors and home-brew shops. The Ju/'hoansi we spoke with in outer villages contrasted the drinking and sexual exchange at Tjumkui with the situation in their home communities. One informant at Dobe, a teenage girl, said: "There is no AIDS here, but I know they have it at Tjumkui. The girls over there told me not to sleep with the boys because they have that disease there. I am afraid of AIDS at Tjumkui."

Nevertheless, when we interviewed at Dobe in 2001 about the situation at Tjumkui, people could name only three people, all women, who they believed had died of AIDS. We were told that one young woman had died, unmarried, at age twenty. The ages of the other two were estimated at thirty-five and forty. The two older women had young children, but there was no knowledge of children's deaths.

In our 2003 survey of Tjumkui, we asked local Ju/'hoan informants to tell us about cases of people who to their knowledge had died of AIDS, promising that strict anonymity would be observed. Name after name was brought forward, both men and women, fourteen in all, with mention of a few possible others. These were people in their twenties, thirties, and forties, struck down in the prime of life, usually with tuberculosis as a co-infection. When we asked Dr. Malita Boschoff (known throughout the region as "Dr. Malita"), the medical officer of health for the administrative region that includes Tjumkui East, what kind of numbers she had, she came up with a figure of seventeen and counting for the number of Ju people who had died of AIDS. The closeness of our tally with hers appeared to strengthen the quality of our data collection and the robustness of our figures.

What does the number seventeen represent as a proportion of the total Ju population, and how does this number compare to corresponding numbers of AIDS deaths in other parts of the region? Assuming that persons aged fifteen to forty-nine years comprise about 50 percent of the total Ju population of Nyae Nyae of 1,800, then the deaths due to AIDS represent 1.9 percent of the population at risk. This compares to a figure of 6.7 percent of AIDS deaths as a percentage of the total population at risk for Namibia as a whole, based on the most recent UNAIDS epidemiologic estimates.

A second part of our July 2003 research consisted of interviewing small groups of women in Tjumkui about their knowledge of AIDS and, where possible, about sexual practices. Sa//gai (name changed), an articulate single woman of twenty-one, had an accurate knowledge of the disease, its mode of transmission, and means of prevention. When asked about how she was coping with problems of dating, she replied: "You must bring your own condom and not just trust the condom of your boyfriend. . . . If your boyfriend refuses the condom, then we know he has that disease and he wants to give it to you."

When we asked if the boy refuses to use a condom, must the girl still have sex with him, a frequent theme in our Owambo interviews, Sa//gai replied, "No, she can refuse and she will refuse."

The term "Goba" is used by Ju/'hoansi to refer to non-San Africans generally. Our informants had strong views about dating Gobas, which was seen as very problematic. "Goba boys will give Ju girls drink after drink to make them drunk," said Sa//gai. "They don't give them gifts like food, or soap, or clothes."

We asked a group of Ju women if they knew of young women who had AIDS: "Yes, a young girl named //Ushe [name changed] only about twelve years old, had a Goba boyfriend; when he died she was tested for HIV and came back positive but her parents tested negative. Then she died. Another member of the same family, an aunt also had a Goba boyfriend. She, too, tested positive, and both she and her boyfriend died."

Even with the seventeen cases noted, the dimensions of the epidemic seemed to be well contained in 2003. However, recent changes in the Namibian economy threaten to make this situation worse, possibly much worse.

The Larger Social Framework of AIDS Risk

Our 2003 fieldwork focused on the drinking-sexuality nexus, but our research quickly opened up additional lines of inquiry. In 2000, ten years after independence, Namibia began to feel the stresses that neighboring Zimbabwe is currently undergoing. Ex-liberation fighters, promised land and jobs when the South West Africa People's Organization (SWAPO) came to power, were loudly expressing their disappointment with the government through marches and demonstrations in the capital. In response, the government of President Sam Nujoma made several moves to address the legitimate grievances of the veterans, moves that directly affected people in remote areas like Nyae Nyae. Thousands of government jobs were opened up to absorb some of the unemployed, including many positions in the Ministry of Environment and Tourism (MET) (formerly the Department of Nature Conservation) for game scouts, road crews, and fencing crews. Tjumkui, in the center of a vast game management area, received many dozens of job-seeking migrants, mostly from the overpopulated and HIV-endemic areas of the north and center of the country. The result has been that, in the estimate of older Tjumkui residents, the number of outsiders in Tjumkui has doubled in the last two years.

A significant proportion of these migrant workers were themselves HIV positive, and some were already sick with AIDS. One reliable source reported that in 2002 alone, no fewer than ten of the recent MET arrivals in Tjumkui died of AIDS.

The Tjumkui Junior Secondary School

A second component in the mix that has brought the AIDS epidemic to the Ju/'hoansi is the Tjumkui Junior Secondary School. In 2003, it had an enrollment of 452 students in Standards 8–10, with forty teachers and auxiliary staff. Students are housed in dormitories and fed what appeared to be a substandard diet on the bare concrete slabs of the dining hall. Nevertheless, when we interviewed students, they appeared to be in good spirits. An attached primary school offers Standards 1–7 to a small number of local day students.

Within the student body, local Ju/'hoansi are matched by a large minority of students from outside the district; the teaching staff are almost all from outside. Interestingly, the preponderance of students from outside the district is explained in part by their parents' expressed desires to have their children spend their most vulnerable years far from the temptations of sex and alcohol in the larger towns of central and northern Namibia. But some of the incoming schoolgirls brought with them a set of attitudes toward sexuality that included seeking liaisons with older men as acceptable practice. One also wonders if becoming caught up in the "sugar daddy" phenomenon is related to the fact that the school attendees are so materially deprived, with poor-quality food and living conditions, and harsh discipline inconsistently applied. Despite the school's stated policies of close supervision of students and against sexual harassment, our Ju informants, young and old, perceived the secondary school as a hotbed of sexual impropriety, with male teachers having sex with their female students. A prominent theme of conversations with Ju informants was the after-school sightings of underage students at shebeens, one of which, the notorious Baby Smile, was located only a few meters from the school's main entrance. The enforcement of liquor laws regarding hours of operation and legal drinking age seemed lax to nonexistent. Thus, added to the forces driving the AIDS epidemic was this volatile mixture of sexually active and materially deprived youth coming into contact with migrant workers with cash and far from home.

This combination is on a scale not seen in Tjumkui since the days of the liberation struggle and the militarization, when the army recruited San for "homeland security" at army bases (Lee and Hurlich 1982). In the 1970s and 1980s, however, HIV/AIDS had not yet appeared in this part of Africa.

Another curious anomaly in school policy has been observed at the times of school vacations. According to informants, no provision is made for students whose home communities are distant from Tjumkui to get transport back home. Nor are they allowed to remain in dormitories until transport is arranged. The result has been that in recent years, some students have been forced to stand in front of the school hitchhiking, on a road that might see only one vehicle per hour, and camp by the roadside overnight until a ride was obtained. The vulnerability of female students to sexual exploitation was so obvious that on one occasion, the district medical officer, Dr. Malita, had to press her ambulance into service to rescue a group of stranded schoolchildren and deliver them to the bus station at Grootfontein, a distance of 300 kilometers.

If girls "fall pregnant," it is school policy to suspend or expel them. The fact that several are expelled each year suggests the magnitude of the problem of unprotected sex. Though certainly not all the pregnancies are the responsibility of teachers, epidemiologically one has to assume that the incidence of unwanted pregnancies is a proxy measure of unprotected sex and an indicator of the possibilities for HIV transmission.

The Old-Age Pension Affair

The provision of old-age pensions might appear at first to be unrelated to the epidemiology of HIV/AIDS. Yet closer examination of the social situation at Tjumkui reveals an unusual link. One of the more enlightened programs of Namibian social welfare, expanded under the postliberation SWAPO regime, is the provision of old-age pensions. In rural populations like the Nyae Nyae Ju/'hoansi, where fewer than 10 percent of adults have waged employment and petty commodity production such as handicrafts is still very limited, the pension for seniors may be the only source of income for entire families. Initially, pension checks were delivered to Tjumkui and picked up there, a difficult trek for outlying villagers. In returning to their homes, pensioners and their relatives had to run the gauntlet of home-brew establishments, and much, if not all, of the pension check could be dissipated if transport home was delayed.

In the mid-1990s, the contract for delivering pensions was awarded to a retired civil servant who saw the difficulties faced by families and instituted a program of delivering the pension payouts directly to villagers and allowing them to purchase essential foods and household goods at fair prices from his truck. By making the long trek to Tjumkui unnecessary, he alleviated a major social problem that was already severe in Tjumkui itself and was in danger of spreading to outer villages as well.

However, in 2002 the contract expired, and when it was put up for bid, it was awarded to a different company. This company stopped the payout trips to rural villages and announced that henceforth pension monies were to be picked up in town. Despite protests, once again pensioners and their families had to make the long trek to town. One observer described a typical outcome: while waiting for a lift home the pensioner and her family would stop at a shebeen, first for one drink, then another and another. After a day or two of waiting, much of the pension money would be gone. In addition, health workers have expressed concern that in the process, family members could be bringing HIV and other sexually transmitted infections (STIs) back with them to the villages.

Craft Buying as Income Generation

Another way in which the rural areas are serviced is through the purchase of handicrafts. The Reverend H. Van Zyl and his wife, Ellie, have been fixtures in the Tjumkui community since the apartheid era. Their obvious commitment to the cause of the Ju/'hoansi has earned them the respect of a range of stakeholders, both Ju and non-Ju. The Van Zyls have combined proselytizing with income generation. For several years they have been conducting monthly craft-buying trips to many of the thirty-five outlying villages of Nyae Nyae. They purchase bows and arrows, ostrich egg–shell jewelry, leather bags, and other items, and craft producers may take the cash or use it to purchase food, tools, household items, and clothing from the inventory on the reverend's truck. Tobacco products, but not alcohol, were available on the buying trips. The result is another way in which cash and resources are being pumped into the rural economy while permitting villagers to avoid the costly trek to Tjumkui.

Storerooms are filled to overflowing with high-quality but unsold handicrafts at the reverend's home, forcing a temporary suspension of the monthly buying trips. Fortunately, Nharo!—a Canadian craft marketing organization run by Paul Wellhauser, of Waterloo, Ontario—carried out negotiations in 2004 with the Dutch Reformed Church mission to purchase and market some of this accumulated inventory in North America. As of late 2004, $50,000 (Canadian dollars) worth of handicrafts was purchased, and another buying trip was being planned.

The *Kashipembe* Crisis

Many of the tensions within the Tjumkui community between long-term residents and recent arrivals came to a head in a series of events in March 2003 that became known as the Kashipembe Crisis. *Kashipembe* is a distilled spirit, a form of moonshine produced by shebeen proprietors in order to increase profit margins. It is colorless and pleasant tasting, and is estimated to be 25 percent alcohol, making it at least ten times more potent than *tombo*, the local home brew. The popularity of *kashipembe*, according to our informants, has made the community's already serious alcohol-related social problems even worse.

The Tjumkui town council, known officially as the Traditional Authority, is chaired by Samkau Toma, cofounder and former head of the Nyae Nyae Farmers Cooperative (later the Nyae Nyae Conservancy) and a leading figure in the films of John Marshall (2003). The Traditional Authority was asked to address the *kashipembe* problem, and it in turn enlisted the aid of the Reverend Van Zyl. When it turned out that a special permit was required to manufacture *kashipembe* and none of the shebeens were in possession of one, the reverend, backed by the town council, went to the police demanding that the laws be enforced. But when the police went around the community confiscating equipment and dumping gallons of *kashipembe* on the ground, the shebeen owners and some of their influential backers, including members of SWAPO, expressed outrage.

A somewhat sinister figure who went by the nickname "Luborsky," after a heroic white SWAPO activist who was murdered during the struggle by the apartheid regime, came from the district capital, Grootfontein, and orchestrated protest meetings targeting Rev. Van Zyl, calling him a racist and demanding that he be driven out of town. Luborsky presented a petition claiming it had been signed by San residents, but it was quickly shown to be a crude forgery. A meeting of residents attended by over seventy people gave strong backing to the reverend and to the stand of the Traditional Authority. With community support, the reverend weathered the attacks, and the situation was defused; however, soon after, the manufacture and sale of *kashipembe* quietly resumed, and *kashipembe* was actively on offer at shebeens during our July 2003 fieldwork.

Local residents saw this as a pivotal battle lost in the fight against drunkenness in Tjumkui, and by extension in the struggle to prevent AIDS from spreading. They regard *kashipembe* as a "date rape" drug, the drink of choice for older men from outside, seducing the Ju women and girls. Francina Simon, an articulate Ju woman and vice chair of the Traditional Authority, said: "There is no way you can stop the shebeens; you must rely on condoms." Another woman added in exasperation: "If you could close the shebeens you would stop AIDS in Tjumkui." Dr. Malita attested that rape is a serious problem and is rarely prosecuted. Under Namibian law, sex with a girl under the age of sixteen, even with consent, is statutory rape. The doctor related several cases of rape in which the victim became infected with HIV, but the families were bribed to keep quiet and not appear in court. She noted, "A Tjumkui Ju/'hoan girl will never force an outside man to use a condom."

The Wider Nyae Nyae Dobe Region

The situation elsewhere in the Ju/'hoan areas is more promising. Although the Ju are certainly poor by world standards, they maintain a strong sense of the value of their culture and lifeways. A Dobe area school dance troupe from /Xai/xai won a national dance competition in Botswana. Outside Tjumkui, on both sides of the border, Ju/'hoan communities do not seem to be suffering the poverty of an underclass in which family and household relations are undermined and women and children are cast adrift to fend for themselves. Both men and women had access to small sums of money from government work programs and from craft production, such as beading and carving. In this situation, if people were poor, there were minimal differences between men and women and between those with higher and lower incomes in terms of their clothes and their shelter. The historical autonomy of women offered the opportunity for forthright sexual negotiations and mobilization to prevent the spread of HIV/AIDS.

The border between Namibia and Botswana had been officially closed from 1965 up to the end of the apartheid era in 1989. It remained closed for the first years of Namibian independence (1989–2003). For the first time in decades, the border is now open to vehicular traffic. Polly Wiessner, of the University of Utah, who visited both sides of the Ju/'hoan world in 2003, commented on the relative prosperity and the absence of heavy drinking on the Botswana side when compared to the situation at Tjumkui.

In 2003, Dr. Elizabeth Yellen visited the Dobe area of Botswana accompanying her parents, longtime Dobe observers, John Yellen and Alison Brooks (Brooks and Yellen 1992; Yellen 1990). Dr. Yellen interviewed the staff at the Qangwa clinic about HIV. Did the clinic test for HIV? They replied that testing did occur, but only on request. When Dr. Yellen asked for a rough estimate of how many HIV tests had come back seropositive, the head nurse responded that to her knowledge, none of the Ju/'hoan patients had ever tested positive (Alison Brooks, personal communication, November 2003).

However favorable conditions may be for the Ju/'hoansi in the Dobe area of Botswana and in Namibian areas beyond Tjumkui, the fact remains that when the majority of Ju/'hoansi leave their villages, for work on road crews, on cattle ranches, and in regional centers, epidemiologic factors alter sharply. The Ju/'hoansi clearly become the "underclass," and their level of risk for HIV/AIDS climbs, as poor women find money through casual sex work or simply seek sexual relations with men who will provide "gifts" of food for themselves and their children. Renee Sylvain, of the University of Guelph, has addressed this topic in her recent writings about the Omaheke Farm San of the Gobabis District of Namibia, 200 kilometers south of Tjumkui (2001, 2002, 2003).

Conclusion

Returning to the focus on Tjumkui and its current problems, here is a follow-up to the shebeen issue. During recent fieldwork, an affable young Goba man introduced himself to us as the AIDS educator for the town of Tjumkui and related all the efforts he was making to get the message out, through the "My Future, My Choice" national AIDS education program for youth, including free distribution of condoms at shebeens. The same man, the district medical officer informed us later, is part owner of one of the shebeens frequented by underage drinkers and is notorious for getting girls pregnant, seven at last count. Not a promising start to the campaign to defeat AIDS.

On the other hand, there have been several signs that do indicate some promise. The Tjumkui Clinic backed by the medical officer, Dr. Malita, distributed 300 female condoms to women, Ju and non-Ju, who willingly accepted them. Condoms are available free from clinics, at shops, and at shebeens and are being used by the Ju/'hoan young men. Some Ju/'hoan mothers encourage their daughters to carry condoms at all times, and they do. A well-established NGO, Health Unlimited, has been working at Tjumkui for almost a decade and has engaged in health education and outreach throughout the Nyae Nyae. Finally, the head of the nursing staff reported on results from Tjumkui of the current nationwide voluntary counseling and testing (VCT) program. At the Tjumkui clinic, seven people tested HIV positive, but of these, six were outsiders and only one a Ju/'hoan.

In August–September 2003, a University of Toronto student, Donna Bawden, spent four weeks in Tjumkui specifically to explore in more detail the involvement of Ju/'hoan men and especially women in the culture of drinking. She confirmed reports of young Ju women frequenting the bars and engaging in sex with men from the outside and added considerable detail to the picture.

Neither the authors of this chapter nor Donna Bawden was able to ascertain how widespread these practices are. Does the subculture of disco, *kashipembe*, and casual sex involve 5 percent, 10 percent, or 50 percent of the young Ju/'hoan women of Tjumkui? How strong are the countervailing forces within the community, such as the Traditional Authority and the church, in their efforts to educate the vulnerable, provide social support, and stop these practices? Are there national and international stakeholders who are prepared to step in and offer assistance in stopping the spread of AIDS? Enforcing liquor laws and providing income generation opportunities would be good places to start. The Kalahari Peoples Fund of Austin, Texas, under the direction of Megan Biesele, has initiated an education campaign in the Ju/'hoan language to alert Ju/'hoansi about HIV/AIDS. Several NGOs have expressed interest in supporting this work. And the revival of craft marketing by the Canadian "fair-trade" organization Nharo! is another hopeful step in the right direction. The answers to the questions raised above will determine whether the AIDS epidemic among the Ju/'hoansi in the next five years rises to national and regional high levels, or whether the famed cultural resilience of the people will come to the fore and pull the Ju/'hoansi back from the brink.

Acknowledgments

This chapter was originally presented as a paper at the annual meeting of the American Anthropological Association, Chicago, November 19, 2003, in a session titled "Updating the San: Image and Reality of an African People in the 21st Century." Financial support for this research was received from the Fogarty Foundation for International Public Health, the University of Toronto, and the City University of New York. The authors wish to thank our Namibian collaborators, Dr. Scholastika Iipinge, Pombili Ipinge, and Karen Nasheya, and our North American collaborators, Megan Biesele, Karen Brodkin, and Robert Hitchcock. Special thanks goes to Donna Bawden, now at the London School of Tropical Health and Hygiene, whose research on the youth culture in Tjumkui in August–September 2003 added valuable detail and insights.

Notes

1. The term "Ju/'hoansi," meaning "real or genuine people," is the self-appellation the people of Nyae Nyae and Dobe want to be known by. It was adopted by a linguistic committee of the Nyae Nyae Farmers Coop in the late 1980s and has become the term of choice among anthropologists and development workers. Earlier terms in use in the 1950s–1980s, such as "!Kung" and "Bushman," were regarded by Ju/'hoansi to be inaccurate or pejorative, or both. Acceptable singular and adjectival forms include "Ju" (person or people) and "Ju/'hoan," pertaining to members of this ethnic group. The term "San" is widely used in southern Africa as an acceptable overall term for the multiple ethnicities formerly covered by the term "Bushman."

References Cited

Brooks, Alison, and John Yellen. 1992. "Decoding the Ju/wasi Past." *Symbols* (September 1992): 24–31.

Draper, Patricia. 1975. "!Kung Women: Contrasts in Sexual Egalitarianism in the Foraging and Sedentary Contexts." In *Toward an Anthropology of Women*, ed. Rayna Reiter, 77–109. New York: Monthly Review Press.

Hansen, J. D., D. Dunn, R. B. Lee, P. Becker, and T. Jenkins. 1994. "Hunter-Gatherer to Pastoral Way of Life: Effects of the Transition on Health, Growth and Nutritional Status." *South African Journal of Science* 89: 559–564.

Lee, Richard B. 1979. *The !Kung San: Men, Women and Work in a Foraging Society.* Cambridge: Cambridge University Press.

———. 2001. "A Fatal Attraction: AIDS and Youth in Southern Africa." *Canadian Journal of Infectious Diseases* 12 (Supplement B): 91.

———. 2003. *The Dobe Ju/'hoansi.* Sausalito, Calif.: Wadsworth/Thomson Learning.

———. 2004. "A Tale of Three Communities: Anthropological Insights into the African AIDS Crisis." In *The University Professor Lecture Series*, ed. Michael Goldberg, 69–85. Toronto: Faculty of Arts and Sciences, University of Toronto.

Lee, Richard B., and Irven DeVore, eds. 1976. *Kalahari Hunter-Gatherers: Studies of the !Kung San and Their Neighbors.* Cambridge, Mass.: Harvard University Press.

Lee, Richard, and Susan Hurlich. 1982. "From Foragers to Fighters: South Africa's Militarization of the Namibian San." In *Politics and History in Band Society*, ed. E. Leacock and R. Lee, 327–346. Cambridge: Cambridge University Press.

Marshall, John. 2003. *A Kalahari Family, Parts I–V.* Cambridge, Mass.: Documentary Educational Resources (Film Series).

Marshall, Lorna. 1976. *The !Kung of Nyae Nyae.* Cambridge, Mass.: Harvard University Press.

Nujoma, Sam. 2003. Speech given in Tjumkui District, July 13.

Preston-Whyte, Eleanor, Christine Varga, Herman Oosthuizen, Rachel Roberts, and

Frederick Blose. 2000. "Survival Sex and HIV/AIDS in an African City." In *Framing the Sexual Subject: The Politics of Gender, Sexuality and Power*, ed. Richard Parker, Regina Maria Barbosa, and Peter Aggleton, 165–190. Berkeley: University of California Press.

Rosenberg, Harriet. 1997. "Complaint Discourse, Aging and Caregiving." In *The Cultural Context of Aging*, ed. Jay Sokolovsky, 19–41. New York: Bergin and Garvey.

Shostak, Marjorie. 1981. *Nisa: The Life and Words of a !Kung Woman*. Cambridge, Mass.: Harvard University Press.

Stein, Zena, and Ida Susser. 2000. "Culture, Sexuality and Women's Agency in the Prevention of HIV/AIDS in Southern Africa." *American Journal of Public Health* 90 (7): 1042–1048.

Sylvain, Renee. 2001. "Bushmen, Boers and Baasskap: Patriarchy and Paternalism on Afrikaner Farms in the Omaheke Region, Namibia." *Journal of Southern African Studies* 27 (4): 717–737.

———. 2002. "'Land, Water and Truth': San Identity and Global Indigenism." *American Anthropologist* 104: 1074–1085.

———. 2003. "Class, Culture and Recognition: San Farm Workers and Indigenous Identities." *Anthropologica* 45 (1): 105–113.

Yellen, John. 1990. "The Transformation of the Kalahari !Kung." *Scientific American* 262 (4): 96–105.

3

Gendered Responses to Living with AIDS

Case Studies in Rwanda

RUTH KORNFIELD AND STELLA BABALOLA

In order to gain an understanding of why HIV prevalence rates remain high and how HIV prevention could be achieved in sub-Saharan Africa, it is necessary to understand how HIV-infected individuals respond to their situation. It is also necessary to understand how those individuals respond so that needed resources can be allocated and made available to people living with HIV and AIDS (PLWHA) as well as to those caring for them. The issue of gender is particularly important to these understandings because in sub-Saharan Africa, HIV is primarily transmitted through heterosexual intercourse, and the epidemic is shared by both men and women. In addition, because of women's increased vulnerability to the infection, for both biological and social reasons, HIV prevalence rates are higher among women than men. Of all persons infected in sub-Saharan Africa, an estimated 58 percent are women and 42 percent are men (UNAIDS 2002a).

The epidemic is exacerbated by inadequate health care and generally low individual health status due to poor economic conditions and limited access to necessary resources, all of which are differentiated by gender (de Bruyn et al. 1998; Farmer et al. 1996; Foreman 1999; Morrell 2001; Schoepf 1988; Setel 1993; Susser 2000; UNAIDS 1999; Vlassoff and Moreno 2002; Whelan 1999). This chapter sheds light on the gendered dynamics of reactions to HIV infection by comparing the responses of men and women living with AIDS in Rwanda and examining the similarities and differences and underlying reasons for these responses. It shows how the process of discovering one's HIV-positive status, living with a highly stigmatized illness and lack of resources, the emotional and sexual reactions, and the social support and health maintenance/survival strategies are mediated by imbalanced gendered cultural, social, psychological, and economic phenomena.

Background

HIV/AIDS is a major problem in Rwanda. By the end of 2001, an estimated 8.9 percent of Rwandans, representing about 500,000 people, were infected with HIV. Proportionally more young women than young men are infected; it is estimated at between 8.9 and 13.4 percent of the female youth aged fifteen to twenty-four years are infected, compared with only 3.9 to 5.9 percent of their male counterparts. Women comprise 58.1 percent of the approximately 430,000 HIV-infected adults, or about 250,000 individuals, and men comprise 41.9 percent, or about 180,000 individuals (UNAIDS 2002a). One peculiarity of HIV infection in Rwanda is that the prevalence is high in both urban and rural areas. From a low level of about 1 percent in the mid-1980s, HIV prevalence rates in rural areas rose rapidly to nearly 11 percent by the late 1990s, probably because the social and political upheaval of the mid-1990s fostered high population movements, widespread use of rape as a weapon of war, and high-risk sexual behaviors in refugee camps (UNAIDS 2002b).

In Rwanda, there is a high level of stigma surrounding HIV/AIDS and a low level of support for those infected and affected by the virus (Kornfield et al. 2002). Antiretroviral treatment is not generally available in the country, and most HIV-infected people have limited or no access to drugs for treating opportunistic infections associated with AIDS. People who are seropositive occupy a very large percentage of beds in the hospitals. Unfortunately, the services are inadequate, and many people cannot afford to pay for them. As a result, an emphasis has been put on home-based care, but there is community resistance to this because of the stigma concerning AIDS and lack of knowledge, as well as limited resources of family members or friends.

PLWHA have been organized into groups called PLWHA associations, which have a legal status allowing them to officially receive food aid and financial grants. Their objective is to improve the conditions of PLWHA through the provision of material resources, moral support, education, and income-generating activities. However, many of these associations are new and are experiencing multiple problems that prevent them from being effective. While Rwanda does have an AIDS control program, there is no systematic functioning national program to care for people living with AIDS. A few nongovernmental organizations (NGOs) and churches implement periodic projects, but these projects rely on foreign donors, with only sporadic funding resulting in lack of continuity of interventions. The result is that PLWHA are basically left on their own to cope with their difficult situation.

Aspects of the geography and social structures of Rwanda have a direct impact on PLWHA. Rwanda is a densely populated, hilly country with a very poor subsistence farming–based economy. Abject poverty among most of the population results in very little surplus food or cash to give to a chronically ill relative or friend. Working on steep hillsides is especially fatiguing for people already weakened by AIDS. Since housing is scattered on the hillsides, home care is difficult because neighbors, who are sometimes family members, live at fairly long distances from each other. Housing conglomerations that were built for refugees after the 1994 war introduced a new village-like community structure. But the people who have moved in are frequently strangers to each other and have no special social bond that fosters mutual assistance.

Descriptions of Rwandan culture are ridden with secrecy, filial jealousy, lack of trust and confidence among neighbors, exploitation of one group over another, stories of poisoning to prevent an individual or his or her immediate family from succeeding for reasons of jealousy, and vengeance (de Lame 1996; Kornfield 2000; Newbury 1988; Ntezimana 2000; Rutembesa 2001; Rwangabo 1993). The genocide and the civil war of the mid-1990s have most likely exacerbated this distrust. This atmosphere of distrust makes it even more difficult for PLWHA, who are already being stigmatized for their condition, to obtain help from relatives, neighbors, and friends.

Gender relations have been shaped by traditional structures that persist in various ways and contribute to women's limited economic access and agency (that is, their capacity to act according to their own desires, assert control over their own lives, and influence others), which in turn contribute to the increase of HIV infection among women. Historically, Rwanda has been a patrilineal (inheritance and family structure through the male line) and patrilocal (marital residence with the groom's family) society (Andre and Platteau 1998; Womenaid International 2003).

Currently, patterns of residence are based on convenience and availability of land, but there still is a tendency for the wife to live on the land given to her husband by his father at the time of their marriage. While in 1999 new legislation (Civil Code 1999) was passed that is supposed to guarantee the right of the wife to this land after her husband's death, there is strong resistance to its application, and many women do not even know the law exists. In addition, the law itself is weak, allowing for various interpretations that could result in nonprotection of the wife or female children's right of inheritance of both movable and nonmovable property. In practice, at the death of a husband, the wife may be allowed to stay on the land, but the final decision is often made by her deceased husband's father or brothers (Kornfield 2000).

Compared to their wives, husbands tend to exercise considerably greater decision-making power within the conjugal family. Customarily, the husband's brothers have sexual rights as well as decision-making power over their brother's wife, especially when he is not present. Furthermore, the levirate, a custom where a woman is expected to marry her husband's brother upon the death of her husband, is still reported to be practiced in Rwanda (Kornfield 2000). The social and political upheavals of the mid-1990s resulted in increased numbers of urban and rural women who are either widows or whose husbands are in prison, resulting in a proportionately larger number of female-headed households. It is estimated that about 130,000 persons suspected of genocide are currently being held in prisons, of which the vast majority are married men. In the three provinces where this study was conducted, Byumba, Gitarama, and Kigali City, 9.2 percent of adults have lost their spouses; 89.7 percent of those who lost a spouse are women. Of the adult female population in these provinces, 14.7 percent are widows, of whom 38.3 percent are between the ages of twelve and thirty-nine (Ministry of Finance and Economic Planning 1999).

Analytical Description of PLWHA, Comparing Women and Men

The following analysis of how the men and women participating in this study dealt with living with HIV/AIDS includes (1) demographic characteristics, (2) living conditions, (3) process of discovery of HIV-positive status, (4) emotional responses, (5) sexual responses, and (6) social support and survival strategies. The data were disaggregated by gender and region. Nonetheless, very few distinct regional differences were found, and these will be mentioned when noteworthy.

Sixty-six case studies of people living with HIV and AIDS were conducted in the three selected provinces. All were areas with high percentages of PLWHA. The data were collected through focus group discussions using Kinyarwanda, the national language of Rwanda; in-depth, open-ended interviews; and field observations during May 2001. PLWHA were interviewed by researchers of their own gender. In total, five focus group discussions were held (three with women and two with men), with a total of fifty-two participants. In addition, six males and eight females with HIV/AIDS, six home-care providers, and six leaders of PLWHA associations were interviewed. For reasons of confidentiality, participants were identified through associations for PLWHA, which generally had a predominantly female membership.

The study participants were comprised of fewer men than women partly because of this selection procedure, and also because men were less willing than women to consent to participate. The reason for their hesitation to participate in the study may have been because of their reticence to personally accept their HIV/AIDS status and therefore to discuss it with others. Field observations were made in households of PLWHA and home caregivers, as well as at PLWHA association meeting places. Discussions were held with several key informants, including medical doctors and counselors who work with PLWHA. In addition, data and insights from the experiences of the first author, who has been living in Rwanda since 1998 conducting research and working on HIV and AIDS care and prevention projects, contributed to the findings and their interpretation.

Demographic Characteristics of the Population Studied

Forty-four females and twenty-two males with HIV/AIDS participated in the study, of which all the females and nineteen of the males provided demographic information. Three males refused to provide this information because of fear of their identities being revealed. The study participants ranged from twenty years of age into their fifties, but the majority were between twenty-nine and forty-nine years old. There was a disproportionate number of widowed women, reflecting one of the results of the 1994 genocide. Twenty-nine women and five men were widows or widowers, respectively. Seven women and twelve men were married, five women and none of the men were separated from their spouses, and three women and two men were never married.

The overall level of education was very low. Nine women and two men had no formal schooling. Twenty-eight women and fourteen men had some primary schooling, and seven women and three men had some secondary education. The majority were subsistence farmers or petty traders, or a combination of both. Only three men and four women did skilled or semi-skilled work. Eight women and two men reported no occupation. All the women had from one to five children under their care, the majority with three to five. Four men had no children under their care, and the rest had from three to five. One man with HIV/AIDS who had three wives had thirteen children for whom he shared responsibility.

Living Conditions

As in other places in Africa (Food and Agriculture Organization 2000), for all the PLWHA interviewed in this study, HIV infection had made preexisting conditions of poverty considerably worse, and in some respects conditions were more difficult for the women because of lack of marital support. For many of the widowed women, the cycle of impoverishment began at the time their husband became sick from AIDS, was exacerbated by their husband's inability to work consistently because of frequent illnesses and general physical weakness, and worsened after their husband's death. By contrast, the men, whose wives had not died or who had remarried after the death of their first wife, continued to receive some help from their spouses. However, as the men became more and more incapacitated, their family income decreased because their wives could not earn as much as they could, nor could their wives keep up with all the necessary farming tasks.

Support from other family members was nonexistent or minimal at best. Many of their families lived in conditions almost as poverty stricken as the PLWHA and had little or no surplus to offer. For others, family and friends had nearly abandoned them altogether, not to mention harboring the unfortunate notion that it would be a waste to use already limited resources on an individual who would soon die rather than on a healthy member of the family who would be able to contribute something in return. Some widows and single women living in urban areas reported that they would not return to their rural families for help for fear of being rejected and/or because they did not want to become a burden. The urban men often were at an advantage because they usually had a plot of land in their rural homestead, so if they returned they would be able to exploit it and not be totally dependent on their extended family.

Due to poor housing conditions, the PLWHA were not able to protect themselves sufficiently from dampness and cold that contributed to the deterioration of their health. Household repairs, such as fixing leaky roofs and broken shutters, work usually done by men, proved a large burden on the women who could not afford to pay a worker, whereas the men, when they had enough energy, were able to do that type of work themselves. The ability to continuously secure lodging was a constant worry for more women with HIV/AIDS than for men with HIV/AIDS because more women did not own their house and were obligated to pay monthly rent that they frequently could not meet. As mentioned above, this precariousness of women was influenced by the patrilocal and patrilineal land tenure systems.

A widow had little agency (capability) in terms of choice of place to live after the death of her husband, as the decision concerning her continued stay in her deceased husband's house was the prerogative of her husband's family. Furthermore, some widows reported that they could not return to their parental home because their brothers were not willing to share the family property with them, although this is contrary to the new legislation (Civil Code 1999). Many PLWHA did not have sufficiently warm clothing or blankets, and many women reported sleeping directly on mats on damp floors crowded with all the children in the household.

Lack of sufficient cooking fuel and sanitary water contributed to weakening physical conditions of many study participants. Women, especially, reported missing meals for a day at a time, sometimes for lack of money to buy food, but also because of lack of cooking fuel. They suffered from intestinal parasites due to unsanitary drinking water. Since the burden of fetching both fuel and water mainly rested with the women, the married men with HIV/AIDS had an advantage over the women with HIV/AIDS, since their wives would fetch fuel and water for them. When the women with HIV/AIDS were too weak, they depended on their children, who frequently were not able to find sufficient quantities of fuel or water. Once the men could no longer work and if their wives could not help them, then they suffered the same way as did the women. These findings echo those of previous studies among PLWHA in Africa. For example, in a study conducted in 1988 (Khoegh et al. 1994), a sample of HIV-positive women in Kigali prioritized their most important needs as housing, employment, and money. In 1991, the same women added food to their lists of current and future needs.

Process of Discovering One's HIV Status

The case studies revealed an evolutionary process of the individuals' self-knowledge of the possibility of their seropositive status as they redefined or reinterpreted the possible meanings of their physical symptoms in light of their own conceptions of HIV and AIDS, their own social and sexual behavior and that of their sexual partner (s), and the advice or opinions of others concerning their symptoms (see Vidall 1996).

The process of discovering the individuals' HIV status consisted of several steps set off by one or more initial cues signaling suspicion of their HIV status. Cues might include, for example, a long history of repeated opportunistic illnesses; a spouse and/or child who had died of AIDS; the experience of miscarriages or infertility of a female with HIV/AIDS or wife of a male with HIV/AIDS; a multipartnering lifestyle on the part of the individual interviewed or of his or her spouse; or the advice by a medical practitioner, friend, spouse, or other relative to be tested. When suspicion became significant enough because of any one or a combination of these cues, then the person went either directly to a screening center to be tested; asked for advice from medical practitioners, a friend, or sister; or was advised by a spouse to go for HIV screening. In a few cases, neighbors who had observed the person's frequent bouts of illness suggested that he or she go for a test.

The initial cue for both the men and women was repeated illnesses over a long period, which signaled suspicion of their status. But the major triggering event was different. The basis of the women's perception of their probable seropositive status was their husbands' extramarital sexual behavior, illness, and ensuing death, where the husbands suspected themselves of being infected based on their own sexual activity and would delay going for a screening test until being advised by their wife or a friend. These differences reflected the gendered differences in perceived or real sexual behavior of the PLWHA.

The contrast of the experiences of two subsistence farmers, a man with HIV/AIDS in Gitarama with that of a woman with HIV/AIDS in Byumba, shows how the difference in the marital roles of men and women influenced the different process they went through before going for an HIV test. The male farmer explained:

First I got sick, but especially we didn't have any children. I thought that it was because of poisoning and I went to a traditional healer for treatment. My wife and I closed our house and went to live at the healer's. We had just spent four years without a child (without getting pregnant) and three years before she had had a miscarriage without another conception. So we decided to try out the traditional healer to ask why we weren't having any children. We spent seven months at the healer's. That was last year [2000] until the month of September. I was so sick that my wife had to bring me what to eat. In order to get what to live on, my wife had to go everywhere with a basket of fruit [selling fruit], because I didn't have the strength to work. I could feel the poison in me. . . . My wife . . . took care of me. Upon leaving the healer to return home I was gravely ill and I arrived just at the point when one said that I was dead. . . . Thanks to the miracles of God . . . after a month I began to get up from bed and little by little walk around, . . . I had no strength and was useful for nothing. I preferred to go for a test to see if it was the virus, and I went with my wife to be tested. They gave us the results and told us we were contaminated.

The female from Byumba, on the other hand, took care of her husband until he died and then went for an HIV screening test herself: "My husband was sick for three years. He had AIDS. He died in September 1998. I took care of him and when I had the symptoms and knew how he had died I went to see the sister [nun] for the test. She tested me and that's how I found out I was seropositive in year 2000. My five-year-old child is also sick."

The case studies indicated a strong tendency, among both men and women, to wait for several months or even years before going for a test. The two main reasons for postponing HIV screening, fear and a pattern of health-seeking behavior that places emphasis on traditional medicine and considers biomedical services as an option of last resort, were not specifically gendered. However, certain aspects of the underlying fear and some of the reasons for seeking treatment from traditional healers were gender specific. Both men and women explicitly expressed the fear of death and suffering, and the fear of being abandoned and the ensuing solitude should their seropositive status become known. Only men directly expressed the fear of losing their dignity and social status. Both men and women patronized traditional healers, *amagendu*, because they considered their symptoms to be caused by poisoning or sorcery (Rwangabo 1993).

For women, however, an additional reason why traditional healers represented an option of choice was because these women perceived their symptoms to be due to an ill-defined set of symptoms called *ifumbi* (Durand 1959; Kamungu 2001; Niang 1999; Rwangabo 1993), which, according to them, could only be cured by traditional medicine. *Ifumbi* does not refer to any known disease as identified in biomedicine and is associated with any kind of discomfort involving the lower abdomen, menstruation, or pregnancy. The symptoms are frequently described as being manifested in the genital areas, but also are believed to affect other parts of the body. They often appear during pregnancy.

The symptoms include almost all those associated with sexually transmitted infections (STIs) such as syphilis or gonorrhea (that is, vaginal secretions, pain during sexual intercourse and during micturition, lower abdominal pain, and swelling and itchiness of sexual organs). A person is considered to be born with *ifumbi*, which is frequently described as some sort of fat worm or round animal in the form of a big blood clot (Niang 1999). Some PLWHA reported that they spent several wasted months under the care of a traditional healer before they were convinced that the treatment was a failure.

For the women, the death of their husbands functioned either as a motivating factor to go for testing, or as a major reason to postpone testing. During the period that they took care of their husbands, they waited, not because they did not think they might be HIV infected themselves, but from a feeling of despair. They explained that there would be nothing that they could do should they be seropositive and foresaw only increasing poverty, as productive work would be neglected because of illness. They also tended to neglect their own health to the advantage not only of their husbands' but their children's as well.

For both the wife of the farmer from Gitarama Province and another female with HIV/AIDS who was a petty trader from Byumba Province, physical distress was originally attributed to reproductive health problems, sterility in the case of the wife of the Gitarama farmer, and missing menstrual periods for the female petty trader from Byumba. This female petty trader took quite a circuitous route before going for her HIV screening test, which included first going to a health center and then a healer for suspected reproductive health problems. She explained:

> I felt OK except that I had just spent nine months without having a menstrual period and when I went to the health center to ask why, they told me it was understandable because I was anemic and, therefore, I didn't have enough blood in my body. And they told me when I don't have blood I can't have my period. But also I didn't think I had AIDS. I fell sick several times and I thought it was *ifumbi* especially since I had only one baby. In the countryside, they say that when you don't give birth to any children and you are still young you suffer from this *ifumbi*. And I also believed that, and I looked for traditional medicine so that I could treat myself and see if I would be cured. You know, I am married with a man who was separated with two wives, and I was married by force. I was sixteen years old and we had had only one child, a girl. Afterward, we separated. Since then I never had sexual relations. I remained faithful for about five years. Afterward, there was a man that I told you about that came and told me that he loved me and is going to marry me. One day he came to visit me. It was in 1993 and we spent the night together. Ah, without lying to you, I just didn't think about AIDS.

The PLWHA reported general nervousness and feared the test results. But those who had already experienced the death of a spouse or had been sick for a long time and had a strong suspicion of their seropositive status were a bit less anxious than were the others. Both the men and women generally went for the test alone because of fear of stigmatization should their positive status be revealed. But women had a greater tendency to take a trusted friend or sister for moral support. While a few of the men reported taking their wife with them, none of the women reported asking their husband to accompany them. For example, one man with HIV/AIDS from Kigali recognized the need for both him and his wife to go for an HIV screening test, but deliberately went to a different clinic from that of his wife because of embarrassment. He also went to several clinics for tests before he would believe the veracity of the results. He explained: "I went to five different testing centers . . . and to a private doctor separately from my wife who went to King Faisal Hospital. It was too embarrassing to go the same place as her. Every place I went to, they kept saying I was positive, but I wanted to really make sure. At each place I gave a different name and age so that they would retest me." Similar barriers to going for HIV testing have been described by Maman and colleagues (Maman, Mbwambo, Hogan, Kilonzo, and Sweat 2001; Maman, Mbwambo, Hogan, Kilonzo, Sweat, and Weiss 2001) and by Temmerman and colleagues (1995) in other African settings.

Emotional Responses to HIV-Positive Status

The situation in which the PLWHA went for their HIV screening test appeared to influence their emotional responses to the discovery of their seropositive status. Those who had already suspected, and had been more or less convinced of, their seropositive status for a long time tended to be more accepting than those for whom the idea was new. The emotional responses to the initial discovery of their seropositive status were similar among the men and women, and consisted of two extremes: one, a quiet resignation as explained, for example, by a male subsistence farmer with HIV/AIDS in Byumba Province: "I knew that I was sick because of these other women that were infected. . . . While waiting for the results I wasn't afraid, I had the courage to receive the results, and when I received them I accepted that this illness really was the reality."

A second strong response was described as feeling like "going crazy" or "wanting to commit suicide," or consisted of isolating oneself without eating or sleeping for a few days. For example, a woman with HIV/AIDS expressed her extreme state of anxiety:

I lost my head and I wanted to commit suicide. I wanted to throw myself in the waterfall, but then I remembered that if a woman throws herself into water, she dies floating in water on her back with her front side exposed to view. And I didn't want people to see me like that and I was afraid. Then I wanted to put rat poison in my porridge and drink it. Then I remembered that I was Christian, that I was baptized, that God can help me and can punish me and I put myself in the hands of God.

In the first reaction, the PLWHA reported having been, in a sense, emotionally prepared for the results because they were already convinced of their seropositive status. In these cases, there was not an initial response of denial or doubt as found among the women studied in Nairobi by Forsythe and Rau (1996), but rather an acceptance, in a sense, of the inevitable. After a while, the initial emotional response diminished, and the PLWHA found various ways to cope with their continuing daily lives. Some who had been HIV positive for quite a while began to treat their HIV-positive status as any other kind of chronic disease they may have had. Similar responses were described by Kantengwa (1997) in a study of HIV-positive clients of a voluntary counseling and testing center in Kigali. The study participants did not seem to express a sense of fatalism as has been found in other studies in central and eastern Africa (Forsythe and Rau 1996), but rather more of a realistic idea of their resources, or lack thereof, and therefore a practical recognition of the little they would actually be able to do about their condition.

Underlying the descriptions given by the men and women of their emotional responses seemed to be gendered differences in the dynamic of feeling and expressing emotions, especially concerning shame, dignity, and trust, and a Rwandan cultural norm restricting the open expression of emotions. Attitudes toward husbands and wives, respectively, were different. Women were very angry with their husbands, blaming them for transmission, while men assumed the blame themselves and expressed shame. But when a man suspected that his wife was the source of transmission, he was humiliated by his wife's assumed sexual "betrayal."

An older man from Kigali sadly described his feeling of humiliation, expressing shame because he married, against the admonition of his first wife and disapproving eyes of his second, a third, younger woman known to be "promiscuous" and whom he blamed for his infection. Another man explained how he had swallowed his pride when he became so sick that he depended on his wife for his food and care, and sheepishly admitted that he "could not criticize her for any extramarital sexual relations she had, since she was contributing money to the family as a result."

The responsibility for their children and lack of economic resources appeared to bear more heavily on the women than on the men with HIV/AIDS. Especially common among the women was a subdued response of fear and sadness with the constant worry concerning the future of their children. They described continual feelings of despair with varying intensity, depending on their current health and capacity to deal with their daily basic needs and those of their children.

Sexual Responses to Being HIV Positive

After becoming aware of their seropositive status, men and women continued to have sexual relations, often unprotected, for pleasure and out of perceived marital obligation, some continuing from seven to eighteen years after having been tested. They mainly stopped because of erectile dysfunction, disgust with their body, and/or because of fatigue or pain experienced during intercourse. Males continued extramarital sexual relations to avoid suspicion in order to maintain their "normal" social identity as defined by their male friends and for fear of losing face. The women, especially those responsible for their own households, had sexual relations in exchange for money in order to support themselves financially.

For both the men and women, giving up sexual relations was difficult. Interviews with the married PLWHA revealed complementarities in gender dynamics concerning sexual marital obligations that contributed to continued sexual intercourse. For example, one male with HIV/AIDS explained, "But if you don't do penetrative sex, then my wife could decide to go back to her family because what would be the reason for her to stay with me." A woman expressed the same idea, "Myself, I have a husband, how can one give up sexual relations between husband and wife?"

The data also suggested that underlying this sense of marital obligation, and for some women a sense of resignation to accepting this obligation, may have been an emotional need to maintain a semblance of normality within their marriage to soften the fear and difficulties of living with AIDS. Also, the response to a natural sex drive by single women was important. An expression of this came from a woman in a focus group discussion who exclaimed, "In order to abstain, how can one control oneself?" And a reply was, "With prayer, I was strong enough not to start having sexual relations again."

The other main reasons for continuing sexual relations were quite different for the men and women and reflected different ways of socializing. The men, who habitually frequented bars mainly to enjoy the comradeship of their male friends, explained they felt compelled to continue extramarital sexual relations so as not to bring on suspicion of their seropositive status and consequently be rejected from their drinking group. They mainly shared a locally brewed banana beer that they drank from a single gourd or bottle, sipping from the same straw as the gourd or bottle was passed from man to man. In Rwanda, this is an important symbol of very valued trust and solidarity. If the other men knew their friend was HIV infected, the infected man was afraid they would refuse to share their straw or not want to be near him for fear of contagion, and they may no longer accept him in their group. This drinking group provided the men with HIV/AIDS with a kind of social support that was very important in their life and which they greatly feared losing. During one focus group discussion, the men also explained that sex was their only means of relaxation. One man exclaimed sarcastically, "We don't go to the soccer game!" Others laughed, and another said, while the rest of the group shook their heads in agreement, "Fun without sex is for children!"

In contrast, some widows and other female heads of household reported engaging in sexual relations for money in order to survive, even though they knew that they were infecting their sexual partners and could be reinfected themselves should their partners be seropositive. An illustration of this was the poignant discussion in one of the female focus groups where one woman said, "If you spend days without eating, and someone offers you 1,000 or 5,000 francs [equivalent to about U.S.$2.00 or U.S.$10.00] to sleep with you, are you going to refuse? [It's] impossible to refuse when you have found a way to relieve your hunger!" The other women cried out all at once, "Five thousand francs! No, no, no, even without a condom I couldn't accept that this money would go somewhere else!" There also were a few cases of reported force, usually of one-time occurrences. For example, one woman from Kigali reported: "I've been sick [HIV-positive] for four years and had stopped all sexual relations. Then one day a man with whom I work took me by force and impregnated me. I cried a lot."

Social Support and Survival Strategies

A most striking report given by both the men and women with HIV/AIDS was the lack of assistance from others, including those who had helped them before their seropositive status had become known. They had no supportive social network, but rather would ask for assistance many times from individual family members, friends, or neighbors before receiving it. Those who received volunteered help were very grateful. Men tended to obtain support from men, and women from women. The women, more so than the men, reported suffering from isolation and often had to simply fend for themselves. Their most continuous source of assistance was from their own small children or sometimes a younger sibling, especially a sister. Associations for PLWHA provided the only organized support and were accessed much more by women than men. Men had a greater tendency than women to rely on friends, and sometimes would have one particular person in whom they could confide and who would give or lend them money periodically. This description of social isolation and rejection related to the stigma associated with HIV in Rwanda is similar to that described in other African countries (Malinga 2002; Nyblade and Field-Nager 2001; Seeley and Kajura 1995; Topouzis and Hemrich 1995).

Neither the men nor the women were able to develop adequate strategies to fulfill their basic needs. They understood the necessity of eating a healthy diet, the advantages of treating opportunistic illnesses early and resting when fatigued, and convalescing to regain their strength, but they were not able to do so. They frequently had to work in fields; do household tasks; walk long distances searching for fuel, water, or food; or do odd jobs when they really were too sick for such tasks and became exhausted.

Women and men used different strategies to obtain cash and food. The strategies employed by women included going to churches or PLWHA associations asking for charity, begging in the street, and selling sex. In urban areas, some of the women with HIV/AIDS reported occasionally borrowing money to buy a basket of produce wholesale that they then sold at a small profit. Unfortunately, they frequently spent all the small profits on food or other immediate necessities and sometimes were neither able to pay back the loan nor keep some money for reinvestment. In Kigali, some of the women, when they had enough energy, did seasonal work in a coffee company, where the manager had taken particular interest in helping PLWHA. The amount they could manage to earn was never sufficient to take care of their ordinary daily needs and those of their children. Many women reported that sometimes they obtained just enough money to pay for transport to the hospital, but not enough to pay for the consultation or buy medication.

Men used different strategies. These included asking for and obtaining bank credit, borrowing money from a special friend or brother in whom they had confided their HIV-positive status, continuing to work at their place of employment until too weak or sick to do so, and continuing to receive some money from their previous employers. One man reported a common way Rwandan shopkeepers help people in need. He obtained credit in-kind, in this case a gallon of oil, from a friend who owned a small shop. He then sold the oil in small quantities, paid back the value, and kept the profit. Some of the married men were able to receive some help from their wives who earned a little money selling small items on the street or even by commercial sex. Remarriage after the death of their wives from AIDS appeared to be another strategy used by men to obtain help.

The strategies to obtain assistance when sick reflected differences in social roles whereby women are expected to be the caregivers. When ill, the married men were cared for by their wives or children. In contrast, married women did not expect their husband to take care of them when ill; a female child or sibling would do so. Only the women reported obtaining help from a female neighbor or reported that they participated in the peer home-care programs of the PLWHA associations. Since the resources of the associations were very limited, help often consisted of a visit where the "care provider" would simply hold the ill woman's hands and talk to her.

The men with HIV/AIDS reported using alcohol as a strategy to relieve anxiety and fear. This was clearly expressed during one of the male focus group discussions: "We [men] drink alcohol to erase the ideas in our head." Another added, "I drink some banana beer each night or else I'm too nervous." One man said, "I must drink for relief even though it's bad for a person who is seropositive." "It is necessary to take beer because it helps you sleep and lets you forget all these problems," another man stated. Drinking in both public places and alone at home provided this relief. As for the women, major outlets for relieving anxiety included prayer and participation in the gatherings of the PLWHA associations, where they were able to share their worries and empathize with each other. They also said that their anxiety would have been greatly alleviated, and the idea of premature death less feared, if they were given money for food and school fees for their children and were able to find anyone who would be willing to provide for their children's future after the death of their mother.

An important coping strategy used by the men to avoid rejection was hiding their seropositive status. The strategy they used reflected the different ways in which men and women in Rwanda socialize. The men hid their seropositive status so that they would continue to be accepted by their drinking groups, while the women had no such informal social group. They, on the other hand, appeared to live in a rather isolated social milieu in which they had one or two women friends they saw from time to time. To avoid social isolation, they joined PLWHA associations, which provided a group of women they could trust and with whom they shared their worries.

As mentioned earlier, joining a PLWHA association was a strategy used much more by women than men. Although both men and women were welcome to join the PLWHA associations, women overwhelmingly dominated their membership. For example, one association in Kigali had 200 female and six male members. In Gitarama, one had fifty women and three men, and another in Byumba had about twenty women with only two men. The associations, sponsored by churches or by local government structures, had very limited funds. Their activities consisted mainly of sporadically distributing small quantities of basic foodstuffs, providing HIV/AIDS education and a place for PLWHA to discuss their problems, organizing home care by PLWHA for each other, and some—mostly unsuccessful—efforts at income-generating activities.

The women's and men's responses to participating in PLWHA associations suggest some underlying psychological differences revolving around humiliation, pride, and the admission of weakness to oneself and others. The women with HIV/AIDS reported that they initially went to the associations to ask for free food and did not express any concern about feeling humiliated doing so. When they discovered that such provisions were either extremely small or nonexistent, they were disappointed. However, they were willing to reveal their seropositive status and risk possible derision in order to obtain some assistance. By taking this risk, they discovered that they received moral support rather than derision and found that the meetings fulfilled an emotional void that they were not able to fill otherwise.

The men with HIV/AIDS, on the other hand, expressed a strong reticence to going to a PLWHA association to "beg" for food for fear of humiliation, and they perceived that the associations had done nothing for their members either. They were also concerned about being ridiculed in front of others. Maintenance of their pride appeared to be very important to them. The following statements sum up the men's responses to these associations. "Men always like to think of themselves as being healthy, so even after he is tested seropositive, he still doesn't want to think of himself differently and join an association thus admitting to himself and others that he is sick" (male, Kigali City). "A person doesn't want to be ridiculed in front of others. No one receives anything from the association. There is no benefit to be in it, that's why the men refuse to be members" (male, Byumba Province). "To always be with people who say, give me, give me and then they give only two kilos of beans. In any case that isn't good" (male, Byumba Province).

Another reason for the lack of participation in PLWHA associations by men reflects a social norm. There is a strong tendency in Rwanda for men and women to separate their social activities. Once an association is perceived as being mainly constituted of females with activities that reflect the traditional roles of the woman (sewing and basket weaving, or caring for other ill people), men tend to be reluctant to join. On the other hand, one quite successful PLWHA association has attracted both men and women by encouraging HIV-positive concordant couples to join and by addressing issues of special concern to them. The success of this association may also be because it is linked to a church mission that is highly respected in the community. The mission has a relatively good hospital and an HIV screening center with a very active and well-liked male HIV/AIDS counselor who facilitates the association.

Conclusion

The differences in responses among men and women to living with HIV/AIDS can be explained by the interplay of imbalanced family, sexual, and friendship dynamics and unequal access to resources. Underlying these differences are strong cultural characteristics pervasive in Rwanda revolving around the value of pride and the strong denigration associated with shame and humiliation. There is a general mistrust of others, leading to strong tendencies to maintain secrecy for fear of reprisals. All of these influenced choices that the PLWHA made when dealing with their particular situation.

An examination of one of the "social locations where patriarchal power is produced and reproduced" (Walby 1990, cited in Morrell 2001), the family and marital relations, reveals that during the process of living with HIV/AIDS, married men began loosing that power. A restructuring of gender relations occurs as the HIV-positive husband became more and more dependent on his wife or wives. Within the family unit, the male with HIV/AIDS lost his vantage point of power when he could no longer adequately meet his economic, sexual, and other obligations defining his role as husband, head of the family, and chief economic provider. As the men with HIV/AIDS became physically weak and more frequently ill, their usual dependency on their wives and/or other female relatives for care when sick, food preparation, and the daily care of their children expanded to a dependence on the women for the duties for which the men themselves were responsible. This increased dependency contributed to their perception of loss of dignity and in sadness and despair.

The women, on the other hand, who, even when already HIV infected and sick, pushed themselves to continue taking care of their husband and children, gained agency over their husband, especially as they took over his duties. Both the married and single women, while initially desperate, turned to each other for support and were extremely courageous in their efforts for survival, and in a sense gained dignity along with a bit of agency, rather than loosing it.

The aspect of stigmatized identity associated with HIV/AIDS defining PLWHA in some cases as "immoral" was more of a concern for women than men. However, when the men admitted they had introduced the infection to their wife or wives, they expressed shame at having done so. The stigma appeared to be related less to the idea of "immorality," and more to the stigma associated with male weakness in face of their stereotypic responsibilities as the "wise, strong husband who is supposed to protect and provide for his family." The aspect of stigmatization associating HIV/AIDS with long suffering and premature death, along with miscomprehensions of the ease of transmission through close proximity or by simply touching an infected person, resulted in the avoidance and abandonment of PLWHA.

Fear of being abandoned contributed to the desire for secrecy similarly for both men and women, but this was played out differently. Overall, however, poverty, common physiological effects of HIV/AIDS, and the general lack of adequate medical services in Rwanda leveled out certain of the differences, such as fear of early death and sadness, and exacerbated poverty, resulting in a quality of life revolving around a struggle for simple survival.

These findings have important programmatic and policy implications. There is a tendency for programs targeting PLWHA to focus on care and neglect prevention. Yet it is clear that both women and men with HIV/AIDS contributed to the sexual transmission of HIV during the years before they knew they were infected, even when they were suspicious of it, as well as after they tested HIV positive. Therefore, it is extremely necessary that prevention and PLWHA care programs be integrated and that such programs recognize in a realistic manner the sexual needs of PLWHA and the varying functions that sexual relations play for men and women. In addition, in order for programs targeting PLWHA for care and HIV prevention to be effective, the above gender differences and similarities must be addressed, providing for practical choices to meet the needs of men and women within their sociocultural and economic contexts.

It is also necessary, however, to avoid reification of gendered responses that could lead to stereotyping male and female characteristics that do not reflect individual men and women, or which perpetuate undesirable inequities. At the same time, programs addressing the needed changes in gender imbalances at the basis of differential access to power and resources must be carried out in order to increase women's agency and reduce their vulnerability to HIV and other sexually transmitted diseases.

Acknowledgments

The study reported in this chapter was implemented with funding from the U.S. Agency for International Development (USAID). The authors are grateful to Chris Barratt and Beth Drabant for their support and insights that helped to guide the study. The authors also acknowledge the support of colleagues at the Johns Hopkins University Center for Communication Programs and the Academy for Educational Development, including Susan Krenn, David Awasum, Jane Brown, Esther Braud, and Berangere de Negri.

References Cited

Andre, C., and J. P. Platteau. 1998. "Land Relations Under Unbearable Stress: Rwanda Caught in the Malthusian Trap." *Journal of Economic Behavior and Organization* 34 (1): 1–47.

Civil Code. 1999. Law No. 22/99 of 12/11/1999 to supplement Book 1 of the civil code and to institute part five regarding matrimonial regimes, liberalities, and successions (articles 18–40). Kigali, Rwanda.

de Bruyn, Maria, Helen Jackson, Marianne Wijermars, Virginia Curtin Knight, and Riet Berkvens. 1998. *Facing the Challenges of HIV/AIDS/STDs: A Gender-Based Response.* Harare, Zimbabwe: KIT and SAFAIDS.

de Lame, D. 1996. "Une colline entre mille ou le calm avant la tempêt: Transformations et blocages du Rwanda rural." Musée de l'Afrique Centrale Tervuren, Belgique. *Annales Sciences Humaines* 154.

Durand, J. M. 1959. *Les Plantes bienfaisantes du Rwanda et du Burundi.* Rwanda: Pères Blancs d'Afrique.

Farmer, Paul, Margaret Connors, and Janie Simmons. 1996. *Women, Poverty and AIDS: Sex, Drugs, and Violence.* Monroe, Maine: Common Courage Press.

Food and Agriculture Organization. 2000. *Food Insecurity and AIDS: A Vicious Circle.* http://www.fao.org/Focus/E/aids/aids2–e.htm.

Foreman, M., ed. 1999. *AIDS and Men: Taking Risks or Taking Responsibility?* London: Panos/Zed.

Forsythe, S., and B. Rau. 1996. *AIDS in Kenya: Socioeconomic Impact and Policy Implications.* Research Triangle, N.C.: UNAIDS/AIDSCAP/Family Health International.

Kamungu, B. 2001. *Analyse Sociologique de la Place du Tradipraticien dans le système des Soins de Santé au Rwanda: Cas de la préfecture de Butare (period post-coloniale). Memoire.* Butare, Rwanda: National University of Rwanda.

Kantengwa, R. 1997. "Le Centre d'Information, de Documentation et de Conseil sur le SIDA (CCCIDC) de Kigali, Rwanda." In *Le dépistage VIH et le Conseil en Afrique au sud du Sahara: Aspects médicaux et sociaux*, edited by A. Desclaux and C. Raynaut, 73–77. Paris: Karthala.

Kantengwa, R. 1997. "Le Centre d'Information, de Documentation et de Conseil sur le SIDA (CCCIDC) de Kigali, Rwanda." In *Le dépistage VIH et le Conseil en Afrique au sud du Sahara: Aspects médicaux et sociaux*, edited by A. Desclaux and C. Raynaut, 73<n>77. Paris: Karthala.

Kornfield, R. 2000. *Evaluation of Training Programme for Social Transformation: Diocese of Kigeme*. Gikongoro, Rwanda. Unpublished report for Tearfund, London, prepared in Butare, Rwanda.

Kornfield, R., S. Babalola, D. Awasum, and B. Quenum-Renaud. 2002. *Living with AIDS in Rwanda: A Study in Three Provinces*. Special Publication No. 22. Baltimore: Johns Hopkins University Bloomberg School of Public Health, Center for Communications Programs.

Malinga, A. H. 2002. "Gender and Psychological Implications of HIV/AIDS for Orphaned Children and Adolescents." Paper presented at the 2002 Women's World Conference, Kampala, Uganda. http://www.makerere.ac.ug/womenstudies/full percent 20papers/Apila percent20Helen percent20Malinga.htm.

Maman, S., J. Mbwambo, M. Hogan, G. Kilonzo, and M. Sweat. 2001. "Women's Barriers to HIV Testing and Disclosure: Challenges for Voluntary Counseling and Testing Programs." *AIDS Care* 13 (5): 595–603.

Maman, S., J. Mbwambo, M. Hogan, G. Kilonzo, M. Sweat, and E. Weiss. 2001. *HIV and Partner Violence: Implications for HIV Voluntary Counseling and Testing Programs in Dar es Salaam, Tanzania*. Washington, D.C.: Population Council Horizons Project.

Ministry of Finance and Economic Planning. 1999. Department of Statistics. *Rwanda Development Indicators* No. 2 (July 1999). Republic of Rwanda.

Morrell, R., ed. 2001. *Changing Men in Southern Africa*. London: Zed Books.

Newbury, C. 1988. *The Cohesion of Oppression*. New York: Columbia University Press.

Niang, C. I. 1999. "Représentations, itineraries therapeutiques et communication concernant les maladies sexuellement transmissibles au Rwanda: Cas de la region sanitaire de Kigali." Unpublished report, Project IMPACT/Rwanda/Family Health International, Kigali.

Ntezimana, V. 2000. *La Justice Belge face au Génocide Rwandais: L'affaire Ntezimana*. Paris: Harmattan.

Nyblade L., and M. L. Field-Nager. 2001. *Women, Communities and the Prevention of Mother to Child Transmission of HIV: Issues and Findings from Community Research in Botswana and Zambia*. New York: Population Council, ICRW.

Rutembesa, F. 2001. "Ruptures socioculturelles et genocide au Rwanda." In *Ruptures socioculturelles et conflit au Rwanda*, 993–123. Cahiers du Centre de Gestion des Conflits 2.

Rwangabo P. C. 1993. *La médecine traditionnelle au Rwanda*. Paris: Karthala.

Schoepf, B. G. 1988. "Women, AIDS and Economic Crisis in Central Africa." *Canadian Forum of African Studies* 22 (3): 625–644.

Seeley, J., and E. B. Kajura. 1995. "Grief and Community." In *Grief and AIDS*, ed. L. Sherr, 73–86. Hoboken, N.J.: John Wiley and Sons.

Setel, P. 1993. "Getting AIDS Is Like Breaking Your Shaft in the Shamba." In *Energy, Disease, and Changing Concepts of Manhood in Kilimanjaro*. Working Paper 168, African Studies Center, Boston University.

Susser, I. 2000. "Culture, Sexuality, and Women's Agency in the Prevention of HIV/AIDS in Southern Africa." *American Journal of Public Health* 90 (7): 1042–1048.

Temmerman, M., J. Ndinya-Achola, J. Ambani, and P. Piot, 1995. "The Right Not to Know HIV-Test Results. *Lancet* 345 (8955): 969–970.

Topouzis, D., and G. Hemrich. 1995. *The Socio-Economic Impact of HIV/AIDS on Rural Families in Uganda*. UNDP HIV and Development Programme Discussion Paper No. 2. New York: FAO/UNDP.

UNAIDS. 1999. *Gender and HIV/AIDS: Taking Stock of Research and Programs*. UNAIDS/99.16E. Geneva. http://www.unaids.org/publications/documents/human/gender/una99e16.pdf.

———. 2002a. *Report on the Global HIV Epidemic 2002*. http://www.unaids.org/Barcelona/presskit/barcelons percent20report/contents.html.

———. 2002b. *Rwanda—Epidemiological Fact Sheets on HIV/AIDS and Sexually Transmitted Infections: 2002 Update*. http://www.who.int/emchiv/fact_sheets/africa.html.

Vidall, L. 1996. "Enseignements anthropogiques d'epériences abidjanaises de maladie." In *Anthropologie et Sida: Bilan et Perspectives*, by J. Benoist and A. Desclaux, 140–141. Paris: Kathala.

Vlassoff, C., and C. G. Moreno. 2002. "Placing Gender at the Center of Health Programming: Challenges and Limitations." *Social Science and Medicine* 54 (11): 1713–1723.

Walby, S. 1990. *Theorizing Patriarchy*. Oxford: Basil Blackwell.

Whelan, D. 1999. *Gender and HIV/AIDS: Taking Stock of Research and Programmes*. International Centre for Research on Women. http://www.unaids.org.

Womenaid International. 2003. *Rwanda: Crimes against Humanity*. http://www.womenaid.org/press/info/humanrights/rwanda percent20hr.html, accessed January 6, 2003.

A Theory of Social Proximity

Accounting for Societal-Level Behavior Change

KATE MACINTYRE AND CARL KENDALL

Prologue

An important man, a vice president of a country, recently died after a long illness, involving multiple hospitalizations in a foreign country. The illness was variously reported through the local and international newspapers as pancreatitis, a heart attack, gout, a chest infection, and an "undisclosed illness." The vice president actually died of complications from antiretroviral (ARV) therapy. His death was yet another of the many HIV- or AIDS-related deaths that remain unspoken of in public. In the initial announcement of his death, the president did not mention the cause of death, merely that the vice president "had been undergoing treatment" at a London hospital. After his death, the press studiously avoided the topic of the cause of his illness or his death. One newspaper had, however, reported during his illness that his doctor in the London hospital was head of the largest HIV clinic in the country.

So, the official word was still silence. Yet everyone from gardeners to taxi drivers to street vegetable-sellers knew the cause of death, just as they know the meaning of the code words and phrases used in newspaper obituaries of the middle-aged. Recall the Hans Christian Andersen story "The Emperor's New Clothes," when a small boy points out the naked emperor, and all the people begin to whisper among themselves. The difference in the context of AIDS in much of Africa is that not enough small boys have spoken out loud yet, so the crowd keeps quiet. The emperor and his chamberlains continue to walk "as if they carried the train [of his clothes] which did not exist."

Introduction

For two decades, researchers have struggled to understand behavior change in the context of AIDS. Theories abound at the level of the individual, but many theories now take into account environmental and structural variables (Parker et al. 2000). However, neither the theories nor the evaluations of these programs have been able to account for the timing of sweeping changes of behavior that occurred, for example, in San Francisco in the mid-1980s, or in Uganda in the late 1980s and early 1990s. None of these theories has attempted to account for the lack of behavior change in communities that are suffering very high levels of disease or death, even when much about the epidemic, including pathways of transmission, are well known and traditional concepts of contagion well established (Green 1999). The urgency from a public health standpoint is obvious: if we can bring communities and whole societies to the point of making these changes, then HIV rates would plummet.

Theories relating how the proximity of the epidemic accounts for behavior change are not new. However, these theories have tended to focus on the sense of the proximity of the epidemic when an individual knows someone with HIV or AIDS (Macintyre et al. 2001). But in societies such as Lesotho, where 40 percent of women attending antenatal clinics are seropositive and deaths from AIDS-related illnesses are everywhere, mechanisms of denial still serve to protect individuals and families from recognition of personal risk.

For this reason, we posit that underlying the success or failure of specific projects is a social and cultural explanation that enables or inhibits behavior change. This explanation we have labeled "social proximity." With social proximity comes a change in the perception of communal as well as personal risk, which triggers a cascade of important changes in behaviors. Social proximity is shaped by a range of influences: the state of the epidemic, history, culture, political economy, institutions, and projects, as well as by individual experience. None of these influences is determinative. The main purpose of this chapter is to define the social proximity of HIV and AIDS, and to begin to hypothesize how this phenomenon may be operating at multiple levels or dimensions to influence behavior change.

Proximity is a contextual variable—an underlying topographical reality—that, like a rubber sheet, can be stretched or squeezed to shape the experience of the multiple epidemics that constitute HIV/AIDS. When proximity, or nearness, to the epidemic is high, it creates increasingly transformative experiences, threatening the survival of both individuals and communities.

When it is low, it permits denial, stigma, and other mechanisms to work to distance the threat. The reason we think proximity or closeness is essential is related to the stigma and subsequent denial, discrimination, and fear raised everywhere by AIDS. Within "social proximity" is the idea that the manner in which people respond to that proximity of illness will dictate how agendas and policies or programs are developed. In other words, we posit that HIV is not considered socially proximate in societies that are still in deep denial.

A theory of social proximity must acknowledge the contributions of Mary Douglas and the role of community as a protective device (Douglas 1994). We revisit earlier ideas of proximity in the social sciences, the notions of otherness and distance, Tobler's first law of geography, and the social construction of illness debated extensively in various sociological and anthropological literatures. We analyze what steps might be taken to shape a theory of social proximity to help explain transformations of the community landscape that support change. We assess how proximity of an epidemic may be affecting communities, and what the specific mechanisms might be.

Evidence for positing social proximity abounds, but due to methodological limitations has rarely been well demonstrated. Evidence has often been treated suspiciously, or with extreme caution. For example, many authorities, including Stall and colleagues (2000), voiced suspicions about the true reasons for the enormous and rapid changes that occurred in San Francisco in the 1980s. At the International AIDS Conference in Amsterdam in 1992, they pointed out that the primary reason for the rapid change—a transformation of community values—was not being measured through traditional evaluation. In published work on the syndemics (that is, associated health problems) of HIV/AIDS, they have looked at the sense of survival, and how the potential loss of community can spur individual behavior change (Stall et al. 2000).

The current debate surrounding the causes of the decline in HIV prevalence in Uganda continues to be stirred by competing notions of what did change, how it changed, and when it changed. Very few authors, in the recent debate around the "ABC" strategies (Abstinence, Be faithful, and Condoms), have asked the next question, which is why did those behaviors change? In the arguments over the moral ground, we have lost the train of thought that asks what were the triggers that made abstinence, or being faithful, or using a condom more possible or the right thing to do. The difficulty of demonstrating social proximity is that evaluations measure (or attempt to measure) the impact of specific projects (often with the individual as the ultimate unit of analysis), while social proximity influences whole populations.

Evaluations—whether externally mandated or utilization focused—attempt to measure direct effects, but an enhanced sense of social proximity might work through indirect mechanisms. This is not an esoteric, obscure, or merely methodological issue. In Kenya recently, a Maasai grandmother rendered a fairly vivid illustration of this notion of proximity. She described how the "bad boys in this community have [already] died of AIDS. Now the disease is coming for their girlfriends and wives, and even the good boys, who are still close to us, are getting sick and dying" (K. S. Oldanyati, personal interview 2003).

Social proximity may help us understand the very different roles that stigma, denial, fear, constraints on access to care, historical reaction, and leadership within communities may be playing in terms of preventing new infections through behavior change or mitigating through institutions and innovations the impact of the epidemic on those already infected.

Background

The use of proximity to describe social and cultural phenomena can be found in various disciplines within the social sciences that have used the idea of proximal relationships to account for social change. Geography, sociology, and anthropology have each employed the use of distance/closeness in a number of theoretical positions. Geographers have used spatial proximity as a key theoretical construct. Tobler (1970: 236) invoked what he called the first law of geography: "Everything is related to everything else, but near things are more related than distant things." The first expression of this law was used to justify heuristic calculations to estimate rates of urban growth, but it has resonated strongly throughout geography and beyond. Much in medical geography is similarly tied to the idea of proximal phenomena being more similar to each other than the more distal. Complex Adaptive Systems theory as explained by Manson (2001) suggests that complexity emerges from simple, local interactions, and these can produce global behavior that can be highly complex and varied.

In sociology, extensive references to various forms of proximity date back to the middle of the twentieth century, when ideas of social and physical proximity were used to explain phenomena related to organizational change and the spread of ideas. J. Clyde Mitchell (1969), Elizabeth Bott (1971), and other early social network researchers were captivated by the idea of homophyly (similarity in social and cultural features) in small groups as a driving force of social action, an interest that continues in the work of Bernard and colleagues (Bernard and Killworth 1973; Bernard et al. 1987), Klovdahl and colleagues (Klovdahl 1985; Klovdahl et al. 1994), and many others. A theory of social proximity also has clear links to Bourdieu's idea that society consists of objective structures and that individuals are "determined" within those structures (1977).

A theory of social proximity also needs to acknowledge how larger social influences penetrate the local. Social demographers such as Watkins, in her investigation into the causes of the European health transition in the sixteenth through nineteenth centuries, laid out a theory of gossip and communication (which was described as a "theory of ideation") to understand how women's fertility rates changed from looking like their immediate neighbors to reflecting the fertility patterns of their nations (Watkins 1991). They explain this significant shift in terms of communication strategies influenced by changing trade routes, expanding markets, and rising urbanization rates. Caldwell (2000) famously posited that the behavior of elites, especially academic elites in Indonesia, was partly responsible for the rapid transition to lower fertility rates in that nation. Rogers (1983), Valente (1995), and other adoption-diffusion scholars recognize in their s-shaped adoption curves how a transition occurs to produce rapid and broad social change.[1]

Another set of social and cultural illustrations of proximity can be found in the medical anthropological literature, which has extensively explored the idea of social nearness and distance in illness and therapy. Green (1999) and others have explored notions of contagion and the role that proximity plays in ideas of disease transmission in local and social constructs. But much of witchcraft is about illness caused "at a distance." Embedded in these ideas is the sense that these forces are more significant for members of the same ethnic group or family. Folk illnesses are another category of illness that is bound by society and culture, rather than geography. The experience of illness as a whole takes place in a bounded cultural and social environment that transforms the experience of illness from a physiological phenomenon to an expression of identity, economics, politics, and culture. This is a reason why proximity must be more than a physical measure of distance, or a response to a given level of the epidemic. Intellectual precedents for the use of proximity within the social sciences abound, but few have been directly applied to explaining behavior change, or the lack of it, in the context of the AIDS epidemic.

Defining Social Proximity

In the context of HIV/AIDS, we define social proximity as operating on several different, and interacting, domains, including individual, intra-household, interhousehold, family, and kin, and at a more communal level. This could involve the immediate surrounding community, neighborhood, village, or religious or ethnic group, or it could operate on a more general regional or national level. At the individual level, we already have some evidence that the personal experience of knowing someone who has died of AIDS may well influence behaviors (Green 1999; Gregson et al. 1998; Macintyre et al. 2001). With increased personal exposure to someone ill or who has died of AIDS-related illness, denial will be overcome. The more denial is reduced, the more likely someone will perceive themselves at risk. At the household or family level, this may reflect the interactions of family members or the impact of illness or death on farming systems, on payment of school fees, and on intrahousehold relationships. At the community level, the growing sense of an epidemic is recognized through the increasing numbers of orphans and vulnerable children, the interactions and knowledge of the illness of neighbors, the transmission of general messages of the threat of AIDS via multiple public channels, and the illness, reactions, and statements of leaders (at both local community and national levels).

It is important to emphasize that the conceptual variable we are discussing here is not just a description of an internal psychological state. Processes of fear, denial, acceptance, and change clearly define psychological states, but those states are themselves created and influenced by a range of cultural features, including interpersonal, subjective, and community variables. Furthermore, these variables have the potential to interact in unusual and nonlinear ways. These states and accompanying behaviors are tested and reinforced in dyadic, family, and community settings. Another phenomenon, described by Douglas (1994), is the sense of how a community protects its members from threat. Much of the early nonresponse to the epidemic by the Reagan administration and its minions in the U.S. government's public health community (as well as much of middle-class America) was the sense that this was a disease of special, "other" populations—gay men and injecting drug users (IDUs)—and not mainstream America. It took a Ryan White to generate a public response. For that reason, we conceptually differentiate between individual and communal proximity.

So, social proximity is conceptualized here as reflecting both personal and communal experiences of the epidemic through AIDS-related illness or death of family members, friends, and/or significant community members such as teachers, business people, shopkeepers, nurses, or politicians. Beyond the actual experiences of death is an equally important element of social proximity and the reactions to those experiences (that is, how the community members react to the illnesses and deaths).

Several features of HIV and AIDS make this study of proximity important. The disease has a relatively long period of asymptomatic infection, which is followed by a potentially complex series of illnesses. This means that even when people do suspect they may be, or find out they are, HIV positive, there are numerous pathways that people or their family, or even their community, may choose to explain these illnesses up to and beyond the death of the person infected. All of this is compounded and complicated by the high, though varied, levels of stigma surrounding HIV and AIDS. The long incubation period is extremely important for this notion of proximity, for without it one can imagine that denial and lack of disclosure would be much more difficult. But it also means that even in countries with extremely high infection levels, denial can continue even as larger proportions of those infected are being told their status (for example, with implications for prevention of mother to child transmission programs). As Heywood (2002: 2) has said: "AIDS, in fact, is very susceptible to concealment and avoidance."

It is worth stating the obvious: an otherwise healthy, young to middle-age adult (even one with a weakened immune system) does not die quickly or easily. A list of a few of the features of what we mean by personalized experience of HIV-related deaths would include: various bouts and recovery periods from opportunistic infections, multiple episodes of diarrhea, increasing levels of anemia, chronic pain, and the symptoms of wasting. Those witnessing deaths from AIDS use the image of people who are being consumed by the illness or illnesses. This would suggest that these bundles of symptoms and illnesses make the personalized illness experience relatively difficult to place. In other words, at what point, without an HIV test, does someone decide that his or her relative has AIDS as opposed to tuberculosis, or malaria, or typhoid? A Malawian doctor, working with those who have HIV, only realized his father died of AIDS-related illness when he saw the death certificate. At the individual level, therefore, it is easy to see why and how denial can be perpetuated.

On the social and care-giving side, the list of characteristics of what households experience is also long but also highly variable: the drop in income as the working-age adults get sick and die, and the rise in the burden on members of the household for more cash for extra food or medicine, for more time for collecting water, for basic cleaning, and for obtaining medicines. After the person's death, the immediate costs of the funeral, and the increased burden of school fees and other essential costs, the family members must then face the emotional burden of grief, depression, or other mental problems in coping with the death of their loved one.

It has been argued that in the earlier stages of the epidemic, the impact of deaths from AIDS on largely rural societies is minimized if many terminally ill patients return from urban areas that experienced relatively high incidence to rural homesteads to die (where there is a low incidence of disease). By definition, if these were largely urban dwellers, then the impact on the rural economies (in terms of general loss of labor) was likely to be relatively low, except in the psychosocial and economic burden placed on members of a household for the duration of the illnesses. Because of the stigma HIV has carried, the cause of these earlier deaths could easily be denied. But certainly now, with the growing toll of deaths, funeral costs, increasing numbers of orphans, loss of agricultural labor, and loss of government personnel such as nurses and teachers, the denial is far less easy, one would hypothesize, to maintain.

Mark Heywood, in discussing why AIDS and apartheid are similar in their ability to hide from public view and "enable" denial to be maintained, writes: "AIDS [like apartheid] displaces people to the margins of society, wraps them in stigma, surrounds them with indignities of illness that make the onlooker want to cower rather than confront. Some might retort that four or five million people [are] a lot of people in hiding, but in our day to day lives we generally only ever notice those directly in front of us" (Heywood 2002: 2).

As this chapter was being written, an electronic mailing list on disclosure was created on the Internet. Managed by the Health and Development Networks Moderation Team (HDN 2004), it was part of the global forum on HIV/AIDS-related stigma. Many of the contributors discussed the role that denial was playing, concerning when, how, and to whom people chose to disclose their status. One doctor described denial among health care professionals, and such denial results in a country such as Argentina, with its well-educated health care workforce, still having the highest prevalence of mother-to-child transmission in Latin America. She spoke of the close link between denial of HIV and two largely taboo subjects—sex and death (Obieta 2004).

Many observers have commented that denial or silence (Caldwell 2000) may be pivotal in changing behavior, because if individuals deny they are at risk, then an important motivation to avoid risky behaviors is absent (Gregson et al. 1998; Linden et al. 1991; Macintyre et al. 2001; Smith 2003). But what has been only rarely examined is the role that denial can play at a community or societal level. Denial is, of course, one of the many consequences of stigma. It is becoming even more important that as mortality rises, we must learn, and learn quickly, what are the interactions between the different causes of stigma (fear, misconception, and notions of sin and morality) and the consequences such as denial of the disease, denial of being at risk, denial of the cause of death, and lack of disclosure to partners, friends, children, or clinicians. Our argument concerning social proximity is that as more people both personally and at a community level feel the impact of AIDS, denial becomes more difficult. Yet how communities respond to the proximity of illness, discuss the deaths, and react to the illnesses will help determine how, when, and among whom behavior changes.

What Has Happened in Uganda?

As a spate of articles suggest, there is a desperation in trying to understand the decrease in the incidence of HIV/AIDS in Uganda (Bessinger et al. 2003; Green, in press; Shelton et al. 2004; Singh et al. 2003). From these publications and other writings, a major debate has ensued about the strategies that have caused this decline. Researchers and many political observers argue whether the ABC strategy is largely responsible. While for strategic, practical public health education, it is vital that we do make progress on understanding whether it was increases in condom use (C) or young women delaying the age of first sex (Abstinence), or whether it was Uganda couples reducing the number of their sexual partners (Being faithful). It will most likely emerge that all these and additional strategies, such as more prompt treatment of sexually transmitted diseases (STDs), have had a role, and that broad-scale behavior change (Korenromp et al. 2000; Stoneburner and Low-Beer 2004; White et al. 2002) in a number of different areas is responsible.

Certainly, many Ugandan commentators believe that the attention to any single strategy takes away from the importance they attach to the whole package of interventions (TASO 2003). What has not (or rarely) been commented on, at least in the recent writings on Ugandan HIV prevalence dating from the late 1980s, is the fact that this decline coincides with the end of a vicious series of political regimes that tore Ugandan society apart for thirty years. The regimes of Idi Amin and Milton Obote, the civil wars, and the war with Tanzania had, by 1986, left an economy in ruins and a society heavily disrupted by migration, war, and disease. Even without AIDS, it would not have been surprising if Ugandan families illustrated more stability after 1986 than before. If this stability translates into increased likelihood of staying with one sexual partner, less mobility, disbanding of at least some of the army, and creating an environment where some degree of self-determination and control was felt by Ugandans, then at least some of the slowing of the spread of HIV can be explained through these societal mechanisms.

Two of the most important studies conducted in Africa on interventions to interrupt HIV transmission are those of Wawer and colleagues (1999) in Rakai, Uganda, and Grosskurth and colleagues (1995) in Mwanza, Tanzania. These studies produced inconsistent findings. Whereas HIV transmission was reduced 42 percent in Mwanza with an intervention that treated clinically diagnosed STDs, an effective, but different, STD intervention in nearby Rakai did not. These studies provide rare data that can be used to model the epidemic. Using a statistical model to simulate HIV and STD transmission rates under different scenarios, White and colleagues (2002) argue that in Rakai, where risk reduction behavior changes were already under way (and where the epidemic and the response were more mature), the effect of mass treatment of STDs was insignificant. In Mwanza, where broad-scale behavior change had yet to begin, treatment of apparent STDs did produce a significant reduction in HIV transmission (Grosskurth et al. 1995). Several scenarios can be envisaged following from this argument. In one, a cascade of behavior changes is precipitated when individuals and communities recognize the broad scale of the threat and begin to feel the proximity of the epidemic. This appears to have been the case in Rakai. In Tanzania, where the epidemic was less proximal, there was room for continuing denial and thus less impact of any nascent interventions to change behavior.

But how and why do this recognition of risk come about? How do people begin to reflect this growing sense of proximity? If we had a good understanding of the mechanisms, causes, and triggers for this reaction to the proximity of the epidemic, perhaps we could design better messages, reach the best or the most appropriate leaders, and use more effective communication strategies to support behavior change. While Uganda had some of the most advanced and certainly most widespread prevention programs in Africa from at least the mid-1980s, it also had a qualitatively different leadership from President Yoweri Museveni down to many other more community-based Ugandan leaders who chose to talk about HIV and AIDS.

One person (Epstein 2003) who has been commenting on the changing profile of the HIV and AIDS epidemic in Africa wrote recently of the difference in the conversations about AIDS by youth in South Africa, compared to her experiences of talking with individuals in Uganda a decade ago. Epstein states that the large, well-funded LoveLife program was ready to train young people to talk openly about sex, but that the program's designers stopped short of discussing death or the pain and reality of AIDS.[2] This continues to leave many young people (the target of the program) very good about discussing sex, but still in denial about their own risk. This situation is contrasted to her conversations with Ugandans in the early 1990s, where many people were ready to talk about the "frightening, calamitous effects of AIDS itself." Ugandan taxi drivers, she recalled, spoke about AIDS because "it was so personal."

Epstein takes the argument a step further and suggests that this openness/closedness to discussing the epidemic may stem directly from the history of the two countries, South Africa and Uganda. While they both have suffered bitter histories of conflict, Uganda did not and does not have a major shortage of fertile land, nor did it have a large settler population that displaced for decades large numbers of indigenous people, put them in squatter camps, and then contracted them to build industry and engage in farming in a systematic, undignified, and segregated way. Other analysts, in particular sociologists, have described the social cohesion of Uganda as being stronger and less disrupted than South Africa's (Low-Beer and Stoneburner 2003). Epstein argues that this cohesion allows Ugandans to talk openly and more realistically about the epidemic.

But another important facet of this argument that suggests that historical and cultural roots may explain the different reactions to the proximity of the epidemic is the very different reactions of the leadership. Nelson Mandela did not mention the gravity, scale, or indeed any details about the AIDS epidemic while he was president, and although he appears to be making up for some lost time with the founding of the Nelson Mandela Foundation and publicly announcing his son's death as due to AIDS, many regard the delay as tragic. People need leaders to speak openly about things that frighten them. Regrettably, his successor also began his term of office by minimizing the impact and questioning the cause of the epidemic.

President Museveni often tells a story of how he first learned how serious a threat HIV/AIDS was to become to Uganda. This is well known, but bears retelling. In 1986, Museveni sent fifty of his generals, with whom he had recently led a rebel force to victory to overthrow the Obote regime, to Cuba for training. Cuba had just instated a policy of testing all foreigners coming to Cuba (and nearly all Cubans) for HIV/AIDS. The story goes that President Fidel Castro personally telephoned Museveni shortly afterward, saying: "Comrade, you have a problem." Apparently, eighteen (36 percent) of these generals tested positive for the virus. Museveni's reaction was to immediately start talking about the problem, and he called a cabinet meeting to inform those closest to him that they were to begin discussing this admittedly difficult problem in all their speeches to their constituents. One general tells the story that "Museveni felt so sorry, so upset, because these were comrades who had fought with him in the bush" (Garrett 2000). It is therefore possible to see this type of proximity, that of the brotherhood among militias, as another characteristic that enabled Ugandans to be more open about the problem. Ugandans could also, from these early days, point to a leader who thought it was an important feature of his leadership to discuss openly the problems of HIV/AIDS.

A contrasting story is of Zimbabwe's President Robert Mugabe, who despite being told in the late 1980s that thirteen out of sixty of his generals who had been sent to China were HIV positive, did nothing. Indeed, Mugabe has either been silent on the subject of AIDS since the early days of the epidemic, or he has been loud and public in his use of stigmatizing language. This contradicts and probably precludes too many dangerous generalizations about the bonds of "militia brotherhood," though it certainly may illustrate the importance of leadership in the reaction to AIDS, particularly in the level of denial portrayed within each country.

Conclusion

Individuals and communities in sub-Saharan Africa are changing in response to the AIDS epidemic. A confusing welter of intervention strategies and approaches argue for one or another explanation of declining prevalence. We have argued that social proximity may be a powerful way of understanding why some people or communities change behavior and others do not. It may be that in some communities, where social proximity to the epidemic is felt and is discussed, interventions are far more likely to work than in those where, due to historical, cultural, or other factors, interventions simply cannot work until there is a greater sense of immediacy and risk to the whole community.

We believe that to understand how a theory of social proximity functions, we need to understand the pathways to denial and lack of disclosure. In all cultures, and for most of the more than twenty years of the epidemic, people have reported on AIDS as being someone else's disease. Almost by definition, the "gay plague," "Gay-related Immune Deficiency (GRID)," and a "disease of prostitutes" or IDUs was beyond most people's immediate and close experience. The early and highly stigmatizing slogans such as the "4 Hs" ("homosexuals, Haitians, hemophiliacs, and heroin users"), or the tag,

"She's got her father's eyes, and her mother's AIDS,"[3] as well as leaders' silence and prudery, all transmitted messages saying that this disease was a disease of "other people" (Crawford 1994).

We posit that the lessening of denial due to the personal and community encroachment of the epidemic may be one of the triggers to behavior change. But without leadership, policy agendas will not reflect this lessening of denial. Leaders at all levels of societies must speak more and do more. It is heartening to hear that in Botswana, initiatives are moving forward to encourage chiefs and administrative leaders to come forward to be tested publicly. However, before we can even begin to explore the larger question about what reduces denial, several more narrow questions need to be asked. What are the main characteristics of the personalized experience, at the individual and, more important, at the communal level? Proximity-related factors have been used over the past decade to highlight how personal and immediate experience may influence behavior change (Gregson et al. 1998; King 1999; Macintyre et al. 2001). Measuring and therefore beginning to account for proximity include characterizing who is experiencing the epidemic and how that experience is being interpreted. How is that experience being translated locally, and how is it being transmitted across families and across communities? Clearly, we are looking at a phenomenon with multiple dimensions, where there are many pathways of direct and indirect effects that may influence which strategies one uses to change behavior.

We do not know how to measure or evaluate "denial," although it may be one of those things that, like obscenity, we think we will know when we see it. But we can hazard a guess that denial will be made up of a mixture of unwillingness to discuss certain topics, discomfort, and outright rejection of evidence. But how do we distinguish between denial (of evidence) versus mislabeling of illness? In addition, we need to develop measures of how proximity is felt at the communal level. Do entire communities feel the pressure of orphans, the numbers of children without school fees, the numbers of street children, or the increasing social and temporal pressure of funerals? How do communities evaluate rumors that well-known public figures have the virus or have died of AIDS, including athletes, politicians, and cultural leaders? If the "chamberlains" continue to carry the royal train of the "emperors," as if it were really there, how do we, as social scientists, contribute to understanding something that people continue to pretend is not there? Is handling HIV and AIDS with "kid gloves" to "avoid stigma" merely making the problem worse?

After the measurement and identification of proximity at individual and communal levels are improved, the next step must be to examine the individual and communal domains that may link these characteristics to changing sexual behavior, through changing perceptions of risk or other mechanisms. Finally, and most important, if proximity itself can be shown to have a direct effect over time on behavior, the practical consequences would be to emphasize interventions that simultaneously focus on proximity and reduce denial, and revisit the ideas around beneficial disclosure. These strategies are already being advocated (Cameron 2000; Timberlake 2000), although they have rarely been substantiated with empirical data.

On a final note, in western Kenya a nickname for HIV translates from Ja-luya to English as "the disease that brought the men home at night." This illustrates, at least in part, what we mean: the behavior change (men coming "home" instead of drinking and sleeping with a girlfriend—at least that is one possible interpretation) appears to be brought about by the disease itself. If anything illustrates the fundamental importance of social proximity, it is this. HIV/AIDS can itself change behavior. Our challenge as social scientists is to understand how, when, and why people respond or do not respond to this social proximity.

Notes

1. Adoption of a new innovation typically begins in a small population of "innovators" and grows slowly until it takes off. The shape of a curve drawn to describe this takes the shape of an S, with time on the X axis and population on the Y axis.

2. LoveLife is South Africa's national HIV prevention program for youth. It was launched in September 1999 by a consortium of leading South African public health organizations in partnership with a coalition of more than 100 community-based organizations, the South African government, major South African media groups, and private foundations.

3. This was the slogan used by the Urban League in the late 1980s to accompany a small African American child on a poster advising that pregnant women in the United States get tested for HIV.

References Cited

Bernard, H. R., and P. D. Killworth. 1973. "On the Social Structure of an Ocean-Going Research Vessel and Other Important Things." *Social Science Research* 2: 145–184.

Bernard, H. R., P. D. Killworth, M. J. Evans, C. McCarty, and G. A. Shelley. 1987. "Measuring Patterns of Acquaintanceship Cross-Culturally." *Ethnology* 27: 155–179.

Bessinger, R., C. Katende, and N. Gupta. 2003. "Multi-Media Campaign Exposure Effects on Knowledge and Use of Condoms for STI and HIV/AIDS Prevention in Uganda." Chapel Hill, N.C.: MEASURE Evaluation Project.

Bott, E. 1971. *Family and Social Networks: Roles, Norms, and External Relationships in Ordinary Urban Families*. London: Tavistock.

Bourdieu, P. 1977. *Outline of a Theory of Practice*. Cambridge: Cambridge University Press.

Caldwell, J. C. 2000. "Rethinking the African AIDS Epidemic." *Population Development Review* 26: 185–234.

Cameron, E. 2000. "The Jonathan Mann Memorial Lecture." Thirteenth International AIDS Conference, Durban, South Africa, July.

Crawford, R. 1994. "The Boundaries of the Self and Unhealthy Other: Reflections on Health, Culture and AIDS." *Social Science and Medicine* 38 (10): 1347–1366.

Douglas, M. 1994. *Risk and Blame: Essays in Cultural Theory*. London: Routledge.

Epstein, H. 2003. "AIDS in South Africa: The Invisible Cure." *New York Review of Books* 50 (12): 44–49.

Garrett, L. 2000. "Allies of AIDS: Among Warring Factions in Congo, Disease Is Mutating." *New York Newsday*, July 9. http: //www.newsday.com/news/health/ny-aids20-africaaids5.story.

Green, E. C. 1999. *Indigenous Theories of Contagious Disease*. Walnut Creek, Calif.: Altamira Press.

———. (in press). "Primary Behavior Change and Reduction of HIV Transmissions: Lessons from Uganda." *Adolescent and Family Health*.

Gregson, S., T. Zhuwau, R. Anderson, and S. Chandiwana. 1998. "Is There Evidence for Behavior Change in Response to AIDS in Rural Zimbabwe?" *Social Science and Medicine* 46 (3): 321–330.

Grosskurth, H., F. Mosha, J. Todd, E. Mwijarubi, A. Klokke, K. Senkoro, P. Mayaud, J. Changalucha, A. Nicoll, G. Kagina, J. Newell, K. Mugeye, D. Mabey, and R. Hayes. 1995. "Impact of Improved Treatment of Sexually-Transmitted Diseases on HIV-Infection in Rural Tanzania—Randomized Controlled Trial." *Lancet* 346 (8974): 530–536.

HDN. 2004. "Health and Development Networks Moderation Team." www.hdnet.org.

Heywood, M. 2002. "Hiding AIDS." *AIDS Analysis Africa* 13 (2): 1–2.

King, R. 1999. *Sexual Behavioural Change for HIV: Where Have Theories Taken Us?* Geneva: UNAIDS.

Klovdahl, A. S. 1985. "Social Networks and the Spread of Infectious Diseases: The AIDS Example." *Social Science and Medicine* 21 (11): 1203–1216.

Klovdahl, A. S., J. J. Potterat, D. E. Woodhouse, J. B. Muth, S. Q. Muth, and W. W. Darrow. 1994. "Social Networks and Infectious Disease: The Colorado Springs Study." *Social Science and Medicine* 38 (1): 79–88.

Korenromp, E. L., H. van Vliet, H. Grosskurth, A. Gavyole, C. Van der Ploeg, L. Fransen, R. Hayes, and J. Habbema. 2000. "Model-Based Evaluation of Single-Round Mass STD Treatment for HIV Control in a Rural African Population." *AIDS* 14 (5): 573–593.

Linden, C., S. Allen, M. Carael, F. Nsengumuremyi, P. Van de Perre, A. Serufilira, J. Tice, D. Black, T. Coates, and S. Hully. 1991. "Knowledge, Attitude, and Perceived Risk of AIDS among Urban Rwandan Women: Relationship to HIV Infection and Behavior Change." *AIDS* 5 (8): 993–1002.

Low-Beer, D., and R. Stoneburner. 2003. "Uganda and the Challenge of AIDS." In *The Political Economy of AIDS in Africa*, ed. Alan Whiteside and Nana Poku, 178–199. London: Ashgate.

Macintyre, K., L. Brown, and S. Sosler. 2001. "'It's Not What You Know, But Who You Knew': Examining the Relationship between Behavior Change and AIDS Mortality in Africa." *AIDS Education and Prevention* 13 (2): 160–174.

Manson, S. M. 2001. "Simplifying Complexity: A Review of Complexity Theory." *Geoforum* 32: 405–414.

Mitchell, J. C. 1969. *Social Networks in Urban Situations: Analysis of Personal Relationships in Central African Towns*. Manchester: Manchester University Press.

Obieta, E. 2004. "Stigma, HIV, and Disclosure." Message posted on HIV/AIDS eForums, http://eforums.healthdev.org/read/messages?id=711#711.

Oldanyati, K. S. 2003. Interview conducted by K. Macintyre, Kajiado District.

Parker, R. G., D. Easton, and C. H. Klein. 2000. "Structural Barriers and Facilitators in HIV Prevention: A Review of International Research." *AIDS* 14 (Supplement 1): S22–S32.

Rogers, E. M. 1983. *Diffusion of Innovations*. New York: Free Press.

Shelton, J. D., D. T. Halperin, V. Nantulya, M. Potts, H. D. Gayle, and K. K. Holmes. 2004. "Partner Reduction Is Crucial for Balanced 'ABC' Approach to HIV Prevention." *British Medical Journal* 328 (7444): 891–893.

Singh, S., S. E. Darroch, and A. Bankole. 2003. "A, B and C in Uganda: The Roles of Abstinence, Monogamy, and Condom Use in HIV Decline." Occasional Report No. 9, December. New York and Washington, D.C.: Alan Guttmacher Institute.

Smith, D. 2003. "Imagining HIV/AIDS: Morality and Perceptions of Personal Risk in Nigeria." *Medical Anthropology* 22 (4): 343–372.

Stall, R. D., R. B. Hays, C. R. Waldo, M. Ekstrand, and W. McFarland. 2000. "The Gay '90s: A Review of Research in the 1990s on Sexual Behavior and HIV Risk among Men Who Have Sex with Men." *AIDS* 14 (Supplement 3): S101–S114.

Stoneburner, R. L., and D. Low-Beer. 2004. "Population-Level HIV Declines and Behavioral Risk Avoidance in Uganda." *Science* 304 (5671): 714–718.

TASO. 2003. "The AIDS Support Organisation (2003)." http://www.tasouganda.org/.

Timberlake, S. 2000. *Opening Up the HIV Epidemic: Guidance on Encouraging Beneficial Disclosure, Ethical Partner Counseling, and Appropriate Use of HIV Case Reporting*. Geneva: UNAIDS.

Tobler, W. 1970. "A Computer Movie Simulating Urban Growth in the Detroit Region." *Economic Geography* 46 (2): 234–240.

Valente, T. W. 1995. *Network Models of the Diffusion of Innovations*. Cresskill, N.J.: Hampton Press.

Watkins, S. C. 1991. *From Provinces into Nations: Demographic Integration in Western Europe, 1870–1960*. Princeton, N.J.: Princeton University Press.

Wawer, M. J., N. K. Sewankambo, D. Serwadda, T. C. Quinn, L. A. Paxton, N. Kiwanuka, F. Wabwire-Mangen, C. Li, T. Lutalo, F. Nalugoda, C. A. Gaydos, L. H. Moulton, M. O. Meehan, S. Ahmed, and R. H. Gray. 1999. "Control of Sexually Transmitted Diseases for AIDS Prevention in Uganda: A Randomized Community Trial." *Lancet* 353 (9152): 525–535.

White, R. G., K. K. Orroth, E. L. Korenromp, R. Bakker, M. Wambura, N. K. Sewankambo, M. J. Wawer, A. Kamali, H. Grosskurth, J. D. F. Habbema, and R. J. Hayes. 2002. "Can Population Differences in Mwanza, Rakai and Masaka Explain the Contrasting Outcomes of the Intervention Trials?: A Modeling Study." Paper presented at the Fourteenth International AIDS Conference, Barcelona, July.

5

Male Circumcision in the AIDS Era

New Relevance of an Old Topic

JUDITH E. BROWN

Adolescent Male Initiation: A Classic Subject in Anthropology

Rites of passage, particularly circumcision and related initiation rites, have long been of interest to anthropologists. My own generation (which began our studies during the 1960s), like generations of anthropologists before and since, spent many hours reading lengthy and detailed descriptions of rites of passage around the world. Those of us headed for fieldwork in Africa studied with fascination the initiation of adolescents, often just a few years younger than ourselves. I myself was off to Liberia, so I read avidly about the Poro (male) and Sande (female) secret societies, with their initiation rites. As the years passed, most of us have been involved with very different avenues of interest and research.

Renewed Interest: Circumcision and the Transmission of Disease

Male circumcision has recently taken on new significance, as studies of HIV prevalence have shown that circumcision may provide some protection against HIV and other sexually transmitted infections (STIs). In Africa, the subject is now widely discussed in professional meetings, health forums, and the popular press.

Early Findings

With the appearance and rapid spread of HIV/AIDS in Africa during the 1980s, medical researchers looked for all possible clues to the physical, microbiological, or behavioral factors that might be facilitating the transmission of the virus. The first scientific reports identifying male circumcision as a possible factor for inhibiting heterosexual transmission of HIV came from Kenya, at the end of the 1980s. First, a retrospective study (in an STI clinic) found uncircumcised men more frequently infected with HIV than circumcised men (Simonsen et al. 1988). The following year, a prospective study of HIV seroconversion reported new HIV infection more frequently in uncircumcised than in circumcised men (Cameron et al. 1989).

Ecological Studies: Society-Level Mapping

Teams of demographers, epidemiologists, and anthropologists began to comb the African ethnographic literature, much of it dating from several decades earlier, to learn which African societies practiced male circumcision. They then mapped and charted that information, along with current HIV prevalence rates.

Bongaarts and colleagues (1989) published the first analysis. For information on male circumcision, the authors used two classic ethnographic surveys of Africa (Murdock 1959, 1967), plus an article on East Africa (Dodge and Kaviti 1965). In all, the data covered 409 ethnic groups in thirty-seven countries, allowing the authors to make country-level estimates of the percentages of men who were and were not circumcised. For HIV seroprevalence, they used World Health Organization (WHO) figures for the capital city of each country. When the proportion of uncircumcised males was plotted against HIV seroprevalence, the figures were highly correlated.

Meanwhile, Moses and colleagues (1990) used the anthropological database of the Human Relations Area Files, and also several other surveys, to determine male circumcision practices for over 700 African societies. For HIV seroprevalence, they used U.S. Bureau of the Census data from 140 urban and rural locations in forty-one countries. The authors produced a map with dots indicating HIV seroprevalence, superimposed on shadings of circumcising and noncircumcising areas. Their conclusion: the exercise supported the hypothesis that lack of circumcision was a risk factor for HIV transmission.

A third society-level analysis (Caldwell and Caldwell 1996) appeared in a more popular article for *Scientific American*. The key map showed a crescent-shaped "AIDS belt" in eastern and southern Africa, where nearly 25 percent of the urban population was infected with HIV. Using overlay maps, the authors explored, and rejected, a variety of hypotheses about why HIV was prevalent in the "AIDS belt," compared with African cultures outside the "AIDS belt":

Widespread sexually transmitted diseases (STDs) (indicated by high levels of sterility)

Late age at marriage

High levels of polygyny

Long postpartum abstinence

Women's financial autonomy

One factor, however, did correlate with HIV prevalence on the maps—lack of male circumcision.

Epidemiologic Studies of Individuals

Meanwhile, during these same years, epidemiologic studies were accumulating evidence on the individual level (and not just at the societal level) that lack of male circumcision was indeed related to HIV infection. Generally, men were asked whether they had been circumcised, and they were tested for HIV. Most of these earlier studies were retrospective—both the circumcisions and the infections had occurred at some unknown time in the past.

One retrospective study did include the reported age at the time of circumcision. In southwestern Uganda, circumcision performed before puberty was found to be associated with less HIV risk, while circumcision after age twenty was not significantly protective. The authors suggested that the reasons for circumcision may have differed in these two groups: circumcision before puberty was usually done for religious or cultural reasons; after puberty, it was often done for health reasons (Kelly et al. 1999).

By the year 2000, more of the circumcision studies were prospective. In these studies, men without HIV infection were classified as circumcised or uncircumcised. All men received equal counseling, preventive education, and free condoms as needed. After a number of months or years, the researchers retested the men to determine the HIV status and the seroconversion rate of each group.

For example, a prospective cohort study of trucking company employees in Kenya found that uncircumcised men had a fourfold increased risk for acquiring HIV infection (Lavreys et al. 1999). A prospective study from southwestern Uganda followed HIV-negative men whose female sexual partners were HIV positive. None of the fifty circumcised men contracted HIV during the course of the study, while 40 of the 137 uncircumcised men did contract the virus. The same study followed HIV-positive men who had

HIV-negative partners: the circumcised men were less likely than the uncircumcised men to transmit the virus to their partners, though this result was not statistically significant (Gray et al. 2000; Quinn et al. 2000). Five review articles have now concluded that the research to date provides compelling evidence of the protective effect of male circumcision against HIV infection (Bailey et al. 2001; Halperin and Bailey 1999; Moses et al. 1998; O'Farrell and Egger 2000; Weiss et al. 2000).

Confounding Factors: Culture and Behavior

Researchers and reviewers often pointed out, however, the limitations common to all these observational studies. The physical effects of circumcision may be confounded with other HIV risk factors—particularly religion, cultural norms, and sexual behavior. For example, if the circumcised men were mainly Muslim (as in several of the Uganda studies), is it possible that they had practiced less risky behavior than the noncircumcised non-Muslims? Had the Muslims perhaps consumed less alcohol, practiced better penile hygiene, and had fewer sexual contacts outside their marriages—whether monogamous or polygynous (Gray et al. 2000)?

Anthropologists and other social scientists have been involved in many of these recent studies, attempting to examine cultural and behavioral variables that may confound the effects of circumcision. For example, in eastern Uganda, risky sexual practices and unhygienic behaviors could not account for the high rate of HIV infection in uncircumcised men. In fact, the circumcised men in this retrospective study reported behaviors that actually may have increased their risk of infection, yet they were less likely to be infected with HIV (Bailey et al. 1999).

Others pointed out that "circumcision" did not always mean the same thing everywhere. In one small area of central Kenya, for example, three distinct styles of circumcision were being practiced in both traditional and clinical settings; these different styles could possibly offer different levels of protection against disease transmission (Brown et al. 2001).

Furthermore, men's yes-or-no answers to the question "Have you been circumcised?" did not always correspond to observations by trained medical personnel, or to the men's own answers at a later interview (Urassa et al. 1997). Such problems with the reliability of self-reports should come as no surprise to anthropologists working in the field of reproductive health (Bleek 1987; Pickering 1988).

Possible Mechanisms of HIV Infection in Uncircumcised Men

Despite the mounting evidence that circumcision provided partial protection against HIV transmission, the international health community remained hesitant about recommending male circumcision as an HIV prevention strategy. One reason was lack of evidence about the biological mechanisms at work. Why should the presence of a foreskin make a man more susceptible to HIV infection? Seven possible mechanisms were commonly suggested in the literature: difficulty in maintaining good hygiene of the foreskin, more genital ulcer disease in uncircumcised men, more inflammations, less hardening of the foreskin or glans, more trauma to the frenulum or foreskin, an environment under the foreskin favorable to bacteria and viruses, and large numbers of HIV target cells on the inner surface of the foreskin.

A recent laboratory study has provided important data, pointing to the last of the mechanisms listed above. The mucosa on the inner surface of the foreskin was found to contain a high proportion of HIV receptor cells, specifically CD4$^+$ T cells, macrophages, and Langerhans' cells (Patterson et al. 2002).

Recommendations for Future Action

Some reviewers have suggested adding safe male circumcision services to existing HIV prevention strategies in high-prevalence areas (Halperin and Bailey 1999; Weiss et al. 2000). In fact, the general African public has not been waiting for researchers to clarify all the issues and questions. Some traditional healers in South Africa, for example, have for some time been recommending circumcision for disease prevention (Green et al. 1993).

In noncircumcising areas, research teams (often with social scientists as members) have investigated the present-day acceptability of circumcision. In western Kenya, for example, in noncircumcising Luo areas, focus group research and interviews have shown voluntary circumcision to be more acceptable among men, women, and health providers than previously thought (Bailey et al. 2000; Bailey et al. 2002). Similar acceptability of male circumcision has also been documented in noncircumcising areas of South Africa (Lagarde et al. 2003) and Botswana (Kebaabetswe et al. 2003).

All these acceptability studies have cautioned, however, that many of the respondents seemed to overestimate the protective effects of circumcision against disease. Authors were concerned about the potential "disinhibiting" effect of male circumcision, if men mistakenly think it offers complete protection against HIV. They recommend that men be clearly informed that condoms and other preventive measures are still needed (Bailey et al. 2001).

Other researchers have expressed reservations about the costs and risks of introducing circumcision services among noncircumcising populations (Gray et al. 2002). To study the feasibility of new services in western Kenya, a pilot study introduced voluntary, safe male circumcision services in a non-circumcising Luo area. In one district, health practitioners in twenty health facilities were trained and equipped to offer safe circumcision services. Consent procedures were developed, and public education was provided on the risks and benefits of circumcision. In that district, during the first twenty-five months of upgraded clinical services, 433 circumcisions were requested and performed, with high rates of patient satisfaction. Meanwhile, in a nearby control district without training or improved services, only 24 circumcisions were reported (Onyango 2002).

The Protective Effects of Circumcision: Randomized Clinical Trials

As mentioned above, all the observational studies linking circumcision and lower HIV infection rates had limitations, particularly the confounding cultural and behavioral variables. Several reviewers began calling for randomized clinical trials before promoting circumcision as an HIV prevention measure (Bailey et al. 2001; Gray et al. 2000; Halperin and Bailey 1999). For a while, however, the ethics and logistics of randomized, case-control studies of male circumcision seemed almost insurmountable.

After long planning, and approval by numerous research review boards, an interdisciplinary team, including anthropologists, began randomized controlled trials early in 2002 in the Luo area of Kenya. At this writing, the study is still ongoing, with the following enrollment and research procedures.[1] Men between the ages of eighteen and twenty-four who voluntarily request circumcision are carefully informed that the researchers do not yet know whether circumcision reduces the chances of infection. The men are counseled at length about various ways to prevent HIV transmission, including condoms (which are provided free to all study participants).

Once their HIV-negative status is confirmed, the young men receive a detailed explanation of the study, and those who agree to participate are then randomly assigned to one of two groups. Young men in the first group are circumcised and followed closely for two years; those in the second group are asked to wait for two years before circumcision, but are also followed closely during the waiting period. The study is designed to compare HIV seroconversion rates in the two groups.

Two other randomized control trials of male circumcision and HIV acquisition, slightly different in design from the Kenya studies, are now under way. One has begun near Johannesburg, South Africa, and the other is soon to start in southwest Uganda (Tramont 2002).

Initiation Rites and Teaching: Can Traditional Forms Be Adapted for Modern Content?

All the studies summarized above are concerned with the physical effects of the circumcision procedure and the way it may affect disease transmission. In addition, anthropologists and health educators are now reexamining traditional circumcision and seclusion rites, particularly the teaching that was considered a key part of the process. In modern African society, teenage boys and young men are often out of school and unemployed, and they do not frequent health facilities. They are thus a difficult group to reach with information and advice, and circumcision may offer a valuable opportunity to do just that. Reproductive health is a key area for teaching, and other modern topics (gender relations, drug and alcohol abuse, physical violence, and mental health) are also being considered.

In Kenya, for instance, many ethnic groups have practiced near-universal male circumcision as far back as anyone can remember, and continue to do so today. Several church organizations, in different parts of the country, have recently begun special teaching programs for adolescent boys as they undergo circumcision. The teaching often includes reproductive topics such as AIDS and other STIs, drugs and alcohol, stress, time planning, and the role of men in the community (Brown 2002; Brown and Micheni 2003).

Other ongoing studies are concerned with the physical aspects of traditional circumcision, in areas where it is still practiced today. How is it done? Is it medically safe? If not, can it be improved? For example, in the Xhosa ethnic areas of the Eastern Cape Province of South Africa, traditional circumcision practices have recently come under medical scrutiny and government regulation. Studies are currently planned to examine the physical effects and any medical complications of traditional circumcision and seclusion. In addition, teaching during the circumcision period may be expanded to include reproductive health topics, violence, and gender issues (Clark et al. 2002).

Anthropologists and Current Circumcision Studies

My own recent work has examined the variety of physical techniques of circumcision currently done in one area of Kenya (Brown et al. 2001), as well as the teaching provided to adolescent boys who go to a hospital for the surgical procedure (Brown 2002). Currently, I am part of a multidisciplinary, multinational team working on present-day male circumcision in a Xhosa area of South Africa. We are focusing on current practices, recent medical complications from the surgical and seclusion procedures, and opportunities for teaching the young men.

In the process, I have learned a good deal about my own discipline and its place among other sciences. At the same time, I have found myself teaching anthropology to colleagues in other disciplines. The observations below are not unique to circumcision studies; the same situations are found frequently these days in applied anthropology and particularly in medical anthropology.

What Are Anthropologists Learning?

Team Research

In classic anthropological field work, a single researcher (with perhaps one or two field assistants) often did the planning, observing, interviewing, and writing alone. In recent circumcision studies, anthropologists work on a day-to-day basis with epidemiologists, nurses, physicians, microbiologists, educators, and statisticians. Team anthropologists are expected not only to understand complex research questions and procedures but also to make unique anthropological contributions to the process and the findings. Anthropologists may nearly lose their professional identity within the large teams. In fact, when attending conferences on male circumcision, anthropologists often discover only by chance that other participants are also trained as social scientists.

Team Publishing

Traditionally, anthropologists have published as single authors or occasionally with one or two colleagues. Single authorship is still the norm in anthropology journals and in the books reviewed there. Circumcision studies, however (like many AIDS-related topics today), have multiple authors—often five or six, and sometimes as many as a dozen. In these cases, individual authors lose some control over the writing and editing process, while still feeling responsible for the accuracy of the final article. Anthropologists, accustomed to sole authorship and control, may find team publishing difficult at first.

Biomedical Style

Biomedical journals and conferences have their own particular styles and rules of courtesy. A short abstract is required for any presentation; it must tell everything, in a particular way. Long introductory statements of theory, literature reviews, or background ramblings bring yawns from an audience and do not get published. Listeners, readers, and editors expect every sentence to be clear and precise. At conferences, speakers are not allowed to exceed their time limits, and they rarely even try. Every slide and every table is supposed to be reduced to the basic essentials. Anthropologists, often trained in other styles of presentation, have to learn these biomedical skills.

What Are Anthropologists Teaching?

Team research and publishing, of course, are not just learning experiences. Anthropologists constantly teach their colleagues the methods and insights of their discipline. Here are some of those lessons, usually much appreciated by our collaborators.

Check Out Your Hunches

It is all too easy, when working as part of a multidisciplinary team, to try out new hypotheses and explanations on other members of the team, and leave it at that. Anthropologists can contribute immeasurably by insisting on talking to the people concerned, in whatever way the team members find comfortable, and for however long it takes.

Asking Is Probably Not Enough

Even asking a man, "Are you circumcised?" has proven far from simple. Researchers have had to teach each other how necessary it is to ask, ask again more carefully, and also examine and observe (Lavreys et al. 1999; Pickering 1988; Urassa et al. 1997). Anthropologists are trained to distrust quick, short answers to questions that may actually be quite complicated. They are willing to take the time to become entangled in complex explanations, to discover unsuspected relationships, and to go far afield to understand the question at hand.

Ignorance Helps

A few years ago, I was trying to understand the different physical styles of circumcision in one small area of central Kenya. I was struggling to make sense of the descriptions given by my male Kenyan colleagues, both nurses and doctors. As I asked more and more questions, I began to suspect that my informants were not very clear themselves on the procedures used by circumcisers outside the hospital. When I asked them to sketch the anatomy and procedures, I realized how inexact their knowledge was.

As men who had grown up in the local society, they seemed unwilling to admit any ignorance about circumcision. As a foreign woman studying a male-only domain, however, I was truly and unashamedly ignorant. I was not expected to know anything in advance about the subject, and it seemed quite acceptable for me to ask questions (as long as I was not too intense about it). So I begged their indulgence and help on getting the drawings right. It worked, and what our team discovered has helped other researchers to recognize their own ignorance (Brown et al. 2001).

Back to the Classics

Our circumcision study in South Africa has also been focusing on current Xhosa practices, recent medical complications and deaths (that may be due to the surgical and seclusion procedures), and opportunities for teaching the young men during seclusion. We have been searching for ways that circumcision can be made safe, educationally effective, and at the same time culturally appropriate.

After the first week of intense observations and interviews, I left my teammates for a weekend and headed for a nearby university library. There I found in the modern stacks some dusty old friends—tattered volumes by anthropologists that I had read thirty years earlier and thousands of miles away. In the chapters on Xhosa male circumcision, every page was alive and relevant. The stages of circumcision rites, which our team had just been struggling to understand, suddenly became clear. Some aspects of traditional adolescent socialization by peers had not been mentioned by modern informants, but they deserved investigation and possibly revival. I returned to my colleagues with a whole list of modern possibilities from the classic anthropological literature.

Conclusion

Modern biomedical evidence is growing that male circumcision offers partial protection against sexual transmission of HIV and other STIs. Anthropologists are part of the epidemiologic research and the controlled clinical trials that are building this evidence.

Anthropologists are also members of teams considering ethical and policy questions about how to proceed. Should male circumcision be offered as a measure to lower the probability of disease transmission? If so, should male circumcision be offered even in societies that never practiced it? What about societies that once practiced circumcision but not any longer? Can male circumcision be offered and understood as an addition to (not a replacement for) other important preventive measures?

Furthermore, in societies where male circumcision is already practiced for boys or adolescents, is the physical operation today accompanied by initiation rites and teaching? If so, can the teaching cover sexual health topics such as AIDS, delaying sexual debut, using condoms, limiting the number of sexual partners, HIV testing, or other areas? Are traditional teachers willing and able to handle these topics?

In sum, male circumcision and initiation rites were key topics of classical anthropology. The subjects are currently proving to be very modern and very relevant indeed.

Notes

1. After this chapter was written, the results of all three randomized controlled trials were published (Auvert et al. 2005; Bailey et al. 2007; Gray et al. 2007; WHO 2006). The trial outcomes in South Africa, Kenya, and Uganda were startlingly similar: the protective effect of circumcision was over 50 percent in all three settings. Male circumcision indeed reduced the young men's risk of acquiring HIV.

These findings led the WHO and other United Nations agencies to endorse male circumcision as an important means of HIV protection—to be added to condom use, reduction in the number of sexual partners, delaying the onset of sexual relations, and HIV testing and counseling.

References Cited

Auvert, B., D. Taljaard, E. Lagarde, J. Sobngwi-Tambekou, R. Sitta, and A. Puren. 2005. "Randomized, Controlled Intervention Trial of Male Circumcision for Reduction of HIV Infection Risk: The ANRS 1265 Trial." *PLoS Med* 2: 1–11.

Bailey, Robert C., Stephen Moses, Corette B. Parker, Kawango Agot, Ian Maclean, John N. Krieger, Carolyn F. M. Williams, Richard T. Campbell, and Jeckoniah O. Ndinyo-Achola. 2007. "Male Circumcision for HIV Prevention in Young Men in Kisumu, Kenya: A Randomised Controlled Trial." *Lancet* 369 (9562): 643–56.

Bailey, Robert C., Richard Muga, and Rudi Poulussen. 2000. "Trial Intervention of Male Circumcision to Reduce HIV/STD Infections in Nyanza Province, Kenya: Baseline Results." Paper presented at the Thirteenth International Conference on AIDS, Durban, South Africa.

Bailey, R. C., R. Muga, R. Poulussen, and H. Abicht. 2002. "The Acceptability of Male Circumcision to Reduce HIV Infections in Nyanza Province, Kenya." *Aids Care* 14: 27–40.

Bailey, Robert C., Stella Neema, and Richard Othieno. 1999. "Sexual Behaviors and Other HIV Risk Factors in Circumcised and Uncircumcised Men in Uganda." *Journal of Acquired Immune Deficiency Syndromes* 22: 294–301.

Bailey, Robert C., Francis A. Plummer, and Stephen Moses. 2001. "Male Circumcision and HIV Prevention: Current Knowledge and Future Research Directions." *Lancet* 1: 223–231.

Bleek, Wolf. 1987. "Lying Informants: A Field Work Experience from Ghana." *Population and Development Review* 13: 314–322.

Bongaarts, John, Priscilla Reining, Peter Way, and Francis Conant. 1989. "The Relationship between Male Circumcision and HIV Infection in African Populations." *AIDS* 3 (6): 373–377.

Brown, Judith. 2002. "Integration of Traditional and Clinical Circumcision in Chogoria Hospital, Kenya." In *Male Circumcision: Current Epidemiological and Field Evidence*, ed. Sam Clark, Willow Gerber, and Imogen Fua, 9–10. Washington, D.C.: Population Services International.

Brown, Judith, and Kenneth Micheni. 2003. "Male Circumcision Education Programs of Kenyan Churches." Abstract 659716. Thirteenth International Conference on AIDS and STIs in Africa, Nairobi.

Brown, Judith E., Kenneth D. Micheni, Elizabeth M. J. Grant, James M. Mwenda, Francis M. Muthiri, and Angus R. Grant. 2001. "Varieties of Male Circumcision: A Study from Kenya." *Sexually Transmitted Diseases* 28: 608–612.

Caldwell, John, and Pat Caldwell. 1996. "The African AIDS Epidemic." *Scientific American* 274: 62–68.

Cameron, D. William, J. Neil Simonsen, Lourdes J. D'Costa, Allan R. Ronald, Gregory M. Maitha, Michael N. Gakinya, Mary Cheang, J. O. Ndinya-Achola, Peter Piot, Robert C. Brunham, and Francis A. Plummer. 1989. "Female to Male Transmission of Human Immunodeficiency Virus Type 1: Risk Factors for Seroconversion in Men." *Lancet* 2: 403–407.

Clark, Sam, Willow Gerber, and Imogen Fua, eds. 2002. *Male Circumcision: Current Epidemiological and Field Evidence*. Washington, D.C.: Population Services International.

Dodge, O. G., and J. N. Kaviti. 1965. "Male Circumcision among the Peoples of East Africa and the Incidence of Genital Cancer." *East African Medical Journal* 42: 98–105.

Gray, Ronald H., Godfrey Kigozi, David Serwadda, Frederick Makumbi, Stephen Watya, Fred Nalugoda, Noah Kiwanuka, Lawrence H. Moulton, Mohammad A. Chaudhary, Michael Z. Chen, Nelson K. Sewankambo, Fred Wabwire-Mangen, Melanie C. Bacon, Carolyn F. M. Williams, Pius Opendi, Steven J. Reynolds, Oliver Laeyendecker, Thomas C. Quinn, and Maria J. Wawer. 2007. "Male Circumcision for HIV Prevention in Men in Rakai, Uganda: A Randomised Trial." *Lancet* 369: 657–666.

Gray, Ronald H., Noah Kiwanuka, Thomas C. Quinn, Nelson K. Sewankambo, David Serwadda, Fred Wabwire Mangen, Tom Lutalo, Fred Nalugoda, Robert Kelly, Mary Meehan, Michael Z. Chen, Chuanjun Li, and Maria J. Wawer, for the Rakai Project Team. 2000. "Male Circumcision and HIV Acquisition and Transmission: Cohort Studies in Rakai, Uganda." *AIDS* 14 (15): 2371–2381.

Gray, Ronald H., Maria J. Wawer, Noah Kiwanuka, David Serwadda, Nelson K. Sewankambo, and Fred Wabwire Mangen. 2002. "Male Circumcision and HIV Acquisition and Transmission: Rakai, Uganda [letter]." *AIDS* 16 (5): 809–810.

Green, Edward C., B. Zokwe, and J. D. Dupree. 1993. "Indigenous African Healers Promote Male Circumcision for Prevention of Sexually Transmitted Diseases." *Tropical Doctor* 23: 182–183.

Halperin, Daniel, and Robert Bailey. 1999. "Male Circumcision and HIV Infection: 10 Years and Counting." *Lancet* 354: 1813–1815.

Kebaabetswe, P., S. Lockman, S. Mogwe, R. Mandevu, I. Thior, M. Essex, and R. L. Shapiro. 2003. "Male Circumcision: An Acceptable Strategy for HIV Prevention in Botswana." *Sexually Transmitted Infections* 79: 214–219.

Kelly, Robert, Noah Kiwanuka, Maria J. Wawer, David Serwadda, Nelson K. Sewankambo, Fred Wabwire-Mangen, Chuanjun Li, Joseph K. Konde-Lule, Tom Lutalo, Fred Makumbi, and Ronald H. Gray. 1999. "Age of Male Circumcision and Risk of Prevalent HIV Infection in Rural Uganda." *AIDS* 13 (3): 399–405.

Lagarde E., T. Dirk, A. Puren, R. T. Reathe, and A. Bertran. 2003. "Acceptability of Male Circumcision as a Tool for Preventing HIV Infection in a Highly Infected Community in South Africa." *AIDS* 17 (1): 89–95.

Lavreys, Ludo, Joel P. Rakwar, Mary Lou Thompson, Denis J. Jackson, Kishorchandra Mandaliya, Bhavna H. Chohan, Job J. Bwayo, Jeckoniah O. Ndinya-Achola, and Joan K. Kreiss. 1999. "Effect of Circumcision on Incidence of Human Immunodeficiency Virus Type 1 and Other Sexually Transmitted Diseases: A Prospective Cohort Study of Trucking Company Employees in Kenya." *Journal of Infectious Diseases* 180: 330–336.

Moses, Stephen, Robert C. Bailey, and Allan R. Ronald. 1998. "Male Circumcision: Assessment of Health Benefits and Risks." *Sexually Transmitted Infections* 74: 368–373.

Moses, Stephen, Janet E. Bradley, Nico J. D. Nagelkerke, Allan R. Ronald, J. O. Ndinya-Achola, and Francis A. Plummer. 1990. "Geographical Patterns of Male Circumcision Practices in Africa: Association with HIV Seroprevalence." *International Journal of Epidemiology* 19: 693–697.

Murdock, George. 1959. *Africa: Its Peoples and Their Culture History.* New York: McGraw-Hill.

———. 1967. *Ethnographic Atlas.* Pittsburgh: University of Pittsburgh Press.

O'Farrell, Nigel, and Matthias Egger. 2000. "Circumcision in Men and the Prevention of HIV Infection: A 'Meta-Analysis' Revisited." *International Journal of Sexually Transmitted Diseases and AIDS* 11: 137–142.

Onyango, Thomas. 2002. "Trial Intervention of MC services in Nyanza Province, Kenya." In *Male Circumcision: Current Epidemiological and Field Evidence,* ed. Sam Clark, Willow Gerber, and Imogen Fua, 8–9. Washington, D.C.: Population Services International.

Patterson, Bruce K., Alan Landay, Joan N. Siegel, Zareefa Flener, Dennis Pessis, Antonio Chaviano, and Robert C. Bailey. 2002. "Susceptibility to Human Immunodeficiency Virus-1 Infection of Human Foreskin and Cervical Tissue Grown in Explant Culture." *American Journal of Pathology* 161: 867–873.

Pickering, Helen. 1988. "Asking Questions on Sexual Behaviour . . . Testing Methods from the Social Sciences." *Health Policy and Planning* 3: 237–244.

Quinn, Thomas C., Maria J. Wawer, Nelson Sewankambo, David Serwadda, Chuanjun Li, Fred Wabwire-Mangen, Mary O. Meehan, Thomas Lutalo, and Ronald H. Gray, for the Rakai Project Study Group. 2000. "Viral Load and Heterosexual Transmission of Human Immunodeficiency Virus Type 1." *New England Journal of Medicine* 342: 921–929.

Simonsen, J. N., D. W. Cameron, M. N. Gakinya, J. O. Ndinya-Achola, L. J. D'Costa, P. Karasira, M. Cheang, A. R. Ronald, P. Piot, and F. A. Plummer. 1988. "Human Immunodeficiency Virus Infection among Men with Sexually Transmitted Diseases." *New England Journal of Medicine* 319: 274–278.

Tramont, Edward. 2002. "Status of Current Clinical Trials (and Related Acceptability Findings)." In *Male Circumcision: Current Epidemiological and Field Evidence,* ed. Sam Clark, Willow Gerber, and Imogen Fua, 6–7. Washington, D.C.: Population Services International.

Urassa, Marc, James Todd, J. Ties Boerma, Richard Hayes, and Raphael Isingo. 1997. "Male Circumcision and Susceptibility to HIV Infection among Men in Tanzania." *AIDS* 11 (1): 73–80.

Weiss, Helen A., Maria A. Quigley, and Richard Hayes. 2000. "Male Circumcision and Risk of HIV Infection in Sub-Saharan Africa: A Systematic Review and Meta-Analysis." *AIDS* 14 (15): 2361–2370.

WHO (World Health Organization). 2006. *Statement on Kenyan and Ugandan Trial Findings Regarding Male Circumcision and HIV: Male Circumcision Reduces the Risk of Becoming Infected with HIV, but Does Not Provide Complete Protection.* http://www.who.int/mediacentre/news/statements/2006/s18/en/print.html.

6

Factors That Influence Ivorian Women's Risk Perception of STIs and HIV

KIM LONGFIELD

Introduction

Côte d'Ivoire, a small coastal nation in West Africa, is among the fifteen countries in the world most affected by HIV/AIDS, with an overall estimated infection rate of 9.7 percent. Estimates hold that between 7 and 10 percent of Ivorian females aged fifteen to twenty-four years are infected with HIV, while rates for males in the same cohort are much lower, at 2 to 4 percent (UNAIDS 2002). Several researchers have argued that HIV cannot be considered in isolation from other sexually transmitted infections (STIs) because they share the same modes of transmission and behavioral risk factors, and STIs may increase susceptibility to and transmission of HIV. Consequently, preventing and treating STIs may help curb the HIV/AIDS epidemic (Grosskurth et al. 1995; National Research Council 1996).

Young women's increased risk for infection can be attributed to several factors, including a lack of essential knowledge about STIs and HIV. Zanou and colleagues (1998) found that although 98 percent of Ivorian youth in their sample had heard of AIDS, only 49 percent of females were able to cite two or more methods of prevention. Likewise, 60 percent of females were unable to cite any symptoms of STIs, and 27 percent of young women in Abidjan, the largest city, said they had never heard of STIs (Zanou et al. 1998).

Other factors such as early sexual onset, physiological susceptibility, high levels of sexual activity, multiple partnerships, the transitory nature of sexual relationships, and low levels of condom use contribute to young women's risk for both HIV and STI infection in West Africa (Calvès 1998; Meekers et al. 2001; Monitoring the AIDS Pandemic Network 2002; National Research Council 1996; Njikam Savage 1998). In 1998, the mean age at sexual debut for Ivorian girls was 15.7 years, and for boys it was 15.0 years (Zanou et al. 1998). The same year, close to 70 percent of Ivorians aged fifteen to nineteen years reported having had a sexual experience, and many reported multiple partnerships (Blanc and Way 1998; Zanou et al. 1998). Several researchers contend that early sexual onset for girls puts them at increased risk for HIV/AIDS since their reproductive and immune systems are immature and more susceptible to infection (Monitoring the AIDS Pandemic Network 2002; UNAIDS 2002).

Even as the AIDS epidemic becomes more pronounced in Côte d'Ivoire, condom use among youth remains low (Kouye et al. 2000; Kuate-Defo 1997; Yelibi et al. 1993; Zellner 2003). Several studies have found that African youth are more likely to use condoms with certain types of partners than others. This is especially true in casual rather than regular partnerships (Agha et al. 2001; Meekers and Calvès 1997a; Van Rossem et al. 2001). Many youth also report using condoms at the beginning of a relationship, but abandoning use once the union becomes more stable or greater levels of emotional commitment are felt (Calvès 1999). Common reasons cited for inconsistent use are fear that partners will suspect one is unfaithful or HIV positive if condoms are proposed, the belief that condoms reduce sexual pleasure, and a perception that condom use suggests a lack of trust in one's partner (Agyei et al. 1992; MacPhail and Campbell 2001; Wilson and Lavelle 1992; Yelibi et al. 1993).

Past research reveals that a variety of partner types are common among youth in sub-Saharan Africa and that different expectations accompany particular types of relationships, including sexual experience, sexual satisfaction, social networking, and marital prospects (Calvès et al. 1996; Gage and Bledsoe 1994; Meekers and Calvès 1997b). Many relationships contain a financial component in which sexual favors are exchanged for monetary or material support (Caldwell et al. 1989; Mensch et al. 1999; Ulin 1992; UNICEF et al. 2002). Although many young women have relationships with peers, some prefer older partners who are better able to provide them support (Gorgen et al. 1993). Still others maintain a regular relationship with a boyfriend while still "going out" with older men (Dinan 1983; Gregson and Garnett 2002). Similar relationships also exist between young men and older women; however, these liaisons appear to be less common (Calvès et al. 1996; Owuamanam 1995).

Little research has been conducted on the influence of relationships and partner choices on sexual decision making and young women's risk perception for STIs and HIV (Gage 1998; Meekers and Calvès 1997b; UNAIDS 1998). Some investigators have argued for improved indices of partner-specific risk perception that reveal differences in self-protective behavior with different types of partners (Poppen and Reisen 1997). Although existing sexual behavior surveys ask participants about "regular" and "occasional" sexual partners, they fail to address characteristics of relationships such as duration, exclusivity, levels of commitment or trust, and the distribution of power between partners (Poppen and Reisen 1997; UNAIDS 1998). This study uses qualitative data from free lists, pile sorts, and in-depth interviews with young women in Abidjan to describe common partner categories, understand the role expectations associated with partners, and examine the influence of partner characteristics on STI/HIV risk perception and risk behavior. Taking into account issues such as relationship dynamics and partner characteristics when designing prevention campaigns can help program planners concentrate their efforts on specific behaviors or types of relationships where risk-taking behavior is high and risk perception is low.

Methods

All participants for this study were youth residing in Abidjan. Data for free lists were obtained from a convenience sample of males and females aged fifteen to twenty-four years who participated in a different study (Kouye et al. 2000). A total of eighty-two partner types were identified, and each term was transferred to an index card for use in pile sorts.

Data from pile sorts (where participants are asked to categorize key terms) and in-depth interviews were obtained from a stratified purposive sample of twenty-four Ivorian women aged eighteen to twenty-two from four major communes (neighborhoods) in Abidjan: Abobo, Marcory, Treichville, and Yopougon (six women from each commune). The known sponsor approach (Patton 1987) was used to recruit women in each cluster and establish researcher legitimacy with participants and communities. Youth presidents (*Presidents de Jeunesse*) in each commune who were approximately the same age as study participants served as recruiters, and snowballing was used to identify women known to recruiters. The study investigator conducted pile sorts and in-depth interviews in private homes belonging to recruiters, participants, and acquaintances of study recruiters in each of the four communes.

Participants were asked to conduct "free" pile sorts and place each of the index cards into piles of similar partner types.[1] The study investigator used Anthropac 3.2 to complete dichotomous variable testing. During the testing, terms that fifteen or more participants identified as "partner types" were collapsed into comprehensive categories, and those that fifteen or more participants did not know were eliminated (Borgatti 1990, personal communication 1999).

In-depth interviews were conducted with each participant immediately following pile sort exercises. Interview questions addressed partner categories and partner-specific risk perception. Participants provided a brief sexual history and indicated into which categories their present and past sexual partners fit. All interviews were conducted in French, lasted approximately one hour, and were audio recorded and transcribed. The text-based software The Ethnograph v5.0 was used to analyze transcripts and highlight similarities and distinctions in participants' comments as well as determine differences in partner categories (Qualis Research 1998).

Results from dichotomous variable testing and in-depth interview analysis were combined to create "supercategories" that describe sexual partners common among young women. Discriminating factors based on social norms, age mixing, terms of address, sexual contact, emotional commitment, and the exchange of money for sex were used to complete componential analysis of supercategories. A final set of nine supercategories and their discriminating factors were used to examine partner-specific risk perception and risk-taking behavior.

Results: Partner Supercategories

Dichotomous testing and componential analysis resulted in nine supercategories used to describe common types of sexual partners. Social, sexual, emotional, and monetary expectations differ for each category, with women giving priority to relationships that contain the greatest amount of sentiment.[2] These supercategories are as follows:

Boyfriend/girlfriend—These sexual partners are common among youth, and they share a strong level of emotional commitment. "Boyfriend/girlfriend" relationships are continuous sexual relationships with differing levels of longevity. However, partners are not married to one another.

Marriage material—These relationships appear to be more permanent than boyfriend/girlfriend relationships, and some couples who fall into this category may or may not already be married; if they are not married, they are considering "marriage material." Partners within this category are considered primary partners because they are given emotional preference over any outside sexual partner.

Spare tire—This type of sexual partner "stands in" for a primary partner who is absent. A "spare tire" usually holds "second place" to a primary partner, may be older than his or her partner, and sometimes provides money or gifts in exchange for sex. Such relationships are generally on a short-term basis and do not involve emotional commitment.

Sugar daddy/auntie—Men who fall within the "sugar daddy" category may or may not be married to their primary partner; however, they also seek young women as outside sexual partners. In general, sugar daddies are in their forties or fifties, have a lot of money or importance within their community, and provide partners with financial or material support. "Aunties" are usually single women, in their thirties or forties, and prefer younger male sexual partners to whom they give gifts. Most study participants thought the basis of these relationships to be monetary rather than sentimental.

Rich fool—"Rich fools" have money occasionally, and young women exploit this type of older partner until the man's funds are exhausted. Some participants said young women exchange sex for money with rich fools, while others said women only "tease" rich fools by making them believe that they will eventually receive sex without ever making good on their promise.

Arm candy—"Arm candy" refers to young, attractive women with whom men of all ages enjoy being seen. Young women participate in relationships with men for emotional, social, or monetary reasons.

One-night stand—"One-night stands" are usually peers who are approached solely for sexual gratification. Sexual encounters are on a temporary basis, and occur only once, and no money is exchanged for sex.

Prostitute—Participants described "prostitutes" as women who regularly have sex with men out of financial desperation and who regard sex as work. They explained that relationships with "prostitutes" are impersonal and temporary, with no emotion shared between partners.

Friend—Participants differed in their interpretation of this partner category; some said sex was a component of such liaisons, while others said relationships with these individuals are based solely on nonphysical friendship. The sexual context of the "friend" category is discussed in this study.

Partner Expectations

Participants identified several expectations for partners, including emotional fulfillment, financial or material support, sexual fidelity, and trust. Different relationships appear to afford more emotional reward than others, and some relationships, especially those of young women with older men, offer the women opportunities for financial gain. Most women spoke of a sexual double standard in which women are expected to be sexually faithful while men are allowed to pursue multiple partners. Overall, participants suspected that men are incapable of sexual fidelity and altered their expectations accordingly: while male partners may pursue outside relationships, women expect to maintain primary partner status, receive emotional priority over other women, and be treated with respect. Couples appear to negotiate several parameters of trust within their relationships, with trust serving as a marker for sexual decision making as well as an indicator of women's risk perception for STIs and HIV.

Emotional Fulfillment and Material Gain

Several study participants spoke about their simultaneous relationships with boyfriends and sugar daddies. They described the emotional expectations linked to partnerships with boyfriends and the material gain expected from sugar daddies. In terms of their relationships with boyfriends, study participants said they look to younger partners for emotional encouragement and support. They also seek young men who are "attentive," "understanding," "faithful," "gentle," "trustworthy," "respectful," and "sincere." Several participants said they obtain emotional gratification from boyfriends who share their own interests and want to grow together emotionally.

Some participants explained that in order for young women to obtain the material goods they need or want, they must partner with older men: "If you want to have a lot of money, you have to do whatever it takes because there aren't a lot of jobs available to girls" (twenty-one-year-old woman, Abobo District).

Participants listed several items young women expect from their sugar daddies, including stylish clothes, jewelry, money for medicine, and cosmetics. Some women also look to their sugar daddies for support for their studies and for payment of school fees. A few participants said they felt "trapped" in their relationships with sugar daddies: even though they may seek to leave the relationship because of their sugar daddy's sexual infidelity, they cannot because they are reliant upon his financial support.

Despite the common perception that young women's relationships with sugar daddies are purely for financial gain, some study participants said they feel what they would describe as "love" for their older partners. They also said they enjoy the mentoring component of these relationships, especially the advice they receive about careers and school and the manner in which their sugar daddies have helped them improve their self-esteem.

Study participants also described the social rewards gained from their partnerships with older men. Some said women with sugar daddies earn respect in their neighborhoods and elevated status among peers. However, others explained that they must act and look more mature in order to "fit the part" of a sugar daddy's partner. One participant explained how young women must "re-create themselves" with clothes and makeup in order to "go out" with sugar daddies.

In addition to the expectations women have of their sugar daddies and boyfriends, some participants spoke about the premise of relationships with spare tires and rich fools. Some explained that women approach spare tires only when they need money or when their preferred partner is unavailable. They added that young women take advantage of these spare tires in much the same way they do rich fools. One participant said, "When a rich fool comes around, you usually make up excuses for why you refuse sex with him. He's only there to give you money" (eighteen-year-old woman, Abobo District).

When asked why rich fools tolerate this kind of treatment, participants explained that they like to be seen in public with young, attractive women because it elevates their social status with peers. In addition, rich fools sometimes tolerate exploitation by younger women because they would like to obtain more emotional commitment from them. One woman explained that her rich fool cares for her a great deal more than she does him. However, she said she is not interested in becoming his "second wife" because she feels that her youth would be wasted on him, and she cannot commit to him emotionally.

Sexual Fidelity

A common topic of discussion with all participants was the cultural standard of sexual prowess for men and sexual fidelity for women. Most women spoke of a sexual double standard common to their past and present relationships. Some also shared how they had become disillusioned with men and their ability to remain sexually faithful to one partner. Even though some study participants had more than two sexual partners at the time of the interview, it appeared that they felt more comfortable talking about their partners' sexual infidelity than their own.

When asked if they knew if their current sexual partners had partners other than themselves, many women said they could not be sure, but they suspected that their partners were involved with other women. Others thought sexual infidelity on a man's part inevitable. "I know that men are never serious about just one woman" (twenty-one-year-old woman, Treichville District).

Several participants agreed that even though men may have more than one partner to demonstrate prowess, women are expected to limit themselves to one sexual partner at a time. Some women explained that even though they could be sure of their own fidelity, they could not know how their partners behave when they are not around. "You could know (your partner), but he could hide things like that from you" (twenty-one-year-old woman, Abobo District).

Many participants appeared to speak from experience. Several discussed how sexual infidelity on a partner's part had ended a relationship or changed its nature. One woman said even the term one uses to describe a partner could change. According to her, if a man has sex with a woman other than his "fiancée," his status would change to that of an "occasional partner."

Trust

Trust was a recurring topic of discussion among study participants. Even though many of the contributions surrounding trust were in terms of sexual fidelity, participants' responses reveal a larger theme: women spoke of trusting their partners emotionally and trusting them to treat them with respect. Trust appears not only to be a marker for the decision-making processes that shape sexual behavior but also an indication of women's perception of risk for STIs and HIV.

Several participants spoke of the level of trust they had in their partners to remain sexually faithful to them. Some said they could not think of any men they could trust because so many of their past partners had been sexually unfaithful. Others felt betrayed when their trust was violated and they discovered that their partner had other sexual partners. Several women used the term "serious" synonymously with sexual fidelity and described how they ended past relationships with men they knew were not "serious" and had outside partners.

Women also described how the sexual activities in which they participate with a partner depend upon the level of trust within the relationship. For example, a few participants said they no longer perform oral sex on their partner or participate in anal sex because they found out that their partners have sex with other women and cannot be trusted. Others said they would not engage in oral sex until they were sure that they could trust their partners not to have affairs. However, several women appeared to think that vaginal penetration was not reliant upon trusting one's partner since it was seen as less intimate than either oral or anal sex.

Some participants spoke of trusting their sexual partners on an emotional level. For example, even though many women suspected that their partners had sexual affairs, they could tolerate such behavior if they were assured that they would remain the preferred partner. One woman said she could accept her partner's outside affairs, but she would not tolerate being his *deuxième bureau* ("second office") or concubine because she wanted to be his "real" partner: "It's me or nothing" (twenty-one-year-old woman, Treichville District).

Another woman said her boyfriend's relationships with other women do not threaten her because she thinks of the women as arm candy and spare tires. According to her, these women do not pose an emotional threat to her, and she is satisfied that her partner gives her emotional priority over them.

Some participants used the terms "trust" and "respect" interchangeably. For instance, one woman said she would feel disrespected by her partner if he paraded his other sexual partners in front of her or her friends and family. She could not trust her partner if he made a mockery of her and flaunted his relationships with other women.

Several women said they trusted their partner because they "knew" him well. For example, some participants said they knew that their partner had outside relationships but they could trust him to limit the number of affairs he had. However, some women said their trust was violated when their partner infected them with an STI, since it meant that he had not limited himself to just a few outside partners. Likewise, some women said they would feel deceived if their partner did not use condoms with his outside partners.

The topic of trust also arose when discussing condom negotiation. Participants explained that proposing condom use with a steady partner could imply a lack of trust in him. According to the participants, if a woman suggests using condoms with a partner, he will automatically assume that she does not trust him and is accusing him of having outside partners. Another area where condoms and trust are implicated is when couples use condoms at the start of a new relationship, but quit using them once an understanding of mutual fidelity or a policy of using condoms with outside partners is established. Finally, some participants said if they found out that they could not trust a partner because he had outside partners, they would reintroduce condoms into the relationship. One woman explained that when she discovered that her partner was having sex with other women, she told him that he either had to give them up or start using condoms with her. Since he decided to keep his outside partners, she insisted that they use condoms together.

Perception of Risk for STIs and HIV

Overall, study participants demonstrated low levels of knowledge and risk perception for STIs and HIV. Although women spoke of risk in a global context and were able to point to partner categories containing an elevated risk for infection, few women seemed to make a connection between general risks for infection and their own behavior. In addition, few participants demonstrated significant behavior change in the face of AIDS, and most seemed to rely on their partners to change their behavior and prevent infection from entering their relationship.

Women's Knowledge of and Exposure to STIs

In general, most participants could cite gonorrhea and HIV/AIDS as STIs, but they were unfamiliar with most other STIs. Some women also demonstrated misconceptions about STIs and their modes of transmission. However, a few participants said they had been infected with STIs in the past, and, as a result, their level of knowledge appeared to be much higher than participants who said they had never been infected. In addition, some women said that some of their past and present partners had tested positive for STIs and sought treatment.

Several women used colloquial terms such as *gono*, *gondo*, *coco*, and *chaude pisse* ("burning urine") to describe gonorrhea. A few participants were able to cite syphilis by its technical name but several knew it by a colloquial term, *chancre mou*. Even though some women could only remember HIV/AIDS at the time of the interview, they said they knew of other STIs but could not recall their names.

Only a few participants said they had ever been infected with an STI; however, several women also said they had never received a gynecological exam, so their true STI status cannot be known. Two women said their current partners had infected them with an STI, but they were unsure of which infection they had. One said she had been diagnosed with STIs on five separate occasions, but since she had had so many sexual partners, she could not determine who infected her. According to her, the STIs for which she had been diagnosed were syphilis and gonorrhea.

The study investigator also asked women about their current and past partners' exposure to STIs. In addition to the two women who said their current partners had infected them with an STI, one study participant said her current partner had tested positive for an STI in the past. Although some women surmised that their partners had never had an STI, they said they could not be sure since they had never discussed it.

Few study participants said either they or their partners had been tested for STIs or HIV. One woman explained that her partner had been tested for HIV under his doctor's recommendation. However, he did not tell her about the test until the results came back negative. Only one participant said she and her partner had been tested for STIs together.

Perception of risk differs according to partner type. When asked to evaluate different partner categories and their risks for STIs and HIV, most participants identified one or two groups they thought at highest risk. Some also pointed out that everyone is at risk for infection despite their partner category. Although some women classified their own partner categories as having an elevated risk, they had difficulty assessing their personal risk for infection or their partner's.

Overall, most study participants said "prostitutes" and sugar daddies were at highest risk for STIs and HIV because they do not have a "fixed" number of partners. One mentioned "prostitutes" as the only type of partner at risk for infection. Several women stated that male partners who give or receive money for sex (such as sugar daddies and spare tires), and women who either receive or give money (arm candy and aunties, respectively) can put one at greater risk for infection because "you never know what they're doing or with whom" (eighteen-year-old woman, Abobo District). Another young woman said, " (With some partners) you can never be sure of where they've been or who they've been with" (nineteen-year-old woman, Marcory District).

Several participants thought they could reduce their risk of infection by avoiding men who have had a number of sexual partners or men they do not "know well." In their opinion, one should know a partner's sexual history and his number of past partners in order to avoid infection with STIs and HIV. These participants also thought that one-night stands or partners one knows "in passing" pose an increased risk for infection.

Some participants said men they would consider marriage material pose less risk for infection because they restrict themselves to fewer sexual partners than other categories of male partners. In addition, such partners only have sex with women they would consider "making a life" with or marrying. Some women added that partners in these categories do not pose a risk for infection when they are sexually faithful to their partners.

Risk Assessment Requires an Analysis of Partner Expectations

According to study participants' comments, evaluating one's risk for STIs and HIV is reliant upon partners' behavior and the expectations one has of sexual relationships. Even though some participants said they recognize their increased risk for infection due to their partners' behavior, they count on their partners to change their behavior outside of the relationship rather than changing the dynamics within their relationship together. Most women spoke of their partners' sexual infidelity as putting them at risk for STIs or HIV infection.

When some participants spoke of reducing their risk for infection, they pointed out actions their partner could take to keep them safe from STIs and HIV. He could limit his number of sexual partners, wear condoms with outside partners, or remain sexually faithful to one primary partner. Some participants surmised that their partner does not wear a condom with he is with his outside partners. In fact, one woman said she knows that her "fiancé" has sexual partners other than herself, and, like other men, he is not "careful" and does not wear condoms when he is with them.

Even though some participants' partners appeared to be making only minor changes in their behavior to prevent STIs and HIV infection, participants' risk perception remained low. For instance, one woman said she was not concerned with her partner's outside affairs because he did not sleep with "professionals," or "prostitutes." Another young woman said her sugar daddy was trying to "arrange his life" and "stop living as before" by reducing his number of sexual partners.

Condom Use

Few study participants said they use condoms consistently with all of their sexual partners. It appears from their comments that condom use is more appropriate with some partners than others, and condoms are used primarily for pregnancy prevention than protection from STIs and HIV. Some women explained that proposing condom use in a steady relationship would insinuate infidelity on their partner's part or indicate a lack of trust on their part. In addition, some study participants spoke of how their partners' sexual infidelity had changed their condom use and convinced them to reintroduce condoms into their relationships even after they had abandoned the use of condoms.

Many women appear to use condoms the first few times they have sex with a partner and then abandon their use once they feel they can "trust" him. Several participants said they used condoms for a short period of time, usually during initial encounters or the first few months of a new relationship. Others elaborated by saying that they wanted to be sure that their relationship with their partner would be "permanent" and their feelings for their partner "sure" before foregoing condom use.

Several participants explained that they rely on condoms more for pregnancy prevention than protection from STIs and HIV. Many women said they use condoms during their "fertile" period in order to prevent pregnancy, or they avoid sexual contact with their partners altogether during these times. A few women explained that when they had "disrespected" their fertile period and not used condoms, they became pregnant as a result. Another participant said she did not use condoms when she was taking the pill, but now that she no longer takes it, she relies on condoms for pregnancy prevention.

Only three women said they used condoms specifically to prevent STIs and HIV. However, another two women said they could not rely on condoms for protection from STIs and HIV since they have had experiences with them tearing in the past. They speculated that condoms available to them are of poor quality and are an unreliable method of protection.

A few women described how a partner's infidelity prompted them to reintroduce condoms into their relationship even after their use had been abandoned. One woman said she insisted on using condoms with her boyfriend after she found out that he had outside partners. According to her, they will stop using condoms once she can trust him to remain sexually faithful and they both have tested negative for HIV. Another woman said she would use condoms with her partner for a "certain amount of time," until she was sure that he understood the necessity of using condoms outside of their relationship. One participant said she used condoms consistently with one of her past partners because she suspected that he was not "serious" and had sexual partners outside of their relationship.

Some participants described how they use condoms with some partners and not others. When asked why she used condoms with her boyfriend but not her sugar daddy, one woman said, "Because I told myself that I can't have unprotected sex with two partners—so I have to protect myself with one of them" (eighteen-year-old woman, Marcory District).

One woman explained that the reverse was true for her, and she insisted on condom use with any partner "in passing" such as a rich fool or sugar daddy. In her opinion, "There are too many diseases out there [not to use a condom]" (eighteen-year-old woman, Treichville District).

Methodological Limitations and Conclusion

As with all studies, this study faced some limitations that must be taken into account when analyzing data and drawing conclusions from study results. Specifically, the shortcomings of this study can be attributed to methods of data collection and analysis, and the challenges inherent with working in a cross-cultural setting. Caution must also be used when interpreting qualitative results. Like all qualitative studies, results from free lists, pile sorts, and in-depth interviews conducted in this study cannot necessarily be generalized to the larger population of Côte d'Ivoire.

In terms of recruiting participants, reliance upon the known sponsor approach may have resulted in some network bias with a sample of women different than those unknown to recruiters or unavailable during recruitment periods. During data collection, the number of terms included in pile sort exercises may have resulted in some participants "lumping" several terms together or others "splitting" terms into very refined categories (Weller 1979; Winch 1993). Some terms were also unfamiliar to participants, indicating that some terms for different kinds of partners are specific to particular areas or communities within Abidjan. The study investigator is reliant upon self-reported data, and underreporting of sexual activity or inaccurate responses regarding risk perception can influence the reliability and validity of study results. A lack of privacy could have also contributed to the underreporting of certain behaviors since the study investigator conducted in-depth interviews in private homes, which sometimes resulted in interruptions by family members.

Finally, the challenge of collecting data in a cross-cultural setting may have influenced study results. The investigator was responsible for all interviews, pile sorts, and transcriptions. Although such a method of data collection ensures consistency in study guide use, interviews conducted, participant selection, and details in field notes, one must bear in mind that the investigator is a nonnative French speaker, and French was a second language for several participants. As a result, language barriers may have compromised some study outcomes. However, all interviews were audio recorded, and the study investigator sought clarification from colleagues when terms or phrases participants used were not readily understood.

Despite these challenges, this study revealed several valuable insights into categories of partners common to young women in Abidjan, expectations associated with partners, and the influence of partner characteristics on STI/HIV risk perception and risk-taking behavior. Results from pile sorts and componential analysis reveal that sexual partners can be divided into nine "supercategories" in order to evaluate partner expectations and relationship dynamics: boyfriend/girlfriend, marriage material, spare tire, sugar daddy/auntie, rich fool, arm candy, one-night stand, prostitute, and friend.

Participants explained that emotional and monetary expectations differ according to each partner category, with priority given to relationships that contain the greatest amount of sentiment. In addition, trust was a recurring topic throughout the in-depth interviews. Even though much discussion about trust centered on sexual fidelity, participants' responses reveal a larger theme in which trust describes an emotional commitment and represents an unwritten contract between sexual partners, establishing the terms of their relationship.

Study results reveal low levels of perceived risk for STIs and HIV among participants. Women spoke of risk in a global context and did not make a connection between general risks for infection and their own behavior. Several women explained how they believed they could avoid becoming infected with STIs and HIV by "knowing their partner well" or by being with men they could trust. Risk perception and risk-taking behavior appear to be influenced by the level of emotional commitment involved in relationships as well as women's level of trust in their sexual partners.

Data also reveal that levels of behavior change in the face of AIDS among study participants are relatively low. Few women reported abstaining from sex or having their male partners use condoms consistently. Most participants appeared to rely on their male partners to reduce their number of sexual partners or use condoms with outside partners in order to prevent infection from entering their relationship.

Study results reveal several opportunities for intervention and appropriate approaches to include in information, education, and communication (IEC) campaigns. Including details about relationship dynamics and partner characteristics in prevention campaigns can help program planners concentrate their efforts on relationships common to young women where risk-taking behavior is high and risk perception low. Likewise, study results demonstrate the association of low levels of discriminatory levels of HIV/AIDS knowledge with high-risk sexual behavior. Programs that encourage women to reduce their number of sexual partners and discourage them from exchanging sex for gifts or money should convey specific types of HIV/AIDS information in IEC campaigns. Messages should include information about safer sex practices, including consistent condom use with all types of partners, partner reduction, and abstinence. In addition, condom promotion campaigns should provide information about the role of condoms in preventing infection from STIs and HIV as well pregnancy.

This study also reveals the influence of sexual partners and relationship dynamics on risk perception and risk-taking behavior. Based on these findings, IEC campaigns should target women in "committed" relationships, where risk behavior is high but risk perception remains low. Messages should emphasize that prevention from STIs and HIV requires more than trusting or "knowing one's partner." In addition, campaigns should stress the need to incorporate risk reduction strategies into committed relationships, rather than relying on partners to prevent STIs/HIV from entering relationships. Finally, interventions for men should be incorporated into program design and complement programs that target women. Campaigns for men should encourage them to reduce their number of sexual partners and incorporate condom use into their secondary and primary relationships.

Acknowledgments

Several individuals are to be thanked for their assistance and contributions to this study. In Abidjan, Côte d'Ivoire, Dr. Basile Tambashe, Tom Scialfa, and other staff members at the Santé Familiale et Prevention du SIDA (SFPS) office provided logistical support. Collaborators from the Focus on Young Adults Project helped collect data from free list sessions, namely Jonathan Dan Veh, Pauline Kouye, and Clemence Noyjan. Mathieu Kei, Idrissa Kone, Michel Konnan-Koffi, Henri Kouassi, and Ibrahime Sory helped recruit study participants for pile sorts and in-depth interviews. Gratitude is also owed to the women in the Abobo, Marcory, Treichville, and Yopougon districts who were kind enough to share their stories.

In the United States, there are several individuals to be thanked for their support during data analysis and report writing. Jane T. Bertrand, Carl Kendall, Patricia Kissinger, Robert Magnani, and Beth Rubin provided guidance as dissertation committee members. Faculty, staff, and students in Tulane's Department of International Health and Development also provided support for the completion of this study. Steven Chapman at Population Services International (PSI) reviewed several drafts of this document and encouraged its publication. Finally, Dinkar Mokadam edited countless drafts and, along with other family members and friends, provided much needed encouragement to finish this project.

Notes

1. During "free" pile sorts, participants are allowed to construct as many categories as they want. For this research, unknown terms were put aside and not included in pile sort categories. After each session, the number on the back of each card was noted as well as its category for analysis.

2. Information from free lists and additional details on partner taxonomies can be found in Longfield (in press).

References Cited

Agha, Sohail, Andrew Karlyn, and Dominique Meekers. 2001. "The Promotion of Condom Use in Non-Regular Sexual Partnerships in Urban Mozambique." *Health Policy and Planning* 16 (2): 144–151.

Agyei, William K., Elisabeth J. Epema, and Margaret Lubega. 1992. "Contraception and Prevalence of Sexually Transmitted Diseases among Adolescents and Young Adults in Uganda." *International Journal of Epidemiology* 21 (5): 981–988.

Blanc, Ann K., and Ann A. Way. 1998. "Sexual Behavior and Contraceptive Knowledge and Use among Adolescents in Developing Countries." *Studies in Family Planning* 29 (2): 106–116.

Borgatti, Stephen P. 1990. Anthropac 3.2. Department of Sociology, University of South Carolina, Columbia.

Caldwell John, Pat Caldwell, and Pat Quiggin. 1989. "The Social Context of AIDS in Sub-Saharan Africa." *Population and Development Review* 15 (2): 185–234.

Calvès, Anne-Emmanuèle. 1998. "Adolescent Premarital Sexuality in Yaoundé: Do Men Have the Same Strategies and Motivations as Women?" In *Sexuality and Reproductive Health during Adolescence in Africa: With a Special Reference to Cameroon*, ed. B. Kuate-Defo, 141–161. Ottawa: University of Ottawa Press.

———. 1999. *Condom Use and Risk Perceptions among Male and Female Adolescents in Cameroon: Qualitative Evidence from Edéa*. Working Paper No. 22. Washington, D.C.: Population Services International.

Calvès, Anne-Emmanuèle, Gretchen T. Cornwell, and Parfait Eloundou Enyegue. 1996. *Adolescent Sexual Activity in Sub-Saharan Africa: Do Men have the Same Strategies and Motivations as Women?* University Park, Pa.: Population Research Institute.

Dinan, Carmel. 1983. "Sugar Daddies and Gold-Diggers: The White-Collar Single Women in Accra." In *Female and Male in West Africa*, ed. C. Oppong, 344–366. London: George Allen and Unwin.

Gage, Anastasia J. 1998. "Sexual Activity and Contraceptive Use: The Components of the Decision-Making Process." *Studies in Family Planning* 29 (2): 154–166.

Gage, Anastasia, and Caroline Bledsoe. 1994. "The Effects of Education and Social Stratification on Marriage and the Transition to Parenthood in Freetown, Sierra Leone." In *Nuptiality in Sub-Saharan Africa: Contemporary Anthropological and Demographic Perspectives*, ed. C. Bledsoe and G. Pison, 148–166. London: Oxford University Press.

Gorgen, Regina, Birga Maier, and Hans Jochen Diesfeld. 1993. "Problems Related to

Schoolgirl Pregnancies in Burkina Faso." *Studies in Family Planning* 24 (5): 283–294.

Gregson, Simon, and Geoff P. Garnett. 2002. "Contrasting Gender Differentials in HIV-1 Prevalence and Associated Mortality Increase in Eastern and Southern Africa: Artifact of Data or Natural Course of Epidemics?" *AIDS* 14 (Supplement 3): S85–S99.

Grosskurth, Heiner, Frank Mosha, James Todd, Ezra Mwijarubi, Arnoud Klokke, Kesheni Senkoro, Philippe Mayaud, John Changalucha, Angus Nicoll, Gina ka-Gina, James Newell, Kokugonza Mugeye, David Mabey, and Richard Hayes. 1995. "Impact of Improved Treatment of Sexually Transmitted Diseases on HIV Infection in Rural Tanzania: Randomised Controlled Trial." *Lancet* 346 (8974): 530–536.

Kouye, Pauline, Kim Longfield, Stephanie Mullen, Ilene Speizer, and Basile Tambashe. 2000. "Les Services de Santé Reproductive: Une Evaluation de l'Utilisation Clinique et des Besoins parmi les Jeunes en Côte d'Ivoire." Paper prepared for the Focus on Young Adults and Santé Familiale et Prevention du SIDA (SFPS) projects, Abidjan, Côte d'Ivoire.

Kuate-Defo, Barthélémy. 1997. "Assessing the Trends and Differentials in Adolescent Sexuality and Reproductive Health through the Lenses of Quantitative and Qualitative Data." Paper prepared for presentation to the U.S. National Academy of Sciences Workshop on "Adolescent Sexuality and Reproductive Health in Developing Countries: Trends and Determinants."

Longfield, Kim. (in press). *Rich Fools, Spare Tires, and Boyfriends: Partner Categories, Relationship Dynamics and Ivorian Women's Risk for STIs and HIV.*

MacPhail, Catherine, and Catherine Campbell. 2001. "'I Think Condoms Are Good but, Aai, I Hate Those Things': Condom Use among Adolescents and Young People in a Southern African Township." *Social Science and Medicine* 52 (11): 1613–1627.

Meekers, Dominique, and Anne-Emmanuèle Calvès. 1997a. *Gender Differentials in Adolescent Sexual Activity and Reproductive Health Risks in Cameroon.* Working Paper No. 4. Washington, D.C.: Population Services International.

———. 1997b. "'Main' Girlfriends, Girlfriends, Marriage, and Money: The Social Context of HIV Risk Behaviour in Sub-Saharan Africa." *Health Transition Review* 7 (Supplement): 361–375.

Meekers, Dominique, Megan Klein, and Leger Foyet. 2001. *Patterns of HIV Risk Behavior and Condom Use among Youth in Yaoundé and Douala, Cameroon.* Working Paper No. 46. Washington, D.C.: Population Services International.

Mensch, Barbara S., Daniel Bagah, Wesley H. Clark, and Fred Binka. 1999. "The Changing Nature of Adolescence in the Kassena-Nankana District of Northern Ghana." *Studies in Family Planning* 30 (2): 95–111.

Monitoring the AIDS Pandemic Network. 2002. *The Status and Trends of the HIV/AIDS Epidemics in the World (Provisional Report July 7, 2002).* Barcelona: Joint United Nations Programme on HIV/AIDS (UNAIDS) and U.S. Agency for International Development (USAID).

National Research Council. 1996. *Preventing and Mitigating AIDS in Sub-Saharan Africa (Summary): Research and Data Priorities for the Social and Behavioral Sciences.* Washington, D.C.: National Academy Press.

Njikam Savage, O. M. 1998. "Adolescents' Beliefs and Perceptions toward Sexuality in Urban Cameroon." In *Sexuality and Reproductive Health during Adolescence in Africa: With a Special Reference to Cameroon*, ed. B. Kuate-Defo, 77–90. Ottawa: University of Ottawa Press.

Owuamanam, Donatus O. 1995. "Sexual Networking among Youth in Southwestern Nigeria." *Health Transition Review* (Supplement 5): 57–66.

Patton, Michael Quinn. 1987. *How to Use Qualitative Methods in Evaluation*. Newbury Park, Calif.: Sage.

Poppen, Paul J., and Carol A. Reisen. 1997. "Perception of Risk and Sexual Self-Protective Behavior: A Methodological Critique." *AIDS Education and Prevention* 9: 373–390.

Qualis Research. 1998. Ethnograph 5.0. Thousand Oaks, Calif.: Scolari/Sage Publications Software.

Ulin, Priscilla R. 1992. "African Women and AIDS: Negotiating Behavioral Change." *Social Science and Medicine* 34 (1): 63–73.

UNAIDS. 1998. *Facing the Challenges of HIV/AIDS and STDS: A Gender-Based Response*. Geneva: UNAIDS.

———. 2002. *Report on the Global HIV/AIDS Epidemic (July 2002)*. Geneva: UNAIDS.

UNICEF (United Nations Children's Fund), Joint United Nations Programme on HIV/AIDS (UNAIDS), and World Health Organization. 2002. *Young People and HIV/AIDS: Opportunity in Crisis*. New York: UNICEF.

Van Rossem, Ronan, Dominique Meekers, and Zacch Akinyemi. 2001. "Consistent Condom Use with Different Types of Partners: Evidence from Two Nigerian Surveys." *AIDS Education and Prevention* 13 (3): 252–267.

Weller, Susan C. 1979. "Structured Interviewing and Questionnaire Construction." In *The Ethnographic Interview*, ed. J. P. Spradley, 173–183. New York: Holt, Rinehart and Winston.

Wilson, David, and S. Lavelle. 1992. "Psychosocial Predictors of Intended Condom Use among Zimbabwean Adolescents." *Health Education Research* 7 (1): 55–68.

Winch, Peter. 1993. *Microcomputer Applications in Qualitative Research*. Baltimore: Center for International Community-Based Health Research, Johns Hopkins University.

Yelibi, S., P. Valenti, C. Volpe, A. Caprara, S. Dedy, and G. Tape. 1993. "Sociocultural Aspects of AIDS in an Urban Peripheral Area of Abidjan (Côte d'Ivoire)." *AIDS Care* 5 (2): 187–197.

Zanou, Benjamin, Albert Nyankawindemera, Jean Paul Toto, Olivier Koko Kossonou, Claude Kamenga, Simon Pierre Tegang, and Jean Paul Tchupo. 1998. "Carte de la Côte d'Ivoire." Paper prepared for Family Health International. Ecole National de la Statistique et Analyse (ENSEA), Abidjan, Côte d'Ivoire.

Zellner, Sarah L. 2003. "Condom Use and Accuracy of AIDS Knowledge in Côte d'Ivoire." *International Family Planning Perspectives* 29 (1): 41–47.

7

Courage, Conquest, and Condoms

Harmful Ideologies of Masculinity and Sexual Encounters in Zambia in the Time of HIV/AIDS

ANTHONY SIMPSON

This chapter draws upon research designed to explore the manner in which mission-educated men in Zambia constructed their sexuality and sexual practices, in order to investigate how these contributed to sexual risk taking and the instability of safer sex practices.[1] It is based on the assumption that a relationship often exists between how a man acts sexually and how he acts in general (see Stoltenberg 2000). My major focus was upon the survivors of a cohort of twenty-four Zambian men educated at a boys' Catholic mission school, which I call "St. Antony's." I taught and first interviewed them in the early 1980s, around the time they completed their secondary education.[2] In 2002, I reinterviewed them in the course of fieldwork that entailed living in some of their homes and participating in their day-to-day life.

Many of the men who were the focus of this study belonged to a Zambian elite. Yet individual men in the cohort occupied various subject positions in relation to local constructions of masculinity that were never single, male-authored achievements, but rather shifting productions in which women and other men necessarily played a number of roles. There can be no simple portrayal of men as uniformly dominant and women as subservient. Constantly shifting power in gender relations could be observed within marriages and households. All the men had lost family members, friends, and work colleagues to AIDS. A number of their school contemporaries had died of what were suspected to be AIDS-related conditions. The men had the information and the means at their disposal to protect themselves and their sexual partners from exposure to the HIV virus. That some at times chose not to do so must be understood within a context where harmful ideologies of masculinity and the vulnerability of men striving to appear as "real" men put them and their partners at risk in intimate sexual encounters.

In 2002, the age range of the men in the cohort was between the midthirties and early forties. They belonged to a number of ethnic groups, primarily Bemba and Tonga, as well as Lala, Ila, Chikunda, Lamba, and Lozi. Though very few men (unlike their wives) regularly attended church, almost all claimed a Christian identity. Religious affiliations included Catholic, Seventh-Day Adventist, United Church of Zambia, Assemblies of God, and various Pentecostal churches. There was a wide range of incomes within the group, some men earning as much as 7,000,000 kwacha a month (about U.S.$1,556) and some as little as 100,000 kwacha (about U.S.$22) a month or less.[3] Occupations included doctors, lawyers, managers, lecturers and teachers, engineers, security guards, and "businessmen" (generally involved in informal trading). Several respondents were unemployed. All were resident in urban or provincial centers. All except two were married. Without exception, respondents reported feeling under enormous economic pressure, especially because they identified the male role as that of the "provider" and were identified as such by their wives and female partners. Several men, whether employed or not, described themselves as "failures" in this regard. Many of the marriages were interethnic. Some wives were in professional employment; some were marketeers and traders. Others were housewives with no employment beyond the household.

For the majority of former students, men's superiority over women was axiomatic. They would cite both "African tradition" and Christianity. In answer to my question whether he and his wife were equal partners, man and woman, husband and wife, Kangwa, for example, raised his voice and gave an impassioned response:

> No, no, we are not equal, no! Of course, we are not equal. The man is superior to the woman. I am superior to my wife. Look, it's obvious. It's obvious! I am the man! I am the man! It's because of the responsibilities that I have. I am there. I have all the responsibilities in the home, in the family. Then there is our tradition in Zambia. Men are superior. Then there is the Bible. Adam was created first! Men are superior! There is no doubt.

It would be wrong, however, not to acknowledge some of the men's self-awareness of the pretense of power, their fear of failing to measure up to prevailing norms of hegemonic masculinity, or their reluctance to forego what has elsewhere been called the "patriarchal dividend" (Connell 2001: 35). For example, describing his sexual exploits, Robert was prepared to acknowledge: "At times men don't really go after women, but women go after men. As for the man, he wants to seem to be the conqueror, or he is afraid of appearing weak." Promise also spoke about this fear of appearing weak, aware that at times, this impelled him to approach women:

> Promise: "When we are talking here, OK, I know the risks; but there are times when I fail to reverse my emotions, especially with those ladies I have known for some time. I have that feeling, 'If I don't do it, then that lady might think I am weak and that I cannot go out [have sex] with her.'"
> Q. "Why do you say 'weak'?"
> Promise: "Well, I mean, it's about strength, strength. My manhood is about strength."

Speaking of a common habit of a husband not letting his wife know his whereabouts, or when he might return to the household, Joshua commented upon the manner in which economic power in a home might place the man beyond question:

> Sometimes, as African men, we tend to want to be dictators. We want to keep our whereabouts secret so that the wife does not know. You see the thinking, "I am the one in employment. I am the one earning the money so why should she ask me? I am bringing everything into the house; she shouldn't question." It is in that line that some men have misused their homes and abused their wives by straying with other women. . . . Then we men want to defend ourselves, shutting up our wives, silencing them.

A number of men explained that they felt they did not match up to local ideals of hegemonic masculinity. Some attributed their late sexual debut, or small number of sexual partners, to shyness. They reported feeling "abnormal." Peter spoke of his lack of sexual experience before marriage and described himself as "somehow lame": "Sometimes I regard myself as somebody who was not normal because I had sex with no one else apart from my wife. And that was after I married her when I was twenty-six. My wife was also a virgin, so we were new in the game!"

Some men, because of difficult life circumstances or religious conversion, had come to revise their earlier notions of women as the "weaker" and "inferior" sex. Henry was not the only one to have come to appreciate his wife's strength in times of crisis. Indeed, losing his job and for a period preferring to live in an alcoholic haze, Henry attributed his recovery to his wife's strength and determined care: "It was a difficult time, but my wife was understanding. She helped me pull through. I was depressed. I used to drink a lot. She used to comfort me [saying], 'No, it's not the end.' During that time, she supported me emotionally and physically."

Henry's wife, Ruth, interviewed separately, considered that it was her husband's responsibility to provide for the family. She judged that her husband had more power in their relationship but not total control: "My husband has the power, but that does not mean that I have to be intimidated. I correct him when he is wrong."

Anthropological Archive

There is a substantial anthropological archive on marriage and the family in Zambia where much can be learned about gender and sexuality in the colonial and postcolonial periods. While there is no intention to posit a unitary, static picture of the recent past or to ignore variations between ethnic groups, observations made in the first half of the twentieth century, the time before AIDS, may offer insights into gender relations in present-day Zambia (see Forster 2001 for similar comments on his ethnography on AIDS in Malawi). Colson (1958) and Richards (1939, 1940, 1982) offered rich ethnographies (cultural descriptions) of marriage and family life in rural households, in particular of relations between husbands and wives in matrilineal societies (where descent is traced through the female line). Among both the Tonga and Bemba, the ethnographers noted the emphasis on men's potency. On the night of the wedding ceremony, the Plateau Tonga man had to prove his potency, and on the following morning his wife had to attest to it. In the Bemba girls' puberty ceremony, *chisungu*, the bridegroom-to-be appeared as a roaring lion, a lion killer, a crocodile, a hunter, a warrior, and a chief. The virility of the bridegroom was emphasized throughout the rite, and the marriage ceremony that followed was "a test of his procreative powers" (Richards 1982: 158).

Colson (1958) noted the emphasis on equality in the husband-wife relationship among the Plateau Tonga, where fertility was regarded as a primary value. Unlike the Bemba, among whom Richards (1982) suggested that companionship in marriage, where it existed, was something of a "happy accident," Colson (1958) noted that Tonga women enjoyed a considerable degree of companionship in marriage. However, the etiquette that governed their relationship subordinated the Tonga wife to the husband. There was an acceptance that when a husband became annoyed with his wife, he was likely to beat her, though women were unlikely to be prepared to take any great measure of abuse. The Tonga man in theory had exclusive possession of his wife, but this was not reciprocated. Adultery was considered a fact of married life; it put neither husband nor wife at risk of mystical harm and need not embitter the relations between them.

Colson (1958) reported that it was common for both husbands and wives to take lovers. In her analysis of *chisungu*, Richards (1982) suggested that the dilemma of a matrilineal society, in which men were dominant but descent was traced through women, was acted out in ritual practice. She hypothesized that so much emphasis was placed upon the duty of the wife to submit to her husband precisely because the maintenance of a stable family group was difficult to achieve. Because of uxorilocal residence (upon marriage the couple move into the woman's household), at least in the early years of marriage, the young man was isolated and lacked influence among his in-laws. Richards (1982) portrayed him as a stranger in his wife's village, honored primarily in his role of genitor (biological father) but not pater (social father). While a man was not seriously criticized for adultery, only his wife could safeguard him in ritual against the punishment of ancestors.

Moore and Vaughan (1994), in their critical reassessment of Richards's work, argued that by the 1950s, a shift in the balance of power in marriage had occurred. Changes brought about largely through men's labor migration to urban centers meant that now it was Bemba women rather than men who needed to be married. More recently, Ferguson (1999) reported that in his fieldwork on the Zambian Copperbelt in the mid and late 1980s, he found domestic life among miners "remarkably similar" to the earlier bleak portrayals of married life on the Copperbelt by Powdermaker (1960) and Epstein (1981). If anything, "hostility and mutual suspicion" seemed to Ferguson (1999: 187) to have intensified: "It was expected that both married men and women would have many sexual partners. . . . While the threat of AIDS was much on men's minds . . . few regarded it as a legitimate reason to forego these affairs (or to use condoms which were in any case not widely available)." In a report of her longitudinal study of low-income households in Mtendere, a compound (neighborhood) in Lusaka, Hansen (1996) noted wives' suspicions and the fact that they did not expect their husbands' undivided attention either economically or sexually.

Manhood and Courage

The men in the cohort of former students had learned in childhood that a key requirement for a "real" man was physical and emotional strength— emotional strength measured, at least in part, by the capacity for silence in suffering and the repression of emotional expression (see Jacobson-Widding's [2000] discussion of Manyika male identity that entailed the silencing of deep-seated emotions). Among peers, manhood was demonstrated first through the ability to produce semen. To fathers, manhood had to be displayed in the manner in which boys performed tasks, in the way they withstood physical punishment, and—to their fathers and other boys—in the way they dealt with the aggression of male peers. Most men reported working on their bodies, developing strength and skill in fighting and such martial arts as karate—activities often encouraged by fathers, uncles, older brothers, and male cousins. For cattle-keeping people, such as the Tonga and Ila, herding activities provided an arena for the performance of manly tasks, especially in herding and the control of animals.

Both as teenagers and now men, former students described to me how they had learned about sex and their sexual debut. Many spoke of childhood play in which their desire to imitate what they considered to be gender-appropriate "adult" behavior resulted in early, nonpenetrative attempts. Several commented that provided the boy was on top of the girl, then they felt they were doing it "properly." As boys, most had experienced peer pressure. Some had been approached by older, more experienced girls; at times, older boys arranged a girl for them. By the time they had completed their secondary schooling, almost all those interviewed had had at least some sexual experience. Indeed, for a considerable number of them, their sexual careers had begun in primary school. For all, "sex" meant penetrative vaginal intercourse. Nothing other than this was classified as "sex." In student initiation rituals, new boys at St. Antony's were required to make speeches in the dormitories, to offer "convincing stories" of their sexual exploits, and to demonstrate how they "chopped girls" (had sex with girls) (see Simpson 2003: 133).[4]

Almost without exception, boys and young men said that ideally they should be the ones to make the first move in sexual encounters (see Simpson 2002 for similar observations recorded in other research among boys and young men in Zambia). The capacity to make this move depended upon a number of qualities, often summed up by the term "courage." The beginning of the process of what was figured as "conquest" depended upon an individual's language skills—the equivalent in British youth parlance of having the ability to "chat up" a girl.

Though it was acknowledged that a girl might signal her readiness through her body language, St. Antony's students considered verbal skills an essential aspect of persuading a girl to engage in sexual activity. In order to achieve his aim, a boy had to demonstrate that he had the courage to speak to a girl and to "convince" her to have sex with him. The importance

of persuasive talk remained a feature for married men in extramarital encounters—though not with those women described as "prostitutes," who,
it was claimed, needed no persuasion beyond the material rewards of beer
and money. However, condom use was most frequently reported in sexual
encounters with "prostitutes."

The personal ideal of the missionary brothers who were in charge of the
school was to live as celibates dedicated to the Virgin Mary. Among the
students, however, virginity was not valued. No one wanted to be called a
"monk" or a "walking stick," a boy who escorted a girl but did not have sex
with her.[5] Girls were "available" either in the surrounding villages or in the
nearby town, though the latter option required sufficient persuasive skills to
gain the necessary permission to leave the confines of the boarding school
for the day or the weekend. In the dormitories at St. Antony's, boys who
were not known to engage in sex with local girls, but who were suspected
of finding "relief" in masturbation, were mocked by those who claimed that
a boy could always find a girl. Sampa, now in his forties, recalled how he
would try to encourage his faint-hearted peers at school—emphasizing that
requirements for success included courage and verbal persuasion:

> Boys would want a girl, but then they would be shy. How to approach
> a girl? That's what it was all about. You need courage to approach a
> girl. At St. Antony's at night, well, you would be trying to get to sleep,
> but you find in the beds near you some of the guys are masturbating. I
> used to say to them, "Why? There are lots of ladies in town but you are
> doing such things!" A lot of boys were masturbating rather than going
> for girls, but if people think you masturbate a lot, then they think you
> are mad. At school the boys really wanted to have sex with a girl. They
> wanted to satisfy themselves but they didn't know how to approach
> girls. I mean, there was a primary school nearby. Well, you could call
> a girl and you talk, but it's not that very day that you make love with
> her. You try to persuade her. You have to be able to talk. You have to be
> very good with words. Very, very good with words! (laughter).

Some boys had been warned by elders that masturbation would lead to
impotence. Among the cohort, as young men, frequency of masturbation
was an issue. Once or twice a month, for some, was considered reasonable; more frequent than that was thought to lead either to a disinterest
in women and or an inability to satisfy them, often because of premature
ejaculation. The young men had thought of masturbation as a means of
"relief" from the build-up of pressure caused by the absence of regular sex.
Like same-sex sex, the general opinion was that masturbation could not

provide much pleasure (see Feldman et al. 1997 for similar views about masturbation among Zambian adolescents). Sampa, like many of his peers, expressed strong disapproval of masturbation. As a boy and a young man, he claimed he had never had a problem finding a girl to have sex with. As a married man, he had resorted to asking his wife to masturbate him only when she was "sick," that is, when she was menstruating:

> Couples masturbating together—ah, that's unacceptable, though there is that masturbation when your wife is sick—maybe it's her period. I mean in that situation I tell my wife, "Can you do this rather than I go and look for other women?" Then she does it, we kiss, and that is all. I mean there it is OK, but not in a situation where she is not even sick and then you tell her to masturbate you. No, that's not in order!

When we had first talked in the early 1980s, HIV/AIDS was only just being mentioned in the media, and what was being said sounded very far removed from the lives of secondary school students in a boarding school in the Zambian bush. The subject rarely emerged in the interviews. AIDS appeared to be a remote threat because initial publicity and campaigns placed great stress on "risk groups" such as "homosexual men," truck drivers, and commercial sex workers. On the point of homosexuality, students and former students were adamant about what they saw as the overwhelmingly heterosexual character of Zambian society. They repeatedly told me, "It's you Europeans who are homosexuals. We African men, we like our women." And in their construction of Zambian society, men were superior and men were in charge. None of us could imagine how AIDS would soon come to dominate everyday life in Zambia.

While there is no intention here to essentialize either men or women, each variously situated in constantly shifting fields of power, a clear profile emerged from men's accounts, irrespective of ethnic identity or religious affiliation, about prevailing ideologies concerning what it meant to be a man. For the majority, this was tied to sexual conquest and sexual performance. These ideologies impacted directly upon the most intimate sexual encounters that were necessarily always socially embedded. Their impact upon the use of safer sex practices in premarital, marital, and extramarital encounters—in particular, the use of condoms—was marked. I concentrate on male condoms here because very few respondents had any experience with female condoms, and there was little enthusiasm for them either among men or women. Several wives had been given female condoms at government clinics, but few couples had actually tried them, and none were using them on a regular basis. The few men who had tried them complained that they were "noisy," and some men feared a loss of control over their semen.

Within marriage, condoms were only used occasionally to prevent pregnancies. Indeed, respondents argued that it would be absurd to use them regularly. Almost all the men's wives were using contraceptive medicine in pill or more usually in injection form. Men gave numerous reasons for not using condoms in premarital and extramarital sex, familiar from other research: the reduction in pleasure, the desire for intimacy, and "wasting" semen, which became "matter out of place" because its proper place was in a woman's vagina (see Mane and Aggleton 2000 for similar observations reported by women of their male sexual partners in Senegal). Using condoms was also likened to impotence—"firing blanks" instead of live bullets. In premarital and extramarital encounters, because many sexual encounters were framed in terms of a type of conquest, performance anxiety at times led some men to forego the use of condoms, a decision men said was usually theirs.

Men revealed a preoccupation with their sexual performance as a demonstration of their strength and power. Several of them attempted to boost their performance by the regular consumption of local aphrodisiacs; the most commonly used was called "gunpowder." Respondents attested to its efficacy, particularly in the number of "rounds" of sex that it enabled the men to experience in one session. In contrast, men explained that condoms threatened their sexual performance and hence the demonstration of masculinity, particularly because condoms reduced both the number of rounds and the speed with which a man could ejaculate. However, some men acknowledged that such speed was not "fair" to women who "took time" and likened such behavior to rape. Two men explained that they had changed their opinions over time, preferring "one slow screw" to several quick rounds.

Sampa explained that condoms had never been popular with him, but not because of the opposition of the Catholic Church to which he formerly belonged. As a secondary school student, while he might use a condom in the first round of sex with older women, for the second and subsequent rounds, he explained, "I would just remove the condom because I was tired." Sampa described himself as very "traditional" on the matter of "dry sex," though he was aware of the reported dangers:

If the woman is tight, ah, that's very nice. I prefer tight and dry. These days they are saying that it is not advisable because of AIDS: the more the vagina is actually tight, the more you risk something, because of the friction. But, as for me, I believe tight cunts are nice. That's when you really feel something nice—the friction—unlike when it's watery. When it's watery, you don't feel anything. These days, women still try to make themselves tight and dry.

Beer

For some men, beer brought both the words and the kind of courage considered necessary to approach a woman for sex. This was the experience of Promise, a married man with several children. He rarely used condoms in extramarital sexual encounters because as far as he was concerned, using a condom was "more or less like masturbating," an activity that met with his strong disapproval:

> When I don't take [drink] beer, then I don't do anything with women. I cannot propose love to a woman when I have not taken beer. I do not have the courage. It's only beer that gives me courage. When I have not taken beer, I don't have words (laughter). But when you are drunk, words will be flowing. You'll find a way! Words are important. I find with ladies, if you tell them the truth, they won't accept [agree] to have sex with you. So you have to tell them you are working and you have a big job. That way they will think I have more money.

Promise reported that once the effects of the beer wore off, the "courage" evaporated, to be replaced—at least temporarily—by anxiety about the possibility of contracting the HIV virus:

> I know myself—and I have heard from my friends. Having slept with a lady openly [without using a condom], you will stay maybe two or three days worried, thinking of what the outcome might be—"Why did I do that?" This applies to me. It's not courage as such. It seems as if at times I lose my consciousness. That's how I would put it, because I stop thinking. All of a sudden you find yourself having sex, "going direct" [without using a condom]. Even while you are doing it, maybe you'll start thinking and you'll realize that you are doing something wrong. But then you think, "Well, I have already done it, so let me continue!" Later again, you will regret it. I mean, sometimes you can have that feeling for a week. A lady can come close to you, but you'll say, "No, no, no!" But later, after some time, you'll forget about what

you had thought at that time—"No, I'm just OK." And then you'll do it again.

Sampa started drinking beer while at secondary school and recognized that this, too, might put him at risk for HIV infection:

Just a few beers, ah, now (laughter) that one is dangerous! You know, if you drink a lot of beer, you will have no power—but just a few beers! With a few beers, still, you can't use a condom. Your power is reduced. If you use a condom, it will take time for you to ejaculate. So you don't use one. And I don't think if the lady is drunk she will even encourage you to use a condom.

Few of the men, whether for or against the use of condoms, had changed their opinions about condom use. As boys and young men, very few had had access to a regular supply of condoms. Even where condoms had been available, not one used a condom when sexual debut occurred in their teens or earlier. In the opinion of most of the men, consistent condom use was neither possible nor desirable. The majority opposed the third term of the ABC—Abstain, Be faithful, use a Condom—campaigns for their children on the grounds that to promote condoms was to encourage "promiscuity."

For some, the option of condom use had been automatically rejected. Hambayi, who had formerly attended a Seventh-Day Adventist church, was not the only one to question the morality of condoms. As a young man, Hambayi had decided against condoms, arguing that they subverted the meaning of sexual relations between men and women, the purpose of which, beyond the pleasure that they gave, was intended by God as the means of human reproduction. God had told Adam and Eve, "Go forth and multiply." Twenty years later, Hambayi was the father of seven children. The pandemic had taken its toll, but Hambayi's position on condoms had not changed, even though he had lost a much-loved brother in circumstances that led him to conclude that he had died of AIDS. Hambayi now stressed what he saw as the unreliability of condoms, though he claimed never to have used them. He was convinced that condoms were "dirty," and he was worried by the idea that his sperm would not be put in its proper place. He maintained the importance of God's injunction in Genesis. This was in spite of agreeing that his wife should now take some form of contraception. His wife, in a separate interview, explained how she had felt no control over the conception of any of their seven children, but would now refuse to have any more. After the seventh child, she had persuaded her husband that they should have no more children because of the economic burden of the children they already had.

For some men, awareness of the prevalence of HIV demanded another kind of courage. Raymond argued:

> It takes courage to have sex with women when you know there is so much AIDS around. Everyone knows that there is AIDS, even the ladies themselves. You are there. You start the game and nobody is even talking about condoms. You need courage—these risks! I know guys who even know that the husband of this lady died of AIDS, but they are still going there and making love—with or without a condom, I don't know, I am not there—but maybe without a condom, "going direct."

At age forty, Hambayi looked back on his youthful sexual encounters and described them as signs of immaturity—"rubbish behavior." He spoke of some of his more successful former schoolmates who, partly because of the "excitement" of money, he judged, engaged in extramarital sex:

> They know the danger. I don't understand why they behave that way. I don't know where they draw that courage from because a normal person would not risk their lives. I don't just know where they draw their courage from. . . . I say it is courage for them to do it because they know the danger already. There is no better word. I feel it is courage. I would say *buyumu yumu* in Tonga. It is courage. When I see the traffic light telling me to stop and I have seen the cops, but I don't want to stop, I must have the courage. What would you call that?

Others commenting on the behavior of their male friends questioned what this "courage" really amounted to. They also knew, as I did, certain men who, unaware of their own status, knowingly engaged in sexual activity with women for whom they judged there was a high probability that they were HIV positive. Some men had told me how "prostitutes" had at times discouraged them from having sex with them by warning them that they were already "dead" women. Men also observed that unprotected sex was not always a sign of "courage" or the result of the influence of alcohol, but at times rather the consequence of anger or despair. Roger explained an episode of unprotected sex after a quarrel with his regular girlfriend:

> She came to see me and, well, we had a big row [quarrel or argument] about something and she left. I was depressed and I just went over to this girl, because I had also been going out with her for a while.

I thought, "Well, let me just go and have a nice time with her," and I think, well, I didn't care then. I just thought, "Well, fine, she's stormed off. That's probably the end of it!" I just didn't care, and I think that's what caught me off guard. So when she got pregnant, I looked back. I could well remember the incident related to that time and I accepted that I was the one responsible.

Conclusion

The sheer scale of the human tragedy unfolding in southern Africa entails taking certain risks in the exploration of links between constructions of masculinity and men's sexual conduct. Concerns may be temporarily pushed into the background as anthropologists engage in efforts to restrict the spread of HIV infection. However, if all representation risks the accusation of being pornography (Kappeler 1986), then investigations into sexuality run a particular risk. It is also crucial to avoid the danger of constructing an "African sexuality," in opposition to some supposed "white" or "European" sexuality. Colonial and postcolonial fantasies of black men's hypersexuality may be perpetuated, and prevailing contests among at least some Zambian men about the meaning of manhood may be screened from view. Involving men may well entail targeting them directly and indeed confronting them about the hegemony of their masculine definitions of sexual behavior (Baylies and Bujra 2000), though this may risk having anthropological research in AIDS prevention efforts becoming merely another form of social control (Clatts 1994).

What has become generally recognized is that the communication of Western biomedical "knowledge" alone will not achieve the aim of curtailing the spread of HIV/AIDS. More needs to be learned about the contexts in which the transmission of HIV takes place and in which health messages are constructed, transmitted, and received (see Heald 2002). Ethnographic data, such as that described in this chapter, can facilitate AIDS prevention efforts by offering local knowledge about the meanings of manhood and their role in the spread of HIV. Research among Zambian men reveals the fragility of their sense of manhood, something that is to be achieved in their performance of masculinity within both public and intimate spheres. Indeed, in both spheres, masculinity may best be seen as a fragile entity, constantly to be reclaimed in its performance.

In 2002, Zambians were fed a daily diet in the news media of mostly depressing statistics and news concerning HIV/AIDS. In urban areas, many witnessed the AIDS "industry" at firsthand and found it hard not to come to some cynical conclusions. This was especially so because of their feelings of powerlessness to access adequate medical help for their family members and, in some instances, for themselves, because of the exorbitant cost of antiretroviral therapy. They needed courage to face the everyday reality of those around them—at home, in the neighborhood, and at work—suffering from AIDS-related conditions. The general perception was that the AIDS crisis was deepening, not getting better, and this led many men and women to conclude that condoms did not safeguard against HIV infection, a deduction officially supported by such bodies as the Catholic church. Added to such suspicions about condoms was the perception among many men that condoms threatened the performance of their manhood in sexual encounters and thereby their achievement of a reassuringly "masculine" identity.

Notes

1. The 2002 research, entitled "Men and Masculinities in the Fight Against HIV/AIDS in Zambia" (R00023493), was funded by the Economic and Social Science Research Council, United Kingdom. Participant observation in Zambian households was augmented by the collection of life history material in interviews. Interviews, conducted mostly in English but also in Bemba, Nyanja, and Tonga, were taped with the interviewees' permission. Anonymity was assured, and I have used pseudonyms at all times throughout this chapter. I am grateful to two local assistants, Dixter Kaluba and Chitalu Mumba, for their assistance in interviewing school contemporaries of the original cohort and wives of former students, and for their insightful discussion of the data. I would also like to thank Jeanette Edwards, Suzette Heald, and David Mills for their comments on an earlier draft of this chapter.

2. The research builds upon work on the concept of manhood in East Africa (Heald 1998, 1999) and explorations of masculinity in Africa (Morrell 1998, 2001; Setel 1999). I draw upon the findings from work conducted in Zambia and Tanzania by Baylies and Bujra (2000) that identified harmful ideologies of masculinity that made men vectors of HIV infection, and by Holland and colleagues (1998) in the United Kingdom that described how heterosexuality systematically privileged forms of masculinity that contributed to sexual risk taking and the instability of safer sexual practices among young men and women. The present focus on men is not to deny the importance of studies that have rightly argued for the need to put women at the center of analysis since they bear the brunt of the multifaceted consequences of the pandemic. Both men and women are at risk, and women are in need of empowerment because of men's violence (Rude 1999) and women's inability to negotiate condom use (Wallman and Bantebya-Kyomuhendo 1996). Many studies have described women's vulnerability to HIV along a number of dimensions, among them biological, economic, social, and cultural. What is perhaps less self-evident in view of the real power exercised by many men in everyday

life in Zambian society is the vulnerability of men, because of the demands placed upon them of particular constructions of masculinity.

3. The rate of exchange fluctuated during 2002, but averaged about 4,500 kwacha to the U.S. dollar.

4. "Chop" was used with the meaning of "to cut with an ax," but it was also used to mean to eat, to consume. In the latter usage, there are numerous parallels with associations between sexual intercourse and eating in Africa and elsewhere.

5. The term "monk" was also used by male undergraduates at the University of Zambia to describe a man who did not have a girlfriend, in contrast to a "mojo," who did.

References Cited

Baylies, Carolyn, and Janet Bujra. 2000. *AIDS, Sexuality and Gender in Africa*. London: Routledge.

Clatts, Michael C. 1994. "All the Kings Horses and All the King's Men: Some Personal Reflections on Ten Years of AIDS Ethnography." *Human Organization* 53 (1): 93–95.

Colson, Elizabeth. 1958. *Marriage and the Family among the Plateau Tonga of Northern Rhodesia*. Manchester: Manchester University Press.

Connell, Robert W. 2001. *The Men and the Boys*. Cambridge: Polity Press.

Epstein, Arnold L. 1981. *Urbanisation and Kinship: The Domestic Domain on the Copperbelt of Zambia 1950–1956*. London: New Academic Press.

Feldman, Douglas A., Peggy O'Hara, K. S. Baboo, Ndashi W. Chitalu, and Ying Lu. 1997. "HIV Prevention among Zambian Adolescents: Developing a Value Utilization/Norm Change Model." *Social Science and Medicine* 44 (4): 4455–4468.

Ferguson, James. 1999. *Expectations of Modernity*. Berkeley: University of California Press.

Forster, Peter G. 2001. "AIDS in Malawi: Contemporary Discourse and Cultural Continuities." *African Studies* 60 (2): 245–261.

Hansen, Karen. 1996. *Keeping House in Lusaka*. New York: Columbia University Press.

Heald, Suzette. 1998 (1989). *Controlling Anger: The Anthropology of Gisu Violence*. London: James Currey.

———. 1999. *Manhood and Morality: Sex, Violence and Ritual in Gisu Society*. London: Routledge.

———. 2002. "It's Never as Easy as ABC: Understandings of AIDS in Botswana." *African Journal of AIDS Research* 1 (2002): 1–10.

Holland, Janet, Caroline Ramazanoglu, Sue Sharpe, and Rachel Thomson. 1998. *The Male in the Head: Young People, Heterosexuality and Power*. London: Tuffnell Press.

Jacobsen-Widding, Anita. 2000. *Chapungu: The Bird that Never Drops a Feather, Male and Female Identities in an African Society*. Uppsala: Uppsala University.

Kappeler, Susanne. 1986. *The Pornography of Representation*. Oxford: Polity Press.

Mane, Purnima, and Peter Aggleton. 2000. "Cross-National Perspectives on Gender and Power." In *Framing the Sexual Subject: The Politics of Gender, Sexuality and*

Power, ed. Richard Parker, Regina M. Barbosa, and Peter Aggleton, 104–116. Berkeley: University of California Press.

Moore, Henrietta, and Megan Vaughan. 1994. *Cutting Down Trees: Gender, Nutrition and Agricultural Change in the Northern Province of Zambia, 1890–1990*. Portsmouth, N.H.: Heinemann.

Morrell, Robert, ed. 1998. "Special Issue on Masculinities in Southern Africa." *Journal of Southern African Studies* 24 (4).

———. 2001. *Changing Men in Southern Africa*. London: Zed Books.

Powdermaker, Hortense. 1960. *Coppertown: Changing Africa, the Human Situation on the Rhodesian Copperbelt*. New York: Harper and Row.

Richards, Audrey. 1939. *Land, Labour, and Diet in Northern Rhodesia: An Economic Study of the Bemba Tribe*. London: Oxford University Press.

———. 1940. "Bemba Marriage and Present Economic Conditions." Rhodes-Livingstone Institute Paper No. 4, Livingstone, Zambia.

———. 1982 (1956). *Chisungu: A Girl's Initiation Ceremony among the Bemba of Zambia*. London: Tavistock.

Rude, Darlene. 1999. "Reasonable Men and Provocative Women: An Analysis of Gendered Domestic Homicide in Zambia." *Journal of Southern African Studies* 25 (1): 7–27.

Setel, Philip W. 1999. *A Plague of Paradoxes: AIDS, Culture, and Demography in Northern Tanzania*. Chicago: University of Chicago Press.

Simpson, Anthony. 2002. *The Measure of a Man*. A report for Save the Children, Sweden. www.rb.se/bookshop.

———. 2003. *Half-London in Zambia: Contested Identities in a Catholic Mission School*. Edinburgh: Edinburgh University Press for the International African Institute.

Stoltenberg, John. 2000. *Refusing to Be a Man: Essays on Sex and Justice*. Rev. ed. London: UCL Press.

Wallman, Sandra, with Grace Bantebya-Kyomuhendo. 1996. *Kampala Women Getting By: Wellbeing in the Time of AIDS*. Athens: Ohio University Press.

8

Attitudes toward HIV/AIDS among Zambian High School Students

DOUGLAS A. FELDMAN, NDASHI W. CHITALU,
PEGGY O'HARA MURDOCK, GANAPATI BHAT,
ORLANDO GÓMEZ-MARÍN, JEFFREY JOHNSON,
KASONDE MWINGA, AND K. SRIDUTT BABOO

Introduction

It might be expected that when a stigmatized disease becomes endemic in a particular society, the social stigma toward people with that disease would decline. But this has not been the case throughout much of sub-Saharan Africa, where a quarter-century after the visible emergence of AIDS, stigma toward and discrimination against persons living with HIV remain strong. In Zambia today, mean life expectancy has dropped from a high of fifty-two years in 1980 to thirty-seven years in 2005. One-sixth of all adults (16.5 percent) in the nation are HIV positive (World Food Programme 2005), a fact that the Zambian government during the 1980s and early 1990s was very reluctant to accept (Moszynski 1999). There are about one million persons living with HIV/AIDS and an estimated 89,000 deaths from HIV/AIDS each year in the country (*World Factbook* 2005).

Hundreds of thousands of children have become orphaned by parents who died from AIDS. An estimated 15.1 percent of all children under the age of fifteen in Zambia are orphans (Kaimana 2005). Recent declines in infant and child mortality rates have been reversed due to AIDS in parts of Africa. Zambia's infant mortality rate increased 30 percent from the beginning of the AIDS epidemic to 1996, and is projected to double by 2010 (Foster 1998). Chronic childhood malnutrition is pervasive, while infant mortality rates are high at 88.3 deaths per 1,000 live births (*World Factbook* 2005). In the early years of the epidemic, wealthy and middle-class Zambians were more likely to become HIV infected than poor Zambians. However, as the disease has spread into all segments of Zambian society, into the shanty compounds of urban Zambia and into the rural villages, poverty has significantly exacerbated the spread and impact of HIV. Poverty caused by having AIDS among survivors leads to a worsening of children's health, as well as increased vulnerability of adolescent survivors to HIV infection (Foster 1998).

Nevertheless, the disease continues to have an impact on those who have specialized professional training in key sectors of the Zambian economy, such as banking, teaching, and management. While many companies in urban Zambia insist on preemployment medical examinations, often including HIV testing, few have developed policies relating to their mandatory test results (Baggaley et al. 1995).

The AIDS epidemic has become an ever-present reality for Zambians. And yet AIDS is rarely discussed. While social conditions are beginning to change with the advent of antiretroviral medications (ARVs), relatively few Zambians still have ever been tested for HIV, as of 2005. Most HIV-infected Zambians remain unaware of their serostatus, unless they have begun to develop end-stage symptoms. When death arrives, the true nature of their illness is infrequently discussed openly by family members. Obituaries and death notices in Zambian newspapers very rarely mention the cause of death if it is HIV related. When AIDS is discussed, it is often talked about within a moralistic, fundamentalist religious framework.

Zambia has been singled out as one of twelve African nations that will receive significant funding from the United States through the President's Emergency Plan for AIDS Relief (PEPFAR). The U.S. $15 billion dollar plan during 2004–2008 will include testing and ARV treatment, HIV prevention (with a strong emphasis on abstinence), and AIDS care (especially for "vulnerable children"). However, PEPFAR had provided ARV treatment for only 22,000 Zambians by March 2005 (PEPFAR 2005). Social stigma is an important factor that has prevented many Zambians from seeking HIV testing and free ARV treatment (Banda 2005; Zambia News Agency 2005a, 2005b).

This chapter describes the attitudes toward HIV/AIDS and people living with HIV/AIDS among 204 male and female public high school students in Lusaka, Zambia. It is part of a larger intervention study carried out by the authors to assess the usefulness of a particular approach in decreasing risky sexual behaviors among sexually active Zambian high school students. The study was carried out from 1997 to 2000, before ARV therapy was introduced in 2004, along with a variety of other PEPFAR-funded programs.

The Zambian Social Setting

Zambia is a nation that has undergone major social transformations during the twentieth century. There are seventy-three tribes or ethnic groups in the nine provinces of Zambia. The major ethnolinguistic groups are the Bemba, Nyanja, Tonga, Lozi, Nsenga, Chewa, Tumbuka, Ngoni, Kaonde, Lunda, and Luvale (Burdette 1988; Hakkert and Wieringa 1986; Siatwinda 1984). Today, English is the language used in the media, schools, and government. Other languages are widely spoken, however, especially Bemba in the north, Nyanja in Lusaka (the capital and largest city) and the east, and Lozi in Livingstone and the west. Social stratification has been rendered quite complex with the advent of sharp class distinctions (especially in the urban areas), of increased regional identification (for example, westerners, northerners), of the presence of other non-Zambian Africans (including in the 1990s an influx of refugees from Zaire, Angola, and Mozambique, and in the early 2000s an intensification of new refugees from Angola and the Democratic Republic of the Congo) and non-Africans in Zambia (especially Asian Indians and British expatriates), and of massive migration patterns that have destabilized tribal residence patterns. Most (86 percent) Zambians live below the poverty line, while the tenth of those households with the highest incomes earn twenty-one times the income of the tenth of those households with the lowest income (*World Factbook* 2005).

Ethnographic research in Zambia has included several important studies. Colson's (1949, 1958, 1974, 1991) body of work on the Tonga, Turner's (1957, 1967) research on the Ndembu, Richards's (1939, 1956) work on the Bemba, and Gluckman's (1955) study of the Lozi have all become classics in the anthropological literature. However, the ethnographic record is uneven, in that there is superb data on some tribes, but poor or little data on others. In recent years, there has been an increase of excellent urban ethnographies in Zambia, including Hansen's (1989) study of Zambian inequality in the workplace, Hansen's (1996) study of housework in Lusaka, and Schuster's (1979) study of professional women in Lusaka.

The extended family and the clan have traditionally been central to Zambian social life. Matrilineal descent has been common in southern Zambia (Colson 1958), while patrilineal descent has been common throughout most of the rest of Zambia. Today, the extended family is still important, although transformed in certain ways. The values placed on strong obligations to kin are maintained despite the breakup of the large coresidential households of relatives, characteristic of the extended family in the rural areas (Burdette 1988). Bridewealth, traditionally a payment to the bride's father uniting the two families together and serving as a means of compensation for the loss of her labor power, continues in modern Zambia, even among persons belonging to tribes that formerly did not emphasize the practice (Epstein 1981; Schuster 1979). Transient marriages and the absence of government assistance ensure the survival of blood kin ties as the major form of social and economic support for both groups.

Polygyny, or having and supporting two or more co-wives, in traditional Zambia was common and widely preferred. Today, the practice is increasingly less frequent, occurring among 18 percent of Zambian married women (Gaisie et al. 1993), especially in rural areas. But the common pattern of married men having a mistress or paying sex workers may serve a similar sociological function (Schuster 1979). A husband and his co-wives in a polygynous household where they are all HIV negative, and where sexual activity stays within that household, are not at greater risk for HIV than a monogamous and faithful couple who are HIV negative. However, in a marital relationship with a rotating mistress or access by the husband to sex workers who do not routinely use condoms, there is a high risk for HIV infection.

Many women in urban Zambia have found it necessary to take marginal positions as traders (Schuster 1982). Squatter settlements have developed throughout urban Zambia. Residents in these settlements are continually threatened with eviction, receive no government services, and live in a habitat with no basic infrastructure (Mulwanda 1989).

Zambia's population increased from 2.6 million in 1950 to an estimated 11.3 million in 2005 (GeoHive 2003; *World Factbook* 2005). The rate of population increase has slowed to 2.12 percent each year (*World Factbook* 2005) because of the increased mortality rate and decreased fertility rate brought about by the AIDS epidemic, and it is likely (based upon prior projections) that there would have been about a million more Zambians by 2005 if AIDS had never occurred. While seroprevalence data are conflicting, varying substantially between antenatal clinic studies and population-based studies (WHO/UNAIDS 2003), one study indicates alarmingly high HIV rates among Zambian adolescents, with older female adolescents (eighteen to nineteen years old) at 22.6 percent, younger female adolescents (fifteen to seventeen years old) at 12.3 percent, and male adolescents (fifteen to nineteen years old) at 4.5 percent (Fylkesnes et al. 1998).

Sexually transmitted diseases (STDs) represent the third most common cause of adult outpatient attendance, with an estimated 300,000 new cases per year. Other common diseases reported to the Zambian Ministry of

Health are malaria, diarrhea, and respiratory infections, including tuberculosis. The AIDS crisis has had a devastating effect upon Zambia's health
care, economic factors, and social infrastructure (Foster 1998; Mutangadura et al. 1998; Timaeus 1998). The number of children surviving on their
own in the streets of Lusaka continues to grow (Baggaley and Needham
1997; Daley 1998; Hastings 1999). Indeed, the HIV epidemic "is having a
devastating impact on Zambia's children who are being robbed of guidance,
emotional nurturing and development and are often left alone to fend for
themselves on the streets" (World Food Programme 2005: 1).

There have been a number of studies conducted among Zambian adolescents focusing on their sexual behavior. Pillai and Barton (1999) found
in a study of 390 females at seven schools that their inability to say "no" to
their boyfriends was associated, as might be expected, with sexual activity. In a study of urban Zambian youth, Kalunde (1997) found that sexual
matters are discussed with close friends of the same sex and peer group, as
with cousins who are of the same age. Grandmothers, but never parents,
sometimes discuss sex with their granddaughters. Many young women do
not regard AIDS as a threat to their lives, and do not even consider it as a
hindrance to sexual relationships. Other STDs are taken even more lightly,
since they are seen as curable.

However, the fear of pregnancy is very real for many sexually active female adolescents (Webb 2000). An estimated two-thirds of unwanted pregnancies end in unsafe abortions. Factors that lead to an abortion are the
boyfriend's unwillingness to accept paternity or assist financially, the stigma
attached to premarital pregnancy, and the desire to stay in school. Webb
(2000) found that about 40 percent of young women who would obtain an
abortion would carry it out either by themselves or with the help of other
nonmedical friends. The most popular methods of abortion are overdosing
on chloroquine, taking traditional herbal medicines, or ingesting washing
powder. In a community-based study in Western Province, Zambia, it was
learned that more than half of the abortion-related deaths were of schoolgirls (Koster-Oyekan 1998). Although abortion is legal in Zambia, most
women resort to illegal abortions since legal abortion services are widely
unacceptable and inaccessible.

Many young women in Zambia engage in "dry sex." In a study of 329
women at an STD clinic in Lusaka, 50 percent had engaged in at least one
dry sex practice (Sandala et al. 1995). The most common practices were
drinking a kind of porridge used to dry and tighten the vagina, removing
vaginal secretions with a cloth, and placing leaves in the vagina to clean it.
Though 10 percent reported swelling or peeling of the vagina when using

a cloth or leaves, there was surprisingly no association between dry sex and increased HIV seropositivity among these women. In a study of a rural community, 73 percent of 312 women reported practicing dry sex, while 40 percent of them did experience vaginal soreness from dry sex (Ashworth 1998).

Some Zambian females at puberty during ritual initiation engage in the practice of elongating their genitalia by manually stretching it, so that it will curl around and grasp the male's penis during intercourse (Feldman et al. 1997). It is not yet known whether this practice is associated with increased risk for HIV among these women or their male partners.

Condom use during the early and mid-1990s was at best usually inconsistent in Zambia, and used more for pregnancy control than HIV/STD control. In rural Zambia especially, condom use is usually only negotiated within some short-term relationships and then not at all consistently (Bond and Dover 1997). Since Zambian women, with very few exceptions, are economically and ideologically dependent on men, they are in a much weaker position to negotiate condom use. In Zambia during the late 1990s and early 2000s, there has been an increase in condom use and a decline in multipartnering among the middle class, elite, urban, and young, but no or little change among the majority of the population who are poor, those who are married couples, and rural Zambians (Agha 2002; Fylkesnes et al. 2001; Slonim-Nevo and Mukuka 2005).

There have been a very limited number of research studies conducted within Zambia that attempted to reduce HIV risk. HIV prevention programs in Zambia have generally suffered from insufficient financial resources, lack of management and organizational skills, the inability to monitor and evaluate program performance, difficulty in generating income, and often lack of culturally appropriate counseling (Leonard et al. 1996). Agha and Van Rossem (2004) conducted an intervention in Zambian high schools with 416 students and found that students at these schools decreased their number of partners, but did not increase condom use. Preliminary data from our study indicates nearly identical findings (Feldman 2000).

Yoder and colleagues (1996) evaluated a radio drama broadcast about AIDS during nine months. At the end of the broadcast, the local population had increased their knowledge about HIV/AIDS, and some reported reducing risky behaviors, though it could not be determined if this was a direct result of the broadcast. Kathuria and colleagues (1998) conducted a community peer education project in three residential areas of Lusaka to reduce HIV and STD transmission. The project included training peer educators, community outreach, community meetings, and condom distribution. Syphilis seropositivity fell at the three sites from a range of 17.4 to 47 percent to a range of 7.3 to 10 percent. There was not a corresponding decline of syphilis in other residential areas of Lusaka.

Kiremire and Luo (1996) evaluated a program directly involving almost 700 former female sex workers in Lusaka, which included AIDS education, condom distribution, counseling, and alternative skills development (such as tailoring, hairdressing, catering, and several other skills that are alternatives to sex work). The program was evidently successful in leading hundreds of sex workers out of their occupation. Nyamuryekung'e and colleagues (1997) conducted an intervention study along the Tanzania-Zambia highway, targeting 1,330 women at seven truck stops. The study, which included providing HIV/STD information, condoms, and drugs for treating STDs, was successful and cost-effective in treating STDs and lowering the risk for HIV. Chiboola and colleagues (1994) evaluated the role of including persons living with AIDS in community-based HIV prevention. They found that persons living with AIDS play a leading role in the process of destigmatization of AIDS at the community level.

Methods and Demographic Considerations

A three-year HIV prevention intervention study was conducted by the authors between September 1997 and August 2000 at an experimental and control public high school in Lusaka, Zambia, to learn how to effectively promote HIV risk reduction among male and female older adolescents (fifteen to twenty years old) in a peer-led workshop setting. An ethnographically informed approach, called the value utilization/norm change, or VUNC, model (developed by the first author), was used that emphasized the cultural values of the students, while challenging some of the norms, attitudes, and beliefs that may impede behavioral change (Feldman 1999; Feldman et al. 1999). The study proved successful in significantly reducing HIV risk among the sexually active experimental students, compared with the sexually active control participants (Feldman 2000).

As part of the overall study, fifteen questions on the lengthy (406-item) baseline written survey were asked of the students about their attitudes toward HIV/AIDS. A total of 204 students (91 in the experimental school and 113 in the control school), including 101 females and 103 males, participated in the baseline survey during September 1998. The study was nonrandom, since it was necessary to recruit more sexually active participants into the study in order to test the hypothesis predicting reduction of HIV risk. A prior screening survey administered in May 1998 to nearly all of the tenth and eleventh grade students at the two schools (n = 1,156) indicated that while most of the males (55 percent) self-reported being sexually active at least once, only 30 percent of the females self-reported being sexually active at least once. For the baseline survey and intervention, selective recruiting increased the proportion of males who had been sexually active at least once to 66 percent and the proportion of females who had been sexually active at least once to 58 percent. A large minority of sexually abstinent students were intentionally included in the baseline survey and intervention, so that participants would not feel stigmatized by nonparticipants within their school as sexually "promiscuous."

Students were recruited from the tenth and eleventh grades only, since many ninth graders are excluded from completing their high school education because they fail a rigorous examination given during their ninth grade, and we needed to follow the control students for more than one year. Also, twelfth graders were excluded from our study, since they would be leaving the school at the end of the year.

Public high school students in Lusaka are by no means representative of older adolescents throughout Zambia. More than half of the Zambian population (57 percent) is rural, living in small towns, villages, and hamlets, and few older adolescents living in rural areas have access to television, radio, telephones, newspapers, or cars that are found more commonly in Lusaka and other major cities. Even within Lusaka, most Zambian youth do not attend high school. Indeed, the mean number of years of education for adolescents not attending high school in a Lusaka sample of out-of-school youth (n = 138) is 7.4 for males and 5.2 for females (Feldman et al. 1997). Public high school is seen as a privilege, and mostly the sons and daughters of the small middle class and some of the wealthy attend. Children of very wealthy Zambians, expatriate whites, and some wealthy Asian Indians are more likely to attend private schools in Zambia. Three indicators of wealth in Zambia are family ownership of a car, a television set, and a refrigerator. In Zambia, passenger cars are owned by 1.5 per 100 population, television sets are owned by 3.2 per 100 population, and refrigerators are similarly uncommon. However, 31.5 percent of the students in our study lived in a household with a car, 92.6 percent lived in a household with a television set, and 68.1 percent lived in a household with a refrigerator. Nevertheless, some students from poor families also attend, especially if they are male, have shown promise in the lower grades, have excelled on the entry test for high school, and the family is prepared to make the financial sacrifice (for example, for school fees, books, uniform) necessary to send one of their children to a public high school. Overall, about twice as many males as females attend public high school.

The baseline survey was in English. While most students speak Nyanja or Bemba at home, instruction and discussion at the public high schools are in English, and all students were fluent in speaking, reading, and writing English. Participants read and signed a voluntary informed consent form approved by the Institutional Review Board (IRB) at the University of Miami before participating in the study, and parents of those students under eighteen years of age were also asked to read and sign a parental consent form before their child could participate in the study. The baseline survey was pretested with eight students.

The fifteen questions that asked about attitudes toward HIV/AIDS used a five-point Likert scale from "strongly disagree" (= 1) to "strongly agree" (= 5) and are listed in table 8.1. The selection and wording of these fifteen questions were developed from focus groups, short-term ethnography, and social network semistructured interviews conducted during the one-year formative research period prior to the baseline survey. These questions or their antitheses reflect statements or themes that were heard from at least some informants during our qualitative research. The wording also reflected terminology used by the students: "homosexuals" rather than "gays," "prostitutes" rather than "sex workers," "AIDS virus" rather than "HIV," "fornication" rather than "premarital sex," "adultery" rather than "extramarital sex," and "an evil sin" rather than "morally wrong."

Kaliondeonde is a local AIDS-like illness that is said to be less severe than AIDS and has been in Zambia and Malawi for generations (Feldman 1993; Feldman and Miller 1998). It is believed to be primarily transmitted by failing to use traditional medication after an abortion or miscarriage, or by having sex with a woman who fails to do so. In two focus groups among students, we had learned that some students believed that Kaliondeonde and AIDS are the same thing, while some believed that they are two separate diseases. Most adults in Zambia also are unclear about the relationship between Kaliondeonde and AIDS, with many believing they are identical. Data from our preliminary research conducted in 1999 indicates that some of the diagnosed Kaliondeonde patients we tested were not HIV positive as we had expected, suggesting that the disease is indeed a unique entity caused by an unknown pathogen.

Statistix was used to perform all statistical analyses. Overall and group-specific mean scores and standard deviations were calculated for each of the fifteen items. Due to the ordinal nature of the data, the Mann-Whitney test was used to assess the significance of differences based upon sex

Table 8.1. Attitudes Toward HIV/AIDS

	Strongly disagree	Disagree	Not sure, mixed opinion	Agree	Strongly agree
Most people with AIDS deserve to die.	84	61	12	29	18
I think people with AIDS should receive compassion and assistance.	1	2	3	77	121
The government should ignore the needs of persons with AIDS.	135	50	10	4	5
In Zambia, male homosexuals are the major cause of the widespread transmission of the AIDS virus.	40	65	83	10	5
People with AIDS should be locked up permanently so they cannot infect others.	91	72	18	13	10
There are many other health problems in Zambia that are much more important than AIDS.	19	54	66	50	14
Prostitutes should all be killed so that they do not infect others with AIDS.	65	104	16	7	12
Homosexuality is perfectly natural and normal, and it should be fully accepted by society.	114	46	18	17	9
Most of the time, condoms don't work in preventing AIDS.	17	36	48	61	42
AIDS orphans should take care of themselves.	109	58	5	16	16
If I learned that someone I know has AIDS, I would avoid coming anywhere near that person.	110	78	9	2	5
Masturbation is an evil sin.	16	21	57	59	50
Fornication is an evil sin.	11	13	32	65	83
Adultery is an evil sin.	13	6	5	64	114
Kaliondeonde and AIDS are the same thing.	20	29	102	32	21

(males versus females), religiousness (very religious versus somewhat religious), and age (fifteen to seventeen versus eighteen to twenty). Similarly, the Kruskal-Wallis test was used to assess differences between more than two groups such as, for example, major tribes (Bemba, Chewa, Lozi, Ngoni, Nsenga, Tonga, and Tumbuka). "Tribe" is the preferred term in Zambia, while "ethnic group" or "ethnicity" is preferred in many other African nations, especially in West Africa.

Results

There was a general consensus among the students that, in principle, people should be compassionate for persons living with HIV/AIDS in Zambia. Nearly all of the students agreed with the statement, "I think people with AIDS should receive compassion and assistance" (mean ± SD = 4.54 ± 0.63). Only 3 (1.5 percent) of the 204 students disagreed or strongly disagreed, and only 3 (1.5 percent) were not sure or had a mixed opinion (see table 8.1). Nearly all disagreed with the statement, "The government should ignore the needs of persons with AIDS" (mean ± SD = 1.50 ± 0.87). Only 9 agreed or strongly agreed (4.5 percent), and 10 (4.9 percent) were not sure.

Students were also aware that HIV/AIDS was very commonplace, and that mere physical proximity to a person infected with HIV was not a danger. Nearly all disagreed with the statement, "If I learned that someone I know has AIDS, I would avoid coming anywhere near that person" (mean ± SD = 1.60 ± 0.83). Only seven agreed or strongly agreed (3.5 percent), and nine (4.4 percent) were not sure.

However, there was less consensus when students were asked to make moral judgments about persons with AIDS. While most disagreed with the statement, "Most people with AIDS deserve to die" (mean ± SD = 2.20 ± 1.34), a sizable minority did not disagree. Forty-seven agreed or strongly agreed with the statement (23.0 percent), and twelve (5.9 percent) were not sure. Also, not everyone was prepared to rule out quarantine camps to stop the spread of AIDS. Most disagreed with the statement, "People with AIDS should be locked up permanently so they cannot infect others" (mean ± SD = 1.92 ± 1.11). Yet twenty-three students agreed or strongly agreed with this statement (11.3 percent), and eighteen (8.8 percent) were not sure.

Furthermore, not all students were sympathetic toward sex workers. Most disagreed with the statement, "Prostitutes should all be killed so that they do not infect others with AIDS" (mean ± SD = 2.00 ± 1.03). But nineteen students agreed or strongly agreed with this statement (9.3 percent), and sixteen (7.8 percent) were not sure. Males (mean ± SD = 1.85 ± 0.98) were more likely to strongly disagree than females (mean ± SD = 2.17 ± 1.06, p = 0.008).

Not all students were compassionate toward AIDS orphans in Zambia. Most disagreed with the statement, "AIDS orphans should take care of themselves" (mean ± SD = 1.88 ± 1.25). But thirty-two students agreed or strongly agreed (15.6 percent), and five (2.5 percent) were not sure.

About half of the students did not see AIDS as a health crisis in Zambia. Nearly as many agreed with the statement, "There are many other health problems in Zambia that are much more important than AIDS," as disagreed with that statement (overall mean ± SD = 2.93 ± 1.07). Sixty-four students (31.5 percent) agreed or strongly agreed, seventy-three (36.0 percent) disagreed or strongly disagreed, while sixty-six (32.5 percent) were not sure. Males were more likely to agree with the statement than females (3.13 ± 1.11 versus 2.73 ± 1.01, p = 0.01).

About half of the students did not think that condoms were effective in preventing AIDS. About as many agreed with the statement, "Most of the time, condoms don't work in preventing AIDS," as disagreed with that statement or were not sure (overall mean ± SD = 3.37 ± 1.23). One hundred three students (50.5 percent) agreed or strongly agreed, fifty-three (26.0 percent) disagreed or strongly disagreed, while forty-eight (23.5 percent) were not sure. Females were more likely to agree that condoms do not work than males (3.56 ± 1.34 versus 3.18 ± 1.09, p = 0.09). Ngoni students were more likely to disagree that condoms do not work than were members of the Bemba, Chewa, Lozi, Nsenga, Tonga, and Tumbuka tribes (2.65 ± 1.14 versus 3.46 ± 1.26, p = 0.006).

Many of the students were not sure what role gay and bisexual men play in HIV transmission (mean ± SD = 2.38 ± 0.94). Slightly more than half (n = 105, 51.7 percent) disagreed or strongly disagreed with the statement, "In Zambia, male homosexuals are the major cause of the widespread transmission of the AIDS virus," while only fifteen (7.4 percent) agreed or strongly agreed. But a sizable number of students (n = 83, 40.9 percent) were not sure or had a mixed opinion. Males were more likely to disagree than females (2.19 ± 0.95 versus 2.58 ± 0.89, p = 0.002). Older students (eighteen to twenty years old) were more likely to disagree than younger students (fifteen to seventeen years old) (2.28 ± 0.92 versus 2.56 ± 0.95, p = 0.028). Most of the students (n = 114, 55.9 percent), however, strongly disagreed with the statement, "Homosexuality is perfectly natural and normal, and it should be fully accepted by society" (overall mean ± SD = 1.83 ± 1.16). Only twenty-six (12.7 percent) agreed or strongly agreed, and eighteen (8.8 percent) were not sure or had a mixed opinion.

Students typically perceived masturbation, premarital sex, and extra-marital sex very negatively. A majority of the students agreed or strongly agreed with the statement, "Masturbation is an evil sin" (mean ± SD = 3.52 ± 1.20), though thirty-seven (18.2 percent) disagreed or strongly disagreed, and fifty-seven (28.1 percent) were not sure or had a mixed opinion. Very religious students were more likely to agree with the statement than less re-ligious students (3.73 ± 1.06 versus 3.25 ± 1.32, p = 0.009). Nsenga students were more likely to disagree with the statement than students from other tribes (2.50 ± 1.57 versus 3.59 ± 1.14, p = 0.013).

Most students agreed or strongly agreed with the statement, "Fornica-tion is an evil sin" (mean = 3.96 ± 1.14), though twenty-four (11.8 percent) disagreed or strongly disagreed, and thirty-two (15.7 percent) were not sure or had a mixed opinion. Younger students were more likely to agree than older students (4.17 ± 1.03 versus 3.84 ± 1.19, p = 0.044). Tumbuka students were more likely to agree than students from other tribes (4.56 ± 0.70 ver-sus 3.90 ± 1.16, p = 0.016). Similarly, most students strongly agreed with the statement, "Adultery is an evil sin" (mean ± SD = 4.29 ± 1.10), while only nineteen (9.4 percent) disagreed or strongly disagreed, and five (2.5 percent) were not sure or had a mixed opinion.

Exactly half of the students (n = 102, 50.0 percent) were not sure or had a mixed opinion about the statement, "Kaliondeonde and AIDS are the same thing" (overall mean ± SD = 3.02 ± 1.05). The other half were nearly evenly split between those who disagreed or strongly disagreed (n = 49, 24.0 per-cent), and those who agreed or strongly agreed (n = 53, 26.0 percent).

HIV Stigma

During focus groups and individual interviews, some students were quite candid about how they felt about persons with AIDS in Zambia. One stu-dent told us: "All AIDS 'victims' should be detained in hospitals. There is no need for them to be sent home, because once they are out of the hospital they are going to misbehave. . . . They shouldn't be allowed to marry. . . . [Two local discos] should be burned [down], because these are places where any-thing goes—drugs, 'prostitution,' alcohol, you name it. It's there! 'Prosti-tutes' should be rounded up and locked up in prisons." Another student went further, saying, "Since there is not yet a cure for AIDS, people with AIDS should be killed to reduce the spread of AIDS, or to stop the spread of AIDS."

People with HIV are often mistrusted. For example, one student asked, "There are some unscrupulous people with HIV who will do anything to infect others. They would go to the extent of putting the virus in ice blocks. Can you get HIV from taking that kind of ice block?"

In spite of the near invisibility of gay and bisexual men in Zambia, there is enormous antipathy toward them. One student said, "I wish scientists and researchers should do some research on those people because I think there is something wrong with them, as God created Adam and Eve." Another seventeen-year-old asked about same-sex relationships: "It is entirely wrong. God created man and woman to produce [children]. So how do people of the same sex produce their babies?" In discussing someone she knows who is gay, a nineteen-year-old female exclaimed, "He's a Christian man. He goes to church. But look at what he's doing, having a homosexual relationship! Isn't that a sin?"

During prior research among Zambian youth conducted in 1992–1994, it was learned that more than half (52.5 percent) of our sample of 276 adolescents believed that AIDS is a punishment from God (Feldman et al. 1997). While Zambian youth live in a social environment where the tragedy of HIV/AIDS is omnipresent, moral judgments are often made condemning those who become sick, sex workers are despised, gay men are vilified, and God is ever wrathful. However, this worldview should not be unexpected. They live, at least at the time of the study, in a world where the schools had no formal curriculum about HIV/AIDS, the media rarely attempted to reduce stigma toward persons with HIV/AIDS, the governmental leadership was mostly silent about the epidemic, and the fundamentalist churches were moralistic against those who "sinned."

Discussion

While most students expressed compassion for persons living with AIDS, many did not. Some believed that people living with AIDS deserve to die, female sex workers should be killed so that they do not infect others, AIDS orphans should take care of themselves, and people living with AIDS should be locked up permanently. Most students have a family member or relative who has died of AIDS. Funerals are commonplace, and most of the hospital beds are taken by AIDS patients. It is, therefore, surprising that the social stigma against AIDS remains so strong within Zambian society. Clearly, while the strong societal norms against premarital and extramarital sex have not substantially changed the sexual behavior of many, if not most, Zambians, the prevalence of AIDS has neither weakened those norms nor diminished the social stigma attached to those norms. Not even the orphaned children of parents who died of AIDS are exempt from the scorn of many of the students.

While it might be expected that less religious students would be more tolerant of female sex workers, the opposite occurs. The less religious students are more likely than the very religious students to believe that sex workers should all be killed so that they do not infect others. It is difficult to interpret this unexpected pattern, other than to surmise that very religious students are more likely to observe the biblical injunction not to kill. Males are more tolerant than females toward sex workers. It is possible that males see sex workers as potential sex partners, and humanize them to that extent, while female students see them as conduits of disease who infect their potential male partners.

While Zambia is a nation plagued by many infectious diseases, including tuberculosis, malaria, STDs, cholera outbreaks, and diarrheal diseases, it is surprising that about half of the students, especially the males, do not rank HIV/AIDS at or near the top of that list. By minimizing the importance of HIV/AIDS in Zambia, many students view HIV/AIDS as affecting only an immoral "other," and make an effective intervention directed at these students more difficult.

The key to safer sex practices among students who remain sexually active is, of course, condom use. However, half of the students, especially the females who were less likely to self-report sexual activity, did not believe that condoms were effective in preventing HIV/AIDS. Focus groups conducted with students before our baseline interview clearly indicated a strong anti-condom bias among many of the students, and a pervasive belief that condoms do not work and that many condoms have holes intentionally put in them. The media, government, and religious leaders in Zambia emphasize that condoms "are not 100 percent effective" in preventing AIDS. When we asked the students during focus groups what percentage is correct, they estimated that condoms are between 50 and 75 percent effective. Research conducted on condom effectiveness, when used properly, indicates a much higher level of between 87 and 98 percent (Davis and Weller 1999; de Vincenzi 1994; Faundes et al. 1994; Hira et al. 1997; Pinkerton and Abramson 1997; Warner et al. 1998), and perhaps about 85 percent effective when typical human error is considered.

Ngoni students were more likely to believe that condoms are effective than were members of other tribes. A focus group of different Ngoni students was asked after the survey to explain why they thought Ngoni students would think this. There was no consensus among the students, but some thought that Ngoni students may be more sexually active, more acculturated in Western thought, or simply more likely to follow the instructions on the condom package.

At the time of the baseline survey, a small group of Zambian gay men and lesbians were attempting to start a gay rights group, named Legatra (Lesbian, Gay and Transgendered Association), in Lusaka. The government openly condemned the group, refused to legally register the fledgling organization, threatened to arrest anyone found to be homosexual, and threatened to deport any non-Zambians who would assist the organization. The government-controlled press ran page-one editorials and news stories attacking and condemning Legatra and homosexuality in general. Similar events occurred in Namibia and Uganda at about the same time (see Lorway's chapter in this volume).

It is within this political and social climate that the intervention occurred. In our study, it was verified through follow-up interviews that two male students and one female student engaged in same-sex sexual behavior. While it may be accurate to assume that about 6 percent or so of the adult male population globally, including Zambia, have a same-sex sexual orientation, the evidence has been clear since the mid-1980s that throughout sub-Saharan Africa, HIV is transmitted primarily through heterosexual transmission (Melbye et al. 1986; Quinn et al. 1986; van der Graaf and Diepersloot 1986). However, it is likely that unprotected sex between men is at least as risky for HIV as unprotected heterosexual sex in sub-Saharan Africa, and that males in Zambia who engage in same-sex behavior on a regular basis without condoms are at high risk for HIV. But, certainly, men who have sex with men (MSM) are not the major cause of HIV transmission in Zambia. The fact that so many of the students in our survey were unsure of this is indicative of widespread misinformation about HIV transmission, perhaps based in the pervasive homophobia in the nation and region. Very few students agreed with the view that homosexuality is natural and normal, and should be fully accepted by society. As expected, most students strongly disagreed with this view.

Religious fundamentalism, perhaps caused by a reaction against AIDS as well as economic and political influence from American-based missionary groups, has grown dramatically in Zambia during the 1990s. Behaviors such as homosexuality, masturbation, premarital sex, and extramarital sex are widely considered "evil" and "sinful." As expected, most students saw masturbation, premarital sex ("fornication"), and extramarital sex ("adultery") as "evil sins." Masturbation among adolescents in Zambia is not very common. In our baseline survey, forty males (40.4 percent) report never having masturbated during the previous five years, while sixty-seven females (67.7 percent) report never having masturbated during the previous five years. Very religious students (the majority of the students considered themselves to be very religious), as might be anticipated, were more likely to see masturbation as an "evil sin" than were less religious students. While Nsenga students were less likely to see masturbation in negative terms than were students from the other major tribes, a focus group of different Nsenga students held after the baseline survey was not able to discern a clear perspective for why this occurred.

Tumbuka students were more likely than students from other tribes to agree that premarital sex is wrong. A postsurvey focus group of Tumbuka students who did not take the survey explained this difference by saying that, traditionally, premarital sex has always been considered wrong, and the Tumbuka have maintained their cultural values. One female student said, "In our tradition it is not right to fornicate. When the girls reach puberty, they are not allowed to mix with boys. This is because as girls grow, they begin to develop feelings and they might want to experiment [with] things. So girls are taught to stay away from boys. They usually tell them fornication is not good because a girl might become pregnant . . . a taboo in our culture."

There is considerable confusion among the students on whether Kaliondeonde is the same thing as AIDS. Half of the students were not sure or had a mixed opinion. There is a need for research on Kaliondeonde to determine the etiology of the illness, the relationship—if any—to HIV-1, and the transmissibility of this AIDS-like disease, as well as an evaluation of the herbal treatments administered by traditional healers. Following this research, health education programs will be needed in Zambia, and in neighboring Malawi where Kaliondeonde is also reported, to clarify the distinction between the disease and HIV/AIDS. It is not clear from our data why the Tonga students in our survey were more likely to agree that Kaliondeonde and AIDS are the same, while Lozi students were less likely to agree.

Conclusion

The pervasiveness of AIDS in Zambia has not resulted, as might have been expected, in a destigmatization of the epidemic. In spite of the reality that HIV is omnipresent in the lives of the Zambian high school students, many distance themselves from it by seeing AIDS sufferers as the "other" and make strong moral judgments against those who are infected with the virus. While Zambian students continue to be influenced to some extent by their tribal cultural heritage, the rapid growth in Zambia of American-based fundamentalist religious doctrine has had a profound effect upon the lives of urban Zambians, especially during the 1990s. In order to bring about sustained change to lower HIV infection, it is not enough to provide accurate information about HIV/AIDS. It is equally important both to challenge their negative assumptions and attitudes against persons living with HIV/AIDS and to challenge their beliefs and norms that conflict with their basic values of good health, long life, family, and community.

Acknowledgments

An earlier version of this paper was presented at the Society for Applied Anthropology annual meeting. This study was funded by the National Science Foundation, SBR-97-10240. We wish to thank the generous assistance of the National Science Foundation; the government of Zambia; the Zambian Ministry of Health; the Zambian Ministry of Education; the administration, teachers, parents, and students of Kamwala High School and Libala High School; the Department of Paediatrics and Child Health at the University of Zambia School of Medicine; and our research assistants: Joe Tembo, Mwaka Choongo, and Martha Banda.

This chapter is dedicated to the memory of Dr. Ganapati Bhat, a co-investigator, who passed away during the writing of this chapter.

References Cited

Agha, S. 2002. "Declines in Casual Sex in Lusaka, Zambia: 1996–1999." *AIDS* 16 (2): 291–293.

Agha, S., and R. Van Rossem. 2004. "Impact of a School-Based Peer Sexual Health Intervention on Normative Beliefs, Risk Perceptions, and Sexual Behavior of Zambian Adolescents." *Journal of Adolescent Health* 34 (5): 441–452.

Ashworth, T. G. 1998. "Family Demography in a Remote Rural Community in Zambia." *Public Health* 112 (5): 313–316.

Baggaley, R. C., P. Godfrey-Fausse, R. Msiska, D. Chilangwa, E. Chitu, J. Porter, and M. Kelly. 1995. "How Have Zambian Businesses Reacted to the HIV Epidemic?" *Occupational and Environmental Medicine* 52 (9): 565–569.

Baggaley, R. C., and D. Needham. 1997. "Africa's Emerging AIDS-Orphan Crisis." *Canadian Medical Association Journal* 156 (6): 873–875.

Banda, P. 2005. "HIV/AIDS: No Need to Hide." *Zambia Daily Mail*, July 3.

Bond, V., and P. Dover. 1997. "Men, Women and the Trouble with Condoms: Problems Associated with Condom Use by Migrant Workers in Rural Zambia." *Health Transit Review* 7 (Supplement): 377–391.

Burdette, M. M. 1988. *Zambia: Between Two Worlds*. Boulder, Colo.: Westview Press.

Chiboola, H., W. Zulu, and M. K. Kelly. 1994. "Role of PLWAs." Paper presented at the International Conference on AIDS, Yokohama, Japan, August.

Colson, E. 1949. *Life among the Cattle-Owning Plateau Tonga: The Material Culture of a Northern Rhodesia Native Tribe*. Livingstone, Northern Rhodesia: Rhodes-Livingstone Museum.

———. 1958. *Marriage and the Family among the Plateau Tonga of Northern Rhodesia*. Manchester: Manchester University Press.

———. 1974. *Tradition and Contract: The Problem of Order*. Chicago: Aldine.

———. 1991. *The History of Nampeyo*. Lusaka, Zambia: Kenneth Kaunda Foundation.

Daley, S. 1998. "In Zambia, the Abandoned Generation." *New York Times*, September 18.

Davis, K. R., and S. C. Weller. 1999. "The Effectiveness of Condoms in Reducing Heterosexual Transmission of HIV." *Family Planning Perspective* 31 (6): 272–279.

de Vincenzi, I. 1994. "A Longitudinal Study of Human Immunodeficiency Virus Transmission by Heterosexual Partners: European Study Group on Heterosexual Transmission of HIV." *New England Journal of Medicine* 331 (6): 341–346.

Epstein, A. L. 1981. *Urbanization and Kinship: The Domestic Domain on the Copperbelt of Zambia 1950–1956*. New York: Academic Press.

Faundes, A., C. Elais, and C. Coggins. 1994. "Spermicides and Barrier Contraception." *Current Opinion in Obstetrics and Gynecology* 6 (6): 552–558.

Feldman, D. A. 1993. "Is It AIDS? Or Is It *Kaliondeonde*?" Paper presented at the American Anthropological Association, Washington, D.C., November.

———. 1999. "Using Ethnographic and Other Qualitative Data to Design an HIV Prevention Intervention in Zambia." Paper presented at the American Anthropological Association, Chicago, November.

———. 2000. "An HIV Prevention Intervention for Zambian High School Students." Presentation at the STD Behavioral Division, Centers for Disease Control and Prevention (CDC), Atlanta, August.

Feldman, D. A., N. W. Chitalu, P. O'Hara Murdock, O. Gomez-Marin, G. Bhat, K. Mwinga, and K. S. Baboo. 1999. "Understanding Normative Beliefs Which Are Impediments to Safer Sex Practices among Zambian Secondary School Students." Paper presented at the International Conference on AIDS in Africa, Lusaka, September.

Feldman, D. A., and J. Wang Miller, eds. 1998. *The AIDS Crisis: A Documentary History*. Westport, Conn.: Greenwood Press.

Feldman, D. A., P. O'Hara, K. S. Baboo, N. W. Chitalu, and Y Lu. 1997. "HIV Prevention among Zambian Adolescents: Developing a Value Utilization/Norm Change Model." *Social Science and Medicine* 44 (4): 455–468.

Foster, G. 1998. "Today's Children—Challenges to Child Health Promotion in Countries with Severe AIDS Epidemics." *AIDS Care* 10 (Supplement 1): S17–S23.

Fylkesnes, K., R. M. Musonda, M. Sichone, Z. Ndhlovu, F. Tembo, and M. Monze. 2001. "Declining HIV Prevalence and Risk Behaviours in Zambia: Evidence from Surveillance and Population-Based Surveys." *AIDS* 15 (7): 907–916.

Fylkesnes, K., Z. Ndhlovu, K. Kasumba, R. Mubanaga Musonda, and M. Sichone. 1998.

"Studying Dynamics of the HIV Epidemic: Population-Based Data Compared with Sentinel Surveillance in Zambia." *AIDS* 12 (10): 1227–1234.

Gaisie, K., A. R. Cross, and G. Nsemukila. 1993. *Zambia Demographic and Health Survey 1992*. Columbia, Md.: Macro International.

GeoHive. 2003. "Historic, Current and Future Population of Africa." http: //www.geo-hive.com/global/poplink.php?xml=idb&xsl=idb&parl=af, accessed October 16, 2003.

Gluckman, M. 1955. *The Judicial Process among the Barotse of Northern Rhodesia*. New York: Free Press.

Hakkert, R., and R. Wieringa. 1986. "The Republic of Zambia." *International Demographics* 5 (5): 1–9.

Hansen, K. T. 1989. *Distant Companions: Servants and Employers in Zambia, 1900–1985*. Ithaca, N.Y.: Cornell University Press.

———. 1996. *Keeping House in Lusaka*. New York: Columbia University Press.

Hastings, D. 1999. "Zambia's Lost Future." *A&U Magazine*, August, 42–45.

Hira, S. K., P. J. Feldblum, J. Kamanga, G. Mukelabai, S. S. Weir, and J. C. Thomas. 1997. "Condom and Nonoxynol-9 Use and the Incidence of HIV Infection in Serodiscordant Couples in Zambia." *Int J STD AIDS* 8 (4): 243–250. Change to: International Journal of STD and AIDS.

Kaimana, G. 2005. "Vulnerable Children Get Lifeline." *Times of Zambia*, July 3.

Kalunde, W. K. 1997. "HIV/AIDS and Sexual Behaviour among Youth in Zambia." *Health Transit Review* 7 (Supplement 3): 91–95.

Kathuria, R., P. Chirenda, R. Sabatier, and N. Dube. 1998. "Peer Education to Reduce STI/HIV Transmission in Lusaka, Zambia." Paper presented at the International Conference on AIDS, Geneva, Switzerland, June–July.

Kiremire, K. M., and N. Luo. 1996. "Practical Interventions in the Prevention of the Spread of HIV among Lusaka's Female Sex Workers—The Case of TASINTHA Program." Paper presented at the International Conference on AIDS, Vancouver, July.

Koster-Oyekan, W. 1998. "Why Resort to Illegal Abortion in Zambia? Findings of a Community-Based Study in Western Province." *Social Science and Medicine* 48 (10): 1302–1312.

Leonard, A., E. Muia, and A. Khan. 1996. "Designing Action-Oriented Research Interventions to Increase the Ability of Community-Based HIV/AIDS Prevention and Care Initiatives to Sustain and Improve Their Programs: Four Examples from Africa." Paper presented at the International Conference on AIDS, Vancouver, July.

Melbye, M., E. K. Njelesani, A. Bayley, K. Mukelabai, J. K. Manuwele, F. J. Bowa, S. A. Clayden, A. Levin, W. A. Blattner, R. A. Weiss, et al. 1986. "Evidence for Heterosexual Transmission and Clinical Manifestations of Human Immunodeficiency Virus Infection and Related Conditions in Lusaka, Zambia." *Lancet* 2 (8516): 1113–1115.

Moszynski, P. 1999. "United Nations Estimates of HIV Prevalence in Zambia Under Attack." *British Medical Journal* 319 (August 7): 338.

Mulwanda, C. 1989. "Squatter's Nightmare: The Political Economy of Disasters and Disaster Response in Zambia." *Disaster* 13 (4): 345–350.

Mutangadura, G., D. Webb, B. Mutsakani, and H. Jackson. 1998. "The Socio-Economic Impact of Adult Mortality and Morbidity on Households in Urban Zambia." Paper presented at the Twelfth International Conference on AIDS, Geneva, June 28–July 3.

Nyamuryekung'e, K., U. Laukamm-Josten, B. Vuylsteke, C. Mbuya, C. Hamelmann, A. Outwater, R. Steen, D. Ocheng, A. Msauka, and G. Dallabetta. 1997. "STD Services for Women at Truck Stop in Tanzania: Evaluation of Acceptable Approaches." *East African Medical Journal* 74 (6): 343–347.

PEPFAR (President's Emergency Plan for AIDS Relief). 2005. "Compassionate Action Provides Hope through Treatment Success, June 13, 2005." Washington, D.C.: Office of the U.S. Global AIDS Coordinator.

Pillai, V. K., and T. R. Barton. 1999. "Sexual Activity among Zambian Female Teenagers: The Role of Interpersonal Skills." *Adolescence* 34 (134): 381–387.

Pinkerton, S. D., and P. R. Abramson. 1997. "Effectiveness of Condoms in Preventing HIV Transmission." *Social Science and Medicine* 44 (9): 1303–1312.

Quinn, T. C., J. M. Mann, J. W. Curran, and P. Piot. 1986. "AIDS in Africa: An Epidemiologic Paradigm." *Science* 234 (4779): 955–963.

Richards, A. I. 1939. *Land, Labour, and Diet in Northern Rhodesia: An Economic Study of the Bemba Tribe.* New York: Oxford University Press.

———. 1956. *Chisungu: A Girl's Initiation Ceremony among the Bemba of Northern Rhodesia.* New York: Grove Press.

Sandala, L., P. Lurie, M. R. Sunkutu, E. M. Chani, E. S. Hudes, and N. Hearst. 1995. "'Dry Sex' and HIV Infection among Women Attending a Sexually Transmitted Diseases Clinic in Lusaka, Zambia." *AIDS* 9 (Supplement 1): S61–S68.

Schuster, I. 1979. *New Women of Lusaka.* Palo Alto, Calf.: Mayfield.

———. 1982. "Marginal Lives: Conflict and Contradiction in the Position of Female Traders in Lusaka, Zambia." In *Women and Work in Africa*, ed. E. Bay, 105–126. Boulder, Colo.: Westview Press.

Siatwinda, S. M. 1984. "Family Health in Zambia." Paper presented at the Union of National Radio and Television Organizations of Africa (URTNA) Family Health Broadcast Workshop, Nairobi.

Slonim-Nevo, V., and L. Mukuka. 2005. "AIDS-Related Knowledge, Attitudes and Behavior among Adolescents in Zambia." *AIDS and Behavior* 9 (2): 223–231.

Timaeus, I. M. 1998. "Impact of the HIV Epidemic on Mortality in Sub-Saharan Africa: Evidence from National Surveys and Censuses." *AIDS* 12 (Supplement 1): S15–S27.

Turner, V. W. 1957. *Schism and Continuity in an African Society.* Manchester: Manchester University Press.

———. 1967. *The Forest of Symbols: Aspects of Ndembu Ritual.* Ithaca, N.Y.: Cornell University Press.

van der Graaf, M., and R. J. Diepersloot. 1986. "Transmission of Human Immunodeficiency Virus (HIV/HTLV-III/LAV): A Review." *Infection* 14 (5): 203–211.

Warner, L., J. Clay-Warner, J. Boles, and J. Williamson. 1998. "Assessing Condom Use Practices: Implications for Evaluating Method and User Effectiveness." *Sexually Transmitted Diseases* 25 (6): 273–277.

Webb, D. 2000. "Attitudes to 'Kaponya Mafumo': The Terminators of Pregnancy in Urban Zambia." *Health Policy Plan* 15 (2): 186–193.

WHO/UNAIDS. 2003. "Reconciling Antenatal Clinic-Based Surveillance and Population-Based Survey Estimates of HIV Prevalence in Sub-Saharan Africa." UNAIDS, Geneva, Switzerland, August.

The World Factbook. 2005. *The World Factbook.* Washington, D.C.: Central Intelligence Agency.

World Food Programme. 2005. "HIV/AIDS and Poor Weather Drive Zambians to the Edge. May 24. http: //www.wfp./org/english/?n=321&elemID=id2462&key=1.

Yoder, P. S., R. Hornik, and B. C. Chirwa. 1996. "Evaluating the Program Effects of a Radio Drama about AIDS in Zambia." *Studies in Family Planning* 27 (4): 188–203.

Zambia News Agency. 2005a. "NZP+ Members Not Accessing ARV's." January 4. http: //www.zana.gov.zm/news/viewnews.cgi?category=7&id=1104839257.

———. 2005b. Teachers in Chipata Shun VCT. January 5. http: //www.zana.gov.zm/ news/viewnews.cgi?category=7&id=1104924825.

9

Myths of Science, Myths of Sex

Homophobia and HIV Vulnerability in Namibia

ROBERT LORWAY

The study of gay and lesbian social movements in southern Africa has received notable attention within contemporary scholarship. In particular, academics have discussed how social actors and groups draw on global and local cultural resources and discourses in their social struggles for legitimacy (Hoad 1999; Phillips 2000). The formation of transnational coalitions has been instrumental in raising human rights concerns of gays and lesbians within civil society networks in southern Africa. However, community-based organizations have had limited success in penetrating public health spheres that confront the urgent threat of HIV/AIDS. The silence around same-sex sexual practices within national HIV/AIDS awareness campaigns has in large part been due to the illegal status of homosexuality, defined as sodomy in criminal codes, in most African countries (IGLHRC 2003). This exclusion from public health discourse has also been greatly reinforced within international health science arenas where narrow and sometimes stereotypical definitions of "African sexuality" are employed.

Gausset (2001) draws a parallel between ethnocentric writings on African sexuality in the late nineteenth and early twentieth centuries and more contemporary anthropological research conducted during the earlier years of the AIDS epidemic in Africa. He attributes the resurgence of ethnocentrism to the state of emergency and "the desire to save lives." According to Gausset (2001: 511), anthropologists who employed cultural HIV risk models have tended to produce understandings of African sexuality as "exotic, traditional, irrational and immoral practices." Bond and colleagues (1997: 46) similarly assert that the urgency of HIV/AIDS produced behavioral knowledge by the West that "was, and often remains, superficial." This lack of careful reflection by social health scientists has lead to exaggerated representations of African heterosexual "promiscuity," produced against imagined notions of a "nonpromiscuous" Western sexuality (see, for example, Bailey and Aunger 1995).

In the southern African region, anthropologists have redressed ideas of the hypersexual African "other" by articulating how the history of colonial economic devastation disrupted "traditional" social relations in African societies, thereby structuring the preconditions for HIV vulnerability (Campbell 1997; Jochelson 2001; Lwanda 2004; Webb 1997). Moreover, the structural adjustment programs of the International Monetary Fund (IMF) and the World Bank during the early 1980s have further exacerbated social inequalities in Africa (Craddock 2004; Lurie et al. 2004). Attending to these larger historical political economic processes, anthropologists have accounted for the disproportionately high prevalence of HIV (and other sexually transmitted infections [STIs]) in African countries, and thus have corrected notions of African sexuality as "uncontrolled and excessive" (Vaughan 1991: 129).

In this chapter, I further dispel stereotypes of African sexuality that underlie current epidemiologic theories of AIDS in Africa. By referring to ethnographic fieldwork with persons involved in alternative (to heterosexual) sexual relationships in Namibia, I expand health scientific notions of African sexuality typically defined in essentialist terms—as "tied to nature" and as "a two-dimensional binary idea of heterosexuality" (Teunis 2001: 173). Through my representations, "sexuality" in Namibia is reconceptualized as uneven, ever-moving, erotic, and strategic engagements of individuals and groups that take shape within "the cultural politics of everyday life" (Werbner 1996: 13). Thus, I challenge epidemiologic constructions that cast sexuality as simply a fixed set of behaviors, practices, or rituals that remain confined within culturally ascribed roles or relationships. Instead, sexuality appears as considerably more flexible. Same-sex desire may take on numerous expressions as persons navigate between multiple shifting cultural contexts. This was very much the case with the young persons who participated in my dissertation research. Their flexible sexual identities allowed them to readily slide between seemingly incommensurable cultural spaces marked by multiple languages, ethnicities, ages, and economic statuses—from the urban life of discos and private parties with foreigners in the capital city, to active participation in the gay rights social movement, to daily community life in outlying townships. Thus, bounded and monolithic notions of culture and sexuality do not lend themselves to HIV risk and vulnerability analysis here.

Although epidemiologists have constructed AIDS in Africa as a Pattern 2 heterosexual epidemic (since the ratio between men and women is close to 1: 1), the possibility that HIV may also be transmitted through same-sex sexuality has remained underexplored (Phillips 2004). Furthermore, this inattention exists in the face of growing documentation by gay and lesbian studies scholars concerning the presence of African same-sex sexual expression (Donham 1998; Epprecht 1998; Gevisser and Cameron 1995; Murray and Roscoe 1998; Niehaus 2002). In this chapter, therefore, I focus attention on the HIV vulnerability of young Namibian males who engage in same-sex sexual practices to consider what is absent from international health science theory on sexuality and AIDS in (southern) Africa. My intention here is not to deny that heterosexual intercourse is a major route of transmission. Instead, I consider the exclusion of same-sex sexual practices as unnecessarily limiting possibilities for HIV epidemic prevention.

Namibian AIDS awareness campaigns, as in most African countries, target persons who are assumed to engage exclusively in opposite-sex sexual practices. As a consequence of this heterosexual assumption, men who have sex with men in Namibia are particularly vulnerable to HIV infection. For example, persons who are incarcerated in Namibia and involved in same-sex sexual behavior are prohibited from receiving condoms despite the growing HIV prevalence within the country's thirteen overcrowded prisons (IGLHRC 2003; Ministry of Prisons and Correctional Services 2000). Furthermore, research efforts in Namibia have left unexplored the areas of male sex work, and same-sex sexual activity among occupants of mining hostels and among soldiers in Namibia's military.[1] In short, there have been virtually no national or regional HIV/AIDS public health campaigns in Namibia that have included any suggestion of same-sex sexual practice in their messages. Ironically, while issues related to same-sex sexuality have been excluded from HIV/AIDS public health discourse, "homosexuality" has been hotly debated in parliamentary arenas, where notions of Namibian authenticity were contested. On March 19, 2001, President Sam Nujoma, in his address to students at the University of Namibia, called for the arrest, imprisonment, and deportation of all gay men and lesbians in Namibia. In a later official address to regional governors, councilors, and traditional leaders at Okahao, Nujoma stated: "Traditional leaders, governors, see to it that there are no criminals, gays and lesbians in your village and regions. . . . We in SWAPO [South West Africa People's Organization] have not fought for an independent Namibia that gives rights to *botsotsos* [criminals], gays and lesbians. . . . If we do not go back to our traditional marriage culture and practices, this killing disease of HIV/AIDS will continue to kill our people" (Shivute 2001).

This chapter traces the effects of state-deployed homophobia as it gets bound up in the contingencies and commitments of local actors in their everyday lives. Drawing on extensive ethnographic fieldwork conducted in Namibia, I focus on the HIV risk practices of young black males living in a Namibian township who identify as gay, bisexual, or transgendered.[2] These youth connect with each other and to broader and transnational lesbian, gay, bisexual, and transgendered (LGBT) communities through the cultural and economic resources of the only sexuality rights nongovernmental organization (NGO) in Namibia, The Rainbow Project (TRP). TRP has provided programming for members around sexuality in the context of human rights. More recently, TRP began to deliver HIV transmission information after several members tested positive and claimed that they had considered AIDS to be a "heterosexual disease" (Ian Swarzt, personal communication 2001).

Despite the HIV-related knowledge transferred through the organization, members continued to experience difficulties in practicing safer sex. Frequent involvement in formal/informal modes of sex work with wealthy foreign and local elites, socially structured gender inequalities, and violent physical, verbal, and sexual harassment greatly undermined individual safer sex negotiating power and health-seeking capabilities. In this chapter, I explicitly draw attention to difficulties in safer sex negotiation within the context of human rights struggles, government sanctioned discrimination, and historically constituted gender and economic inequalities.

Methodology

My ethnographic study in Namibia focused on the daily lives of young black males and females living in the Windhoek municipal township known as Katutura. My point of entry, however, was gained through TRP, which is located in the central business district of Windhoek. At the time of my second arrival in Namibia (2002), TRP's membership totaled 190 persons. Through TRP's facilitation, I established contacts with members who, in turn, introduced me to individuals who did not associate with TRP (but who also lived in Katutura). Within the first three months, I established ninety-three contacts, who assisted to varying degrees with the interpretation of findings throughout the research process. Of these contacts, sixty-two persons (thirty-one males and thirty-one females) agreed to participate in more formal, in-depth interviewing and ethnographic follow-ups. The remaining thirty-one persons continued to act as "informal" contacts and were consulted with on a less regular basis. I specifically refer to the findings concerning the males (ages eighteen to twenty-six) who participated in this study.

Sexual and gender identities employed by participants were frequently altered depending on the social context. During TRP political meetings, local press engagements, and formal interviewing, persons identified as gay, bisexual, or transgendered. Labels such as *moffie* (effeminate male), "drag queen," "bottom/top," and "straight" were used more during informal social gatherings.[3] Although some *moffies* employed female names and identified themselves as sexually receptive during anal sex, others identified as being "gay men" who engaged in penetrative as well as receptive sexual practices. Traditional words that referred to gender nonconformity, such as *eshenge* and *!gamas*, tended to circulate within Katutura society among community elders.[4] Eight males who engaged in bisexual behavior, and who did not directly associate with TRP, identified as "straight" men. However, bisexual behavior was not limited to these men, but was also practiced by persons who appeared more effeminate. In fact, sexual relationships were commonly reported between effeminate men and "butch lesbians" (as they were sometimes called). Thus, gender and sexual identities did not always signify sexual practices that were predictable for a Western ethnographer.

Open-ended structured interviews were conducted initially at the center, but later took place in coffee shops, restaurants, parks, and homes as I came to know participants well. Although the interview guides were pilot tested with staff and TRP volunteers, open-ended structured interviewing did not consistently provide rich detail about sexual risk behavior and involvement in sex work as expected. Formal interviewing did, however, become useful for emphasizing the research objectives to participants. Once the tape recorder was shut off, persons tended to talk more freely. As greater rapport developed outside the formal interview setting, participants explained sexual risk practices in greater detail. Thus, ethnographic follow-up, participant observation, and field-note writing yielded the most significant findings.

After several months, I was welcomed in participants' daily social lives. This allowed me to witness several factors that significantly contributed to HIV risk, such as alcohol and drug use, violence, stigma, gender inequality, and homophobia. Participants and contacts explained sexual risk-taking practices in terms of these factors during informal conversations. I also spent considerable time observing interactions between participants and their friends and family at local discos in the capital city, and at shebeens (unlicensed drinking establishments), parties, and funerals in Katutura. Tape-recorded qualitative interviews (which elicited life histories of "coming out" and sexual risk taking) were conducted during the day, while participant observation and note taking took place at night, as I moved about the streets of Katutura and the capital city with participants, from house to house, shebeen to shebeen, disco to disco.

In consultation with TRP staff, it was decided that the interviewing process could provide the opportunity both to correct any misinformation about HIV transmission and to respond to outstanding questions concerning HIV/AIDS. Because participants claimed that anal sex required more lubricant than was afforded by the free condoms distributed by the Ministry of Health and Social Services, small satchels of lubricant, paid for by TRP, were provided during ethnographic work. Persons were also directed to TRP's HIV/AIDS resources, where they could receive further information, free condoms, and lubricant for future need. TRP staff conducted workshops on STIs, and held safer sex information sessions based on the findings of this research. Together, we organized a safer sex weekend called "Let's Talk About Sex, Baby," which, in addition to presenting HIV educational materials, allowed us to formulate strategies concerning how to effectively conduct further HIV/AIDS work with persons engaged in same-sex sexual practices within a political climate that sanctioned homophobia.

State Homophobia and Health-Seeking Behavior

In southern Africa, what has come to be known as the "Book Fair Dramas" in Zimbabwe sparked modern LGBT social movements during 1995 and 1996 (Gevisser and Cameron 1995; IGLHRC 2003). Following the barring of the Gays and Lesbians of Zimbabwe (GALZ) exhibition at the Zimbabwean international book fair in 1995, Zimbabwe president Robert Mugabe delivered his now infamous hate speech, suggesting gays and lesbians were worse than "dogs and pigs" (IGLHRC 2003: 12–15). As Palmberg (1999: 66) maintains, this rhetoric placed homosexuality "on the agenda for the whole subcontinent." In Namibia, SWAPO government ministers, echoing Mugabe, launched verbal attacks against Namibian gays and lesbians. Since 1995, an extensive parliamentary and public debate ensued in Namibia. Minister of Home Affairs Jerry Ekandjo, in 1998, attempted to have anti-homosexuality legislation drafted. Although unsuccessful in his attempts, Ekandjo later publicly announced to police graduates: "The constitution does not guarantee rights for gay and lesbians. . . . We must make sure we eliminate them [gays and lesbians] from the face of Namibia. We must combat all such unnatural acts, including murder" (Anonymous 2000).

As the state crafted "homosexuality" as a threat to national survival, homosexuality became linked to a multitude of emergent social problems and tensions of the postcolonial era, such as criminality, national identity/authenticity, globalization, and neocolonialism. For example, during his official address to SWAPO supporters outside the Okuryangava Women's Center, Nujoma stated: "The enemy is still trying to come back with sinister maneuvers and tricks called lesbians and homosexuality and globalization. . . . They colonized us and now they claim human rights, when we condemn and reject them. In Namibia, there will be no lesbian and homosexual left. Those who want to do that [continue with homosexual activities] must pack up and go back to Europe" (Maletsky 2001).

This ongoing homophobic rhetoric did not, however, operate without meeting local resistance. In February 1997, a gay and lesbian social movement mobilized in response to ongoing discrediting remarks made by government officials. The initial collective of more than fifty persons (TRP) drew its membership from preexisting gay and lesbian groups in Windhoek.[5] Most of the members identified as white and "colored." They were generally well traveled in Europe and North America, well credentialed, and employed in middle-range income jobs as teachers, lawyers, NGO directors, or local embassy representatives. A sizable number of the core organizers were non-Namibian. Sister Namibia, a feminist lobbying and advocacy group sponsored by German and Dutch development foundations, organized the first meetings. In 1998, TRP received operational funding and program directives from several European-based international development foundations.[6] Under the watchful eye of this international human rights network, the emergent gay and lesbian social movement was established through what Appardurai (2001: 17) would refer to as an organized effort "to globalize from below."

During the barrage of hate speeches, leading officials from Amnesty International, international lesbian and gay associations based in Europe and North America, and local and international NGO networks released a flurry of press statements condemning SWAPO politicians' remarks. The gay and lesbian struggle in Namibia received considerable media attention in national and international newspapers, television, and radio (including the BBC), and was featured strongly in South African, Dutch, and German newspapers and magazines. Politically savvy local activists and academics commanded several public forums in Windhoek that directly challenged, and at times ridiculed, the remarks made by President Nujoma and his ministry. But because the international human rights community carefully guarded the Rainbow community, such open castigation did not meet with any official arrest, imprisonment, or deportation.[7] However, many young black men and women living in poorer townships like Katutura experienced immediate antihomosexual feedback within their communities. State-articulated homophobia penetrated Namibian society at the most intimate levels of social life. One twenty-year-old male explained how he came to feel increasingly marginalized during the hate speeches:

> When the president made that speech, my mother said, "He's doing the right thing. When they start to arrest or deport people I will personally bring you to the police or to whoever will do the job!" I was hurt. I was scared. So I moved to my grandmother's place from my mother's. My grandmother sent me to the shops and the people were saying, "Sam is saying you must go out of our country, you must be deported." I felt like . . . I wish we [he and his two best friends] could just go somewhere. I felt like we had nowhere to go.

As contestations concerning homosexuality worked their way through township culture, tensions also took shape within local fields of ethnic identity politics. The president's condemnations of homosexuality were accompanied by a call for a return to "traditional" practices (Menges 2001). However, many viewed the president's mention of "traditional" as referencing Owambo and Herero ethnic identities. Thus, the queer social movement also provided a platform from which gay and lesbian persons from other ethnic groups (particularly Nama/Damara) could protest the tribalism associated with the homophobic rhetoric.[8] Those who identified as Owambo or Herero and engaged in same-sex sexual practices experienced extreme isolation and stigmatization within their communities. Two TRP members in their early twenties who identified with Nama/Damara ethnic groups commented on how these issues became articulated among their peers:

> From the [heterosexual] Damaras, you won't really get discrimination or sharp words, you will just get, "Hey ladies, where are you going," or "Can I fuck you tonight," or "Did you hear what the president said?" But the Owambo [heterosexual people], they go deep into your skin and they work their way out with words.
>
> The Owambo and Herero people [some of them] are also *moffies* like us, but they are just hiding it. . . . They are very scared. Our friends who are Owambo and Herero guys, if they get drunk they will get like this, "girlfriend" [said in campy way]. But if he is sober, he is very masculine.

Participants described their encounters with antihomosexual discrimination as occurring within institutional, community, and familial settings.

It should be noted that the regulatory power of the police, the church, and the medical system intruded on community and private spaces, thus driving local social processes of stigmatization. Take, for example, one young male who described his experiences of harassment by the paramilitary police, known as the Special Field Forces (SFF), at the height of the homophobic government rhetoric:

> We were at a shebeen in Katutura, me and my friends . . . even the one who is a drag queen. We were having our drinks. We were sitting there. After a while we decided to go to my aunt's place because she was selling some beer and on our way to the house while we entered we just saw a car coming with the lights off and they [SFF officers] stopped and said that all of us would have to come out from the yard. Then my aunt said, "No they are staying here!" And then one said, "Yah, it's *eshenges* [Oshiwambo word for effeminate man]; *eshenges* are not allowed in Namibia!" Then they began to speak in Owambo and my friend said, who was also Owambo, "I am Owambo *eshenge*" and they started to beat him and my aunt said she was going to call the LAC [Legal Assistance Centre, a nonprofit public interest law center] and they drove off. We filed a report after that, but nothing happened.

Christian associations, which wield great symbolic capital in Namibian society, also took cues from government hate speeches. To fully understand the social weight of church condemnation of homosexuality, it must first be recognized how Christian regulatory power has come to operate with great efficacy in Namibian society. During apartheid, the church was one of the few spaces where racial segregation could be transcended. Moreover, antiapartheid political strategies drew on liberation theology to mobilize the universalizing discursive potential of Christian ideologies (Katjavivi et al. 1989). Many of the most prominent antiapartheid leaders were also prominent church leaders. Thus, Christian ideology and the state have become inexorably linked in Namibia. In postapartheid Namibia, significant national and community solidarity continues to come through participation in church ritual and social activity. At the time of the hate speeches, many church leaders took up the issue of homosexuality in public sermons with local congregations.[9] Twenty-year-old John discussed his feelings of devastation when he faced discrimination in his church:

> I grew up as a Pentecostal churchgoer. At the moment the hate speeches started in church, pastors, the deacons, the elders started

preaching that homosexuality was a sin. And every Sunday when I go to church, there was a thing about homosexuality as a sin. It was after the human rights weekend; it was a pressure for me. I couldn't stand it. Usually I would be singing in the choir. I moved away from the church because my mum was an elder in the church and people were saying, "Oh that elder's son is a gay person." The choir would have worshiping practice and they would move from house to house but would not tell me and they said, "No you are a gay, you are not supposed to sing in the worship." It made me sick for a while, you are so depressed; it is as if God is chasing you away. The way the pastors preach, the way the elders would speak, I would feel that God doesn't want me and I am excluded from the human race.

Most participants perceived the state health care system, which shares overlapping history with Christian missionary work (Wallace 2002; Walter 1996), as supporting the government's discriminatory remarks. This greatly inhibited the effort of TRP to promote HIV and other STI testing practices. When I asked twenty-year-old John if he would ever consider going for an STI test, he quickly said "No!" and explained: "If you go to the health officer and tell them about your sexuality they will say that 'Oh you sleep with a man, that is not allowed.' I once had a health officer tell me when I wanted some condoms, 'Oh you are a gay man. You also use condoms?' Also with health officers, it is not confidential, the nurses will tell their husbands and then everyone will find out."

Participants who were unemployed, worked part-time, and came from poorer households consistently expressed apprehension toward the medical community.[10] These participants discussed two main concerns. First, they perceived health care practitioners to be untrustworthy when it came to matters of privacy and confidentiality. Second, they were fearful of being mistreated if they disclosed their sexuality to practitioners. Those participants who were employed full time, however, stated that they fully trusted their physician. Moreover, they had gone for regular STI and HIV testing, and were open about their sexual identity with their health care practitioner. Twenty-two-year-old Romeo explained this marked contrast to me:

If you have the money you can have a family doctor at one of the private hospitals. Most of my friends don't have the money and have to use the state hospital and use whoever is on call. So, of course, they won't disclose their sexual identity. My friends don't even like to go to doctors because they are afraid that their HIV status will come out. I feel the nurses will make fun of you if you have something down there [points to genitals]. One of my friends had an STD. . . . They [the nurses] called each other around him to look at him and referred to him as a *moffie*. That is why people are afraid to go.

This story of the man who was ridiculed by nurses had widely circulated within the closely knit Rainbow community. What is of great concern here is not only if, in fact, nurses and physicians disclosed identity regularly (although LeBeau et al.'s [1999] research suggests a prevalence of breeches in confidentiality by health care practitioners in many regions of Namibia) but also that persons perceive themselves to be at great harm. Such perceptual barriers become concrete as they prevent poorer persons from accessing health resources. Furthermore, fear of identity disclosure is understandable when one considers the overcrowded environment of the state hospital where private matters of health status are frequently shouted aloud between staff. Thus, as institutional homophobia becomes re-created at the most intimate levels of perception, fear of stigmatization diminishes the likelihood of individuals engaging in health seeking and protection behavior.

"Struggle for Manhood" and Safer Sex

Fear of social stigma also frames patterns of HIV vulnerability for young effeminate males in their sexual relationships with local men identified as "straight." The social isolation resulting from sexual identity concealment intensifies difficulties for effeminate males when negotiating for safer sex with socially dominant "straight" men. Campbell (2003: 32), in her research on miners, masculinity, and HIV risk in South Africa, refers to the social construction of masculine identities as "bringing together the concepts of bravery, fearlessness . . . and going after women." In her theorization of masculinity, which builds on the work of Moodie and colleagues (1988), multiple notions of manhood are socially constituted in the mines and get drawn into self-conceptualizing and felt as "identity" (Campbell 2001). I would suggest, in the case of my study, that masculine identity formation proceeds through a less stable and more ambivalent social process. Among male participants in this project, securing a sense of manhood also moves by alternating between seizing on to and disavowing, even violently negating, what is differentiated as feminine.

Through this struggle for manhood among males in Katutura, dominance tends to be asserted by "straight" men over bodies identified and discredited as *moffies* during male-male sexual encounters. In such situations, the safer sex negotiating capacity of effeminate males becomes greatly constrained.

Ron, who sometimes dressed in drag when he attended discos in the capital city, referred to his gender and sexual identity as follows:

> I am a man, a homosexual. I'm gay and I am sleeping with men and I am fucking men. I am fucked by men, also. In some cases, I am a *moffie*. I have a "straight" boyfriend in [Katutura]. He is very aggressive, very violent. I told him I don't like to be fucked all the time and I said, 'sometimes I must do it [penetrate you],' and he got so worked up at the club. He was beating me with brooms and champagne glasses. He would not go 50/50.

He continued by saying:

> Sometimes straight guys, they won't want to use the condom and you say no and you get a smack on the face. . . . When he hits me . . . I think he loves me . . . I know that he loves me. I feel that someone cares for me. I don't get love at all, [or] affection in my family. My father is very violent. I didn't come out to him, but he knows from the start that I am a *moffie*. But if I came out to him he would beat me.

Participants and informal contacts asserted that it was common for "straight" men and *moffies* to engage in sexual relationships in Katutura. According to *moffies*, men were "straight" when they had girlfriends or wives and appeared to conform to other culturally ascribed gender roles. Although the *moffies* had attended numerous workshops and information sessions at TRP, their safer sex negotiating abilities were greatly restricted by "straight" men who insisted on sex without condoms. But what makes these young *moffies* particularly vulnerable to HIV is that their struggles remain deeply hidden. Familial and community mechanisms of support and accountability are generally unavailable to them. Nineteen-year-old Derek explained the difficulties that he and his friends experienced concerning safer sex negotiations with "straight" men:

> We don't date *moffies*, each other . . . it is only "heterosexual" guys, so most of them approach us at the clubs. We have sex sometimes at his house but usually in the veld [field] or in the toilet. I have slept with about 60 percent of the guys in that shop [he points to the nearby community bar]. They have girlfriends also. If we sleep with a guy, it is only us *moffies* who know. We only tell each other. The "straight" guys do not socialize with us, they approach us only when they are drinking or are drunk. We do not sleep together in the day, mostly we sleep

with each other at night. It is difficult to make them wear a condom when they are drunk. . . . Although my family knows that I am a gay, I don't talk about my sexuality with them.

Jason maintained that sexual practices between "straight" men and *moffies* were related to fear of HIV infection:

Most of the men I know who have girlfriends are saying that they prefer to have sex with us *moffies* because they don't want to catch STDs cheating on them, or HIV, or pregnancy. Most of them think they can even have sex with men without a condom because they think it is less risky than sex with a woman. Mostly, some of the things are happening while in the night, or when the wife is gone. You can stay for the weekend [people frequently go to the farms to visit relatives], but some of them they will prefer it during the day and they will call you up and say, "Go and meet me there. I would like to take you." Some of the girlfriends will talk to you, you must just know how to talk to them so that you don't make them suspicious.

The idea that sex with men was somehow safer than sex with women was a common misconception among participants and informal contacts. As one twenty-year-old male told me, "Some of the 'straight' guys think that we *moffies* are virgins because we are tighter than women." Such beliefs stand in contrast to the early mislabeling of AIDS as a "gay disease" in Pattern 1 countries. In an interview with two self-identified "straight" men who had sex with *moffies*, they told me:

[Calin]: I believe that you can't get HIV from having sex with a *moffie* because there is no mixing of fluid there [points to anal region]; it is dry.

[Peter]: I see it as more risky with a woman . . . because there is blood connected. In a man I do not know where the blood is connected. In a woman you are directly connected.

Thus, epidemiologic constructions of AIDS in Africa have become reconstituted, in unexpected ways, through local myths of male-male sex as safer sex. "Straight" men were not, however, the only persons who believed that anal sex was somehow safer than vaginal sex. Such myths of anal sex also traveled through the community of *moffies*, particularly among those who were younger. Note the following responses when participants were asked, "What is more risky—sex with men or with women?"

[Christina, eighteen years old]: With a woman, it is riskier . . . from people having sex to get babies. You are more likely to get STDs from a woman because HIV comes through sexual intercourse.

[Lorin, nineteen years old]: I think it is more risky in heterosexual sex . . . because in biology in school we would have the diagram and the anatomy [of a vagina]. You could see that all the way inside [a woman] it is wet. It is like full of membranes. But men don't have as many membranes [in their anus].

[Tuli, eighteen years old]: I feel sex is safer with [other] *moffies*. I feel I am not doing it like the heterosexuals are doing it, in the front like the girls are doing. It is different. With it [anal sex] I am not really sure what is happening there.

When participants did wear condoms, they frequently used oil-based lubricants (unaware of the damage caused to the latex). In general, participants used Vaseline, Dove or Dawn hand cream, baby oil, and cooking oil. One person even used Dark and Lovely hair cream. Only two male participants and four (out of thirty-one) informal contacts knew the difference between water-based and oil-based lubricants. This lack of knowledge points to public health officials' failure to bring discussions of lubricant use (and anal sex) into HIV-awareness campaigns.[11] To begin to address this safer sex issue, which emerged during the interviewing process, TRP staff, TRP members, and I organized information sessions on the differences between water-based and oil-based lubricants.

Two problems were identified during this community meeting. For one, some members could not afford water-based lubricants. Second, the lubricant was not readily portable if one was going out for the night or to a disco. Although we did locate one drugstore that carried pocket-sized satchels of lubricant, most drugstores in Windhoek did not carry them. Moreover, they were not readily accessible for persons who lived in the townships. It was therefore decided that a water-based lubricant would be given out during interviews and supplied by TRP for free once the project was completed. However, these health safety measures are ineffective in the context of gender inequality, where *moffies'* decision-making capacities are greatly limited by "straight" men who do not attend HIV information sessions at TRP.

Sex Tourism

In addition to HIV educational training, members attended TRP's sexuality programs, during which they were taught how to distinguish between gay, lesbian, bisexual, and transgender sexualities. Although some had never heard of these categories previously, they both claimed and resisted these identities as they creatively reinterpreted them through their daily lived experiences (Lorway 2003). In addition to attending regular educational and social meetings, members frequently borrowed books, movies, and magazines from TRP that were produced in Germany, the Netherlands, the United Kingdom, the United States, and South Africa. As members consumed global queer culture, overly idealized notions of Western countries as "homophobia free" formed. But because Western people seen as images of sexual freedom were dressed in affluence, the aesthetic of gay liberation appeared far out of reach for those who endured daily struggles with poverty. Relationships with foreigners, however, were recognized as one of the few means of not only escaping economic oppression but also achieving the (Western) aesthetic of sexual freedom. The "wonderful success stories" that moved within the community of *moffies* were of those *moffies* who had married foreigners and were able to leave Namibia.

During the height of the hate speeches, TRP became a focal point of international attention. This NGO was imbued with letters and e-mails of support from across the globe. Moreover, gay and lesbian foreigners visiting and working in Namibia came to be closely affiliated with TRP. There was, therefore, plenty of opportunities for local and foreign gay men to socialize. Relationships between foreigners and locals, which were generally marked by financial unevenness, took on numerous forms. For some participants I interviewed, relationships with foreigners strictly provided them with opportunity for economic gain, as Larry explained: "I have dated a lot of older white men for financial reasons. This is a very common thing around here . . . especially with the young black guys. They only date white guys for the financial aspect."

Most participants, however, did not agree with this explanation. For many who experienced the daily struggles of discrimination and isolation, foreigners were the objects of their desire for achieving social as well as economic mobility. Thus, I distinguish these forms of sex tourism (Farmer 1992; Kempadoo 1999) from what Preston-Whyte and colleagues (2000) refer to as "survival sex." In the context of Namibia's Rainbow community, sexual exchanges must also be understood as existing beyond straightforward definitions of economic survival (as "survival" took on numerous and divergent meanings for participants). This supports Larvie's (1999) assertion that male sex work is not always governed by necessity and cannot be understood only as formalized rational monetary exchanges. Therefore, in the ethnographic case studies below, I highlight the symbolic complexities of sex tourism as mediated by desire, emotion, eroticism, and pleasure. These personal economies produce particular ambiguities during exchanges involving sex that do not fit strict, predictable monetary schemes. Such ambiguities somewhat parallel Bloor's (1995: 85) description of male sex work in Glasgow as a

> highly diverse phenomenon and, while some respondents pursued the same businesslike and directive approach as female prostitutes, many others did not. Some respondents, for example, would mingle socially with their [clients] in bars and discos, making no clear distinction between private and commercial sexual relationships. Similar ambiguities could be encountered at the lavatories and parks where prostitutes . . . often failed to make clear to their sexual contacts that payment was expected.

The following ethnographic case studies bring together a range of sociocultural themes, situating them within the globalizing context of informal sex tourism. These case studies are intended to illustrate how sometimes conflicting cultural processes collide in the daily lived experiences of persons in ways that complicate agency during safer sex negotiations.

Travis is a twenty-year-old black man who identified himself as being gay and Damara. Dressed up in the most fashionable attire, he was often criticized by fellow TRP members for dressing beyond his means. His hair was painstakingly straightened to emulate particular European styles he viewed in TRP magazines. Growing up, he told me, he did not have many troubles because of his "difference." However, he did remember at times being called names like *!gamas* by other children (which he explained was a mildly derogatory term that referred to a goat that possessed both genitalia).

During one meeting we had at a library, Travis brought along his photo album and showed me pictures of former boyfriends. His first boyfriend, when he was sixteen, was a Roman Catholic priest in his early fifties. Next he showed me a picture of a local man—"He's a Boer [Afrikaans word for white farmer]"—who was his boyfriend for several months. He went on to show me other pictures of boyfriends. They were all similar in two respects. They were white, and they were considerably older than him. He explained that he desired white men. He liked foreigners in particular, he stated. "They know how to treat you right and take care of you. The black guys just want to take from you, they are so dependent."

Several months later, Travis seemed upset. He had caught his current partner in bed with someone else—"another black guy," he exclaimed. It was someone who had been a longtime friend. Travis stated that he no longer wanted to date white men, even though they had money. He declared one day, "I would rather be poor!" It was particularly difficult for Travis to find work because he had come out rather publicly about his sexuality during Nujoma's hate speeches. He asked, "Who would hire me now?" He was quite angry with his ex-boyfriend for having treated him like a "common street prostitute." Although he liked that his former partner had money, took him to dinner, and bought him gifts, he was with him "for love," he explained. For this reason, Travis had been faithful to his partner. After two months in their relationship, he had trusted his partner enough to have unprotected anal sex. Travis said during an interview: "I always practice safer sex, but sometimes you trust your partner and you are faithful but the other person is not. They are faithful in front of you. I left that relationship because I became so scared of HIV."

Travis was greatly concerned about getting HIV. It was certainly close to home for him. Two of his sisters had already tested positive and were dying of AIDS. One day he showed me the official papers that permitted him to adopt his sister's newborn HIV-positive baby. Thus, leaving his wealthier boyfriend was a difficult decision to make because of the financial difficulties that he experienced. As I got to know Travis further, he told me that occasionally he had sex for money with "foreigners" he met at local discos. "It was exciting," he said, "to be wanted like that—it makes you feel attractive and good about yourself." One evening, Travis showed up at the disco with a considerably older man (a wealthy foreign businessman). He approached me and smiled as he said, "I'm his 'chaperone' for the weekend." But he was not a "prostitute," he maintained, because he did not do it all the time, and he was really looking for "love that is lasting."

When I first met nineteen-year-old Winston, his appearance was striking. He wore bright purple eye shadow and matching lipstick and nail polish. He also wore a leopard print cowboy hat that looked as if it were out of a Madonna video. Winston, who identified himself with the Owambo ethnic group, had come to live in Katutura to get away from the severe homophobia pervasive in his community in northern Namibia. During an interview, he described his tumultuous journey that brought him to live in Katutura.

My father hated me, sometimes beating me. He is not supporting me anymore. My mother understands [my sexuality], but she cannot do anything because they are men [father and brothers]. My family, when they found out about me, thought I had a mental illness. My father put me in the mental hospital for two months. I remember the psychologist was giving me a pill and injections every day. I do not know what was in it. . . . My parents signed the forms to put me in there. But there was nothing wrong with me except that I was gay. I was locked in a room with only a toilet. I escaped from there and came to TRP. That is where I learned that I was a gay.

My uncle's friend he . . . he was the one who raped me. He is not a gay; he is married. He used a gun and I was stabbed twice. My father wanted to solve the problem in the family . . . but . . . he [the rapist] had pointed the gun at my head and he stabbed me here twice [he shows me the large scar]. Sometimes, I want to go to Owamboland [northern Namibia] to visit my mother, but I cannot because of my father.

As I came to know Winston well, he mentioned that he had taken cocaine on several occasions and was supplied with it by two wealthy gay foreign health practitioners who worked in Windhoek. He also mentioned that, on occasion, he had sex with "butch lesbians," as he called them. "They sometimes would fight over me when I am at the shebeen [he laughs]." Winston maintained that most of the time he practiced safer sex whether it was with men or women. His knowledge of HIV transmission was excellent. However, it was difficult sometimes to practice safer sex because of drugs and "how they made you feel." He stated:

Dagga [marijuana] and cocaine, make you want to do things. Cocaine is very expensive. Sometimes you get it from your partner, usually the rich gay people, especially the white. Some of my friends work on the street. The rich people will take you home and they will give you cocaine and then you give them to your friends to try.

I love to date white men, I think that there is never a white man that is not cute [he said glowingly]. I was involved with a man from the USA. I was involved with him for two years. He was a priest. I was finishing my Standard 10 [grade 8]. I was fifteen years old. I was staying with him at the mission. He liked to have sex. He used to preach in the church and after, when he returned, we would have our sex. When the nuns came around, he pretended to be very holy [Winston laughed loudly].

Dion is a twenty-six-year-old gay man who identified as both Damara and Owambo. He worked in the hospitality industry but made very low wages, despite his long working hours. On his days off, he generally spent his time looking after his daughter and his sister's children. When I first met Dion, he was quite upset over the imminent break-up between him and his boyfriend. After being together for a year, his boyfriend's work contract was completed, and he was, therefore, due to depart for his home in Europe. Dion told me that his partner was very handsome and made good money as a health specialist. He assured me, however, that his "soon-to-be ex-boyfriend" would still help him out financially when he returned home. It was incredibly difficult for Dion to support his mother, sister, and the children on his meager wages.

When asked how he felt about the president's hate speeches, Dion described them as very upsetting: "Because of the homophobic remarks of the president, most of us want to leave here, go to South Africa, to Europe, and those who have the money do."

He also described how his social support circles began to dwindle after the series of announcements were made: "I have been very close to Owambo guys. So they knew I was gay. But after the hate speeches I could see that they were starting to withdraw from me, moving away slowly but surely. Many are cousins to me, but they don't want to be seen with me and go out with me clubbing like they use to."

Dion told me a painful story of when he moved in with his first boyfriend from Katutura:

I was involved with this guy and we went out for more than a year, he would stay at my house, and I would stay over at his. So we said, "Why don't we move in together" . . . and we did. We visited his church. His brother-in-law was also a member of the church, but he did not greet us. In the middle of the ceremony, my lover decided to move up to the front to confess [his homosexuality]. The pastor put his hand on his head and started praying for him. I was still sitting there and I saw his brother-in-law stand up and move towards me. He asked me to get out of the church. I asked "Why?" And he said, "Just get out of the church!" This is during the service! So I got up, I stood up. My lover is in the front confessing and on my way out he [the brother-in-law] picked up a chair and hit me with the chair [breaking the collar bone]. I fell down and I got up again and ran out of the church. I went with my best friend down to the police station and the investigator later

said, "You know why he beat you?" I said no. "Because you are a gay."
To this day the investigator did nothing.

Because of financial burdens, Dion worked for a local informal dating
service where gay foreigners were fixed up with local men. The operator
of this enterprise often held parties in his home for locals and foreigners
where drugs and alcohol were made available. As Dion told me, he had
tried cocaine and "poppers" (nitrite inhalant drugs) with some of his friends
when he went downtown. But, for him, alcohol was the greatest influence
for engaging in unsafe sex: "When you are drunk . . . you won't believe it.
The condom is lying close to you . . . very nearby, but you just don't go and
take it. Maybe even in your pocket but you don't go for it! You just want to
'do-it' and that's it. You are that high when you pick up people at the club
especially."

In follow-up interviews, Dion discussed how one of his former boyfriends
from Katutura had shown extreme physical violence toward him and had
attempted to stab him when he tried to end their relationship. When they
did finally break up, his boyfriend tested positive for HIV. Because Dion had
had unprotected sex with this man, he was fearful of taking an HIV test: "I
hear they say 'take the challenge, go for a test,' but I have made mistakes.
'Cause I believe that if I am positive, every little sore will worry me, even if
I have a normal headache. I believe that people often die from the worry. It
just eats them up and eats them up until they are thin."

Conclusion

As homophobic discourses circulate through Namibian society, local, national, and global ideas of sex are reconstituted within the shifting cultural
identity politics of everyday life. In the Windhoek urban area, safer sex negotiations often break down unevenly for persons in same-sex sexual relationships around notions of gender, class, and ethnicity. In particular, the
wider social scene of gender inequality is replayed during intimate safer sex
negotiations where masculinities dominate feminine forms, placing *moffies*
at great risk for HIV infection. The concealment of same-sex sexual practices, as means of coping with anticipated stigmatization, renders struggles
with discrimination, violence, and sexual harassment invisible. Against this
backdrop of oppression, relationships with foreigners are desired in their
potential for social as well as economic liberation. Such relationships get
appraised at so high a value that unsafe sex may be considered worth the
risk.

Campbell (2003: 185) suggests that "it is vital that long-term measures [that] bring about sweeping social improvements in sexual health, are accompanied by short-term measures." The push by TRP for the legalization of sodomy and the wider recognition of gay and lesbian human rights is paramount to the mitigation of health-related problems in the Rainbow community. However, to effectively address the urgency of the AIDS epidemic, more immediate community-based intervention measures must take place in order to inhibit the spread of HIV through male-male sexual transmission. The difficulty here is in defining "the community." Presently, HIV programming is conducted on an ongoing basis with members who have adequate knowledge of HIV transmission. The question for intervention work remains: how does one reach those men who neither directly associate with TRP nor attend its HIV awareness programs? Including "straight" men in this intervention work poses great difficulty, given the secrecy that surrounds male-male sexual practices in Namibia. Short-term community-level intervention strategies, therefore, must begin to explore how safer sex information can move through such secretive social networks without risking public exposure.

Within the postcolonial context of nation (re)building, the "truth" of Namibian sexuality—as "traditionally heterosexual"—is produced through the silencing of alternative practices and identities. The resulting exclusion of "homosexuality" from Namibian public health translates, in unexpected ways, into local myths of male-male sex as safer sex. Therefore, international and national public health constructions of African sexuality are somehow implicit in the structure of HIV vulnerability for the individuals I came to know.

In this ethnographic study of male-male sexual behavior in Namibia, gaps in public health discourses operate as material forces that produce detrimental effects within local sexual risk-taking perceptions and practices. To redress the invisibility of homosexuality in the health science literature on AIDS in Africa (Phillips 2004), social scientists must further analyze how sexuality is intimately bound up in contemporary moral and political economies. By including long-term and intensive ethnography within methodologies, health researchers working with marginalized and hidden communities can further unravel the complexities of sexuality, culture, and social inequality and rework de-contextualized epidemiologic categories of sexual behavior.

Notes

All names of interviewees in this chapter are pseudonyms.

1. For a discussion of male-male sex and HIV risk among miners in South Africa, see Niehaus (2002). Extending the theories of Campbell (1997) and Moodie and Ndatshe (1994) on masculinity (and sexuality), Niehaus (2002: 79) emphasizes how male-male sexual expression comes through a "renegotiation of pre-existing masculinities."

2. In 2001, I was invited to Namibia to participate as a presenter in an HIV/AIDS research capacity building project involving the University of Namibia, the University of Toronto, and Columbia University (sponsored by the Fogarty Foundation). I began preliminary doctoral fieldwork during this seven-week period. In July 2002, I returned to Namibia, where I continued my ethnographic research until June 2003.

3. The word *moffie*, according to Cage (2003), originated from the slang word "morphy" used by sailors to refer to the transvestite prostitutes working in Cape Town harbor. Among my informants, *moffie* was used more generally to refer to males or females who did not conform to gender conventions. Although this term was frequently used pejoratively by outsiders, the Rainbow community claimed this word as a way to signify community solidarity and resist discrimination.

4. The Nama/Damara word *!gamas* also signified intersexed status, that is, "hermaphroditism" (participants did not consistently define this word). Some participants explained that when they were younger, other children used this word, which referred to a goat or cow that possessed both genitalia, to belittle them. When community elders employed the word *!gamas*, it was generally not meant to be derogatory. *Eshenge* was translated as "gay" in the section of the *Namibian* newspaper written in Oshiwambo. Participants who identified as Owambo referred to *eshenge* as the "traditional word" for homosexuality. For a more extensive documentation of indigenous terms for same-sex practices in Namibia (early-twentieth-century Southwest Africa), see Falk (1998). Many of the words that Falk mentioned were unfamiliar to interviewees or were not considered as relating to gender/desire nonconformity.

5. Social Committee of Gays and Lesbians (SCOG), which existed before the anti-homosexual government announcements, primarily organized local parties and other socials events. After Mugabe's hate speeches in 1995, SCOG gave rise to Gays and Lesbians of Namibia (GLON), which focused on constitutional and legal matters, as homosexuality became the subject of a larger debate in southern Africa. According to former organizers I interviewed in August 2001 and September 2002, GLON quickly dissolved due to a lack of unified vision.

6. These donor agencies included the Swedish International Development Association, the Heinrich Böll Foundation of Germany, and Mama Cash and HIVOS of the Netherlands.

7. There was, however, a highly publicized immigration case involving local activist Elizabeth Khaxas's partner, Liz Frank (former antiapartheid activist and German national). Frank's initial attempt to gain permanent residence in Namibia was rejected on the grounds of her lesbian relationship (Hancox 2000).

8. Although ethnologists may consider Nama and Damara ethnic groups to be distinct in terms of cultural history, my research participants generally conflated the two

on the grounds of linguistic similarity. Both Nama and Damara languages are mutually intelligible dialects of Khoekhoe, a central Khoesaan language (Vossen 1999).

9. The Council of Churches in Namibia (CCN) did eventually support the protection of constitutional rights of gays and lesbians in 2001. However, it has continued to maintain that homosexuality is a sin.

10. Of the thirty-one male participants I interviewed, fourteen were unemployed, ten were employed full time, and seven had part-time employment. However, only four of the ten males employed full time were paid wages that elevated their standard of living above the Namibian poverty level.

11. I conducted a series of workshops with eighty-eight students (sixty female and twenty-eight males) at the University Center for Studies in Namibia (TUCSIN; northern branch). These participants, who identified as "straight," also reported to using oil-based lubricants (Vaseline or hand cream) during anal and vaginal sex.

References Cited

Anonymous. 2000. "Jerry in New Anti-Gay Rant." *Namibian*, October 2.

Appadurai, Arjun. 2001. "Grassroots Globalization and the Research Imagination." In *Globalization*, ed. Arjun Appadurai, 1–21. Durham, N.C.: Duke University Press.

Bailey, Robert C., and Robert V. Aunger. 1995. "Sexuality, Infertility and Sexually Transmitted Disease among Farmers and Foragers in Central Africa." In *Sexual Nature, Sexual Culture*, ed. Paul R. Abramson and Steven D. Pinkerton, 195–222. Chicago: University of Chicago Press.

Bloor, Michael. 1995. *The Sociology of Transmission*. London: Sage.

Bond, George C., John Kreniske, Ida Susser, and Joan Vincent. 1997. *AIDS in Africa and the Caribbean*. Boulder, Colo.: Westview Press.

Cage, Ken. 2003. "From Moffietaal to Gayle—The Evolution of a South African Gay Argot." Paper presented at the International Association for the Study of Sexuality, Culture, and Society, Johannesburg (Sex and Secrecy Conference), June 22–25.

Campbell, Catherine. 1997. "Migrancy, Masculine Identities and AIDS: The Psychosocial Context of HIV Transmission on the South African Gold Mines." *Social Science and Medicine* 45 (2): 273–281.

———. 2001. "Going Underground and Going After Women: Masculinity and HIV Transmission amongst Black Workers on the Gold Mines." In *Changing Men in Southern Africa*, ed. Robert Morrell, 275–286. New York: Zed Books.

———. 2003. *Letting Them Die: How HIV/AIDS Prevention Programmes Often Fail*. Bloomington: Indiana University Press.

Craddock, Susan. 2004. "Beyond Epidemiology: Locating AIDS in Africa." In *HIV/AIDS in Africa: Beyond Epidemiology*, ed. Ezekiel Kalipeni, Susan Craddock, Joseph R. Oppong, and Jayati Ghosh, 1–10. Malden, Mass.: Blackwell.

Donham, Donald L. 1998. "Freeing South Africa: The 'Modernization' of Male-Male Sexuality in Soweto." *Cultural Anthropology* 13 (1): 3–21.

Epprecht, Marc. 1998. "The 'Unsaying' of Indigenous Homosexualities in Zimbabwe: Mapping a Blind Spot in an African Sexuality." *Journal of Southern African Studies* 24 (4): 631–651.

Falk, Kurt. 1998 [1925–1926]. "Homosexuality among the Natives of Southwest Africa." In *Boy-Wives and Female Husbands*, ed. Stephen O. Murray and Will Roscoe, 187–196. New York: Palgrave.

Farmer, Paul. 1992. *AIDS and Accusation: Haiti and the Geography of Blame*. Berkeley: University of California Press.

Gausset, Quentin. 2001. "AIDS and Cultural Practices in Africa: The Case of the Tonga (Zambia)." *Social Science and Medicine* 52: 509–518.

Gevisser, Mark, and Edwin Cameron, eds. 1995. *Defiant Desire: Gay and Lesbian Lives in South Africa*. New York: Routledge.

Hancox, Toni. 2000. *Constitutional and Human Rights Unit Annual Report*. Windhoek, Namibia: Legal Assistance Centre.

Hoad, Neville. 1999. "Between the White Man's Burden and the White Man's Disease." *GLQ: A Journal of Gay and Lesbian Studies* 5 (4): 559–584.

IGLHRC (International Gay and Lesbian Human Rights Commission). 2003. *More Than a Name: State-Sponsored Homophobia and Its Consequences in Southern Africa*. New York: IGLHRC.

Jochelson, Karen. 2001. *The Color of Disease: Syphilis and Racism in South Africa, 1880–1950*. New York: Palgrave.

Katjavivi, Peter, Per Frostin, and Kaire Mbuende, eds. 1989. *Church and Liberation in Namibia*. London: Pluto Press.

Kempadoo, Kamala. 2000. Introduction. In *Sun, Sex and Gold: Tourism and Sex Work in the Caribbean*, ed. Kamala Kempadoo, 3–33. New York: Rowman and Littlefield.

Larvie, Patrick. 1999. "Natural Born Targets: Male Hustlers and AIDS Prevention in Urban Brazil." In *Men Who Sell Sex: International Perspectives on Male Prostitution and HIV/AIDS*, ed. Peter Aggleton, 159–177. Philadelphia: Temple University Press.

LeBeau, Debie, Tom Fox, Heike Becker, and Pempelani Mufune. 1999. *Taking Risks—Taking Responsibility: An Anthropological Assessment of Health Risk Behavior in Northern Namibia*. Windhoek, Namibia: Ministry of Health and Social Services.

Lorway, Robert. 2003. "Inventing Namibian Queer Selfhood in the Era of HIV/AIDS." Paper presented at the International Association for the Study of Sexuality, Culture, and Society, Johannesburg, June 22–25.

Lurie, Peter, with Percy C. Hintzen and Robert A. Lowe. 2004. "Socioeconomic Obstacles to HIV Prevention and Treatment in Developing Countries: The Role of the International Monetary Fund and the World Bank." In *HIV/AIDS in Africa: Beyond Epidemiology*, ed. Ezekiel Kalipeni, Susan Craddock, Joseph R. Oppong, and Jayati Ghosh, 204–212. Malden, Mass.: Blackwell.

Lwanda, John Lloyd. 2004. "Politics, Culture, and Medicine: An Unholy Trinity? Historical Continuities and Ruptures in the HIV/AIDS Story in Malawi." In *HIV/AIDS in Africa: Beyond Epidemiology*, ed. Ezekiel Kalipeni, Susan Craddock, Joseph R. Oppong, and Jayati Ghosh, 29–46. Malden, Mass.: Blackwell.

Maletsky, Christof. 2001. "Madness 'On the Loose,' Says Nujoma." *Namibian*, April 23.

Menges, Werner. 2001. "Rights Group Fears Effects of President's Statements." *Namibian*, April 6.

Ministry of Prisons and Correctional Services. 2000. *Annual Report.* Windhoek: Republic of Namibia.

Moodie, Dunbar T., and Vivienne Ndatshe. 1994. *Going for Gold: Men, Mines, and Migration.* Berkeley: University of California Press.

Moodie, Dunbar T., Vivienne Ndatshe, and British Sibuyi. 1988. "Migrancy and Male Sexuality on the South African Gold Mines." *Journal of Southern Africa Studies* 14 (2): 228–256.

Murray, Stephen O., and Will Roscoe, eds. 1998. *Boy-Wives and Female Husbands: Studies in African Homosexualities.* New York: Palgrave.

Niehaus, Isak A. 2002. "Renegotiating Masculinity in the South African Lowveld: Narratives of Male-Male Sex in Labour Compounds and in Prisons." *African Studies* 61 (1): 77–97.

Palmberg, Mai. 1999. "Emerging Visibility of Gays and Lesbians in Southern Africa: Contrasting Contexts." In *The Global Emergence of Gay and Lesbian Politics: National Imprints of a Worldwide Movement,* ed. Barry D. Adam, Jan Willem Duyvendak, and André Krouwel, 266–292. Philadelphia: Temple University Press.

Phillips, Oliver. 2000. "Constituting the Global Gay: Issues of Individual Subjectivity and Sexuality in Southern Africa." In *Sexuality in the Legal Arena,* ed. D. Herman and C. Stychin, 17–33. London: Athlone Press.

———. 2004. "The Invisible Presence of Homosexuality: Implications for HIV/AIDS and Rights in Southern Africa." In *HIV/AIDS in Africa: Beyond Epidemiology,* ed. Ezekiel Kalipeni, Susan Craddock, Joseph R. Oppong, and Jayati Ghosh, 155–166. Malden, Mass.: Blackwell.

Preston-Whyte, Eleanor, Christine Varga, Herman Oosthuizen, Rachel Roberts, and Frederick Blose. 2000. "Survival Sex and HIV/AIDS in an African City." In *Framing the Sexual Subject: The Politics of Gender, Sexuality and Power,* ed. Richard Parker, Regina Maria Barbosa, and Peter Aggleton, 165–190. Berkeley: University of California Press.

Shivute, Oswald. 2001. "Round-up Gays, Urges Nujoma." *Namibian,* April 2.

Teunis, Niels. 2001. "Same-Sex Sexuality in Africa: A Case Study from Senegal." *AIDS and Behavior* 5 (2): 173–182.

Vaughan, Megan. 1991. *Curing Their Ills: Colonial Power and African Illness.* Cambridge: Polity Press.

Vossen, Rainer, ed. 1999. *The Tonology of Khoekhoe (Nama/Damara).* Cologne, Germany: Rüdiger Köppe.

Wallace, Marion. 2002. *Health, Power and Politics in Windhoek, Namibia, 1915–1945.* Basel, Switzerland: P. Schlettwein.

Walter, M. Bernita. 1996. *Service That Heals: Health Care Services of the Catholic Church in Central and Northern Namibia.* Windhoek, Namibia: Roman Catholic Church.

Webb, Douglas. 1997. *HIV and AIDS in Africa.* Chicago: Pluto Press.

Werbner, Richard. 1996. "Multiple Identities, Plural Arenas." In *Postcolonial Identities in Africa,* ed. Richard Werbner and Terence Ranger, 1–25. London: Zed Books.

10

HIV/AIDS Prevention

Strategies for Improving Prevention Efforts in Africa

ELIZABETH ONJORO MEASSICK

Introduction

This chapter addresses constraints hindering HIV/AIDS prevention in Africa, examines some reasons behind program failures, and lists components for successful HIV/AIDS prevention strategies. It also discusses research needs for developing effective interventions and the role of anthropological research in developing policies to support effective HIV/AIDS interventions. The chapter focuses on HIV prevention in Africa, which presents a unique and daunting array of challenges.

HIV/AIDS prevention issues, especially in Africa, are complex. Working in the HIV/AIDS field has led me to appreciate more fully that nothing is as simple as it looks, and to develop deeper respect for others whose views may differ from my own. It is not a matter of who is right or wrong, but what important lessons each person might bring to the effort. At times, failure is an important contribution toward a more effective course. For example, the continued increase in new HIV infection demonstrates that current prevention strategies need to change. I want to convey my sense of how urgent it is today to work toward a dialogue that moves beyond opinion and personal agendas, toward a course based on what different people understand to be their true needs, and reflecting what works and does not work to prevent HIV/AIDS. To move forward effectively, HIV/AIDS policy should be based on sound scientific evidence.

A central concern and conundrum we face in the fight against HIV/AIDS is the challenge of finding the appropriate prevention strategies and a cure to reduce human suffering and of rekindling the hope for the next generation in the face of AIDS. In order to design effective prevention strategies, we need to incorporate myriad circumstances and a wide range of cultural contexts that are truly complex, even when they appear straightforward and simple. The suggestions presented below address only a few details in the rich kaleidoscope of human cultures and customs. Perhaps paying more attention to some of them might guide us down a more fruitful path.

Current Status of HIV/AIDS

More than a quarter-century into the HIV/AIDS pandemic, there is no cure in sight and no preventive vaccine, and the repeatedly high incidence of infection on every continent continues unabated. At the end of 2003, UN-AIDS (2003a) reports five million new infections globally. Those are exactly the same figures reported in 2002. Does this mean that efforts to reduce new infections in 2002 and 2003 achieved no success? The reality is that current prevention efforts worked earlier on in the epidemic, but in the past few years they have had very little effect on reducing HIV incidence world-wide. Perhaps the disease has changed, calling for new strategies. New and more effective prevention strategies are urgently needed to slow the spread of HIV/AIDS.

Nevertheless, 2003 has brought hope where little existed in the past. The United States' President's Emergency Plan for AIDS Relief (PEPFAR) and the World Health Organization's (WHO) "3 by 5 Initiative" are efforts that generate much hope (UNAIDS 2003c). Successful implementation of the two HIV treatment programs means more infected individuals than ever before stand to gain access to treatment. In addition, the Global Fund to Fight AIDS, Tuberculosis, and Malaria is also currently funding HIV treatment and care. The expansion of treatment will bring many benefits of extended longevity to Africa. With improved life expectancy, many parents stand a better chance to care for their children longer, reducing the number of children being abandoned or moving into orphanages and into the streets. Living longer will also provide time for parents to impart survival skills to their offspring. In addition, communities will be better able to maintain their skilled labor force and economic productivity.

Treatment reduces the rate of infection (Porco et al. 2004). People receiving treatment are less infectious compared to those who are infected but are not receiving antiretroviral treatment. However, even though treatment does reduce the ability to infect others, it does not completely eliminate the virus from the body. As more people get treatment, especially in Africa where HIV drugs are already flooding the black market, there should be caution regarding the possibility of increases in resistance to the medications (Anonymous 2003b; Anonymous 2004a; Redfern 2003). Additionally, the long-term effects of most HIV medications are not yet known. Some of the earlier drugs first offered in the market are now used much less frequently because they cause high liver toxicity and maintain low mutation thresholds. But we do know that many patients no longer have to take twenty or more drugs each day to stay alive.

Even with these serious concerns, we must remain hopeful that the spread of HIV can be overcome somehow and that lessons from the past twenty years can provide insights on how to prevent and treat HIV and AIDS more effectively. With nearly 40 million people currently infected with HIV worldwide, Africa alone saw 3.2 million new infections in 2003 (UNAIDS 2003a). According to Floyd (2003), those under twenty-four years of age are increasingly at risk (Kaiser Daily HIV/AIDS Report 2003). The challenge is clear: Africa must take urgent and dramatic steps to save its future. Its leaders must step up and take the necessary responsibility to fight the spread of HIV/AIDS in their countries.

As a public health professional, I see HIV as a public health issue. As an anthropologist, I see HIV/AIDS as complicated by the cultural reality of human behavior. Tackling the disease requires both cultural and public health understanding. To take it a step further, the disease also needs to be understood in regional, historical, and socioeconomic contexts (UNAIDS 2003b). Obviously, hope for those already infected must be medically driven through treatment and care. Effective prevention, however, has to be rooted in the underlying causes—the dynamics of human behavior, especially sexual practices and drug use.

There is no question that work in the field of HIV/AIDS leaves many medical and public health professionals with few victories, and many families feel frustrated as they face the daily realities of death and despair. Anthropological research—research into patterns of human cultures and customs—can offer insights in the battle against HIV/AIDS. To attain these insights, anthropological discussions regarding human behavior and its effect on health outcomes must transcend the typical discourse of academic anthropology and enter into the wider arena of public health, where it can inform prevention efforts based on sound science. Such research can be a critical component of the knowledge base necessary to inform public policy regarding HIV/AIDS, and to develop more culturally appropriate sustainable and effective prevention and treatment programs capable of halting the advancement of the disease.

A Brief Encounter with Hope and Despair of an African Family Living with HIV/AIDS

In August 2003, as we sat in a small round hut in rural Uganda, the frail proud father introduced us to his three children, a twelve-year-old girl and his two boys, ages seven and five. In the father's eyes, you could sense that we, a transitory group of U.S. professionals visiting HIV programs in Africa, somehow symbolized hope. The sound of our vehicles had spread curiosity among the neighbors; soon his brother-in-law was sitting among us, while the curious eyes of children stared from a distance. This man whose home we were visiting and his wife both have symptomatic HIV disease. The wife is due to start antiretroviral (ARV) therapy soon, but the man must wait until his tuberculosis (TB) is under control. They were both registered in The AIDS Support Organization (TASO) initiative (Anonymous 2004c), which provides them with free tuberculosis treatment, and they will soon start receiving ARV therapy. This man had lost a lot of weight and was obviously very weak. He has been on TB medicine for a month and must continue for a while to get stronger before he can begin ARV therapy. Although he is weak, his determination is evident and his focus clear as he says, "I want to start on ARVs soon, so I can get strength back to take care of my children." His piece of land lay untilled, because of his and his wife's illness. He is not sure how his family will survive until he feels strong enough to get back to work.

The story of this family depicts the hopelessness and economic devastation that accompanies AIDS. Having grown up in a poor rural African village, I empathized with the family's poverty and the importance of their optimism that treatment would help the parents survive to care for their children. Without the hope for ARV therapy, their three children would soon become orphans left to fend for themselves, putting their future at great risk (Anonymous 2003f; Camillo 2003). Combining a life with HIV and the struggles of poverty undoubtedly seems like too much to bear each and every day.

While the man and his wife await treatment, his brother-in-law, like many others in the village, is too scared to get tested. An HIV diagnosis is a status still severely stigmatized even in Uganda, one of Africa's most progressive countries in HIV/AIDS education, prevention, and treatment. The tragedy is that HIV is a preventable disease, and this couple could have been spared this devastating illness. Now their only hope is a lifetime of dependence on ARV therapy, and the benevolence of foreign countries to provide and deliver it at no cost. Meanwhile, infections continue to occur in Uganda, as in many African countries, due to human behaviors: stigma, fear, and lack of knowledge (Anonymous 2002; Nyblade et al. 2003). Regardless of how one looks at it, each new infection is failed prevention.

As I fought back tears while listening to this proud man who spoke in such a humble voice, I could not help telling myself that we have failed to design prevention strategies that effect wide behavior change. Even under their difficult circumstances, this couple is considered lucky, by local standards, because they are part of a select few enrolled under the TASO initiative, while so many others are not.

ARV therapy may or may not prolong the lives of this couple and others like them, but it is the best option currently to respond to HIV infection and AIDS. Unquestionably, the best long-term weapon against HIV/AIDS is prevention, yet we have failed to research and design effective strategies for Africa or any place else, for that matter. Families continue to be torn apart and more children left helpless every day as their parents die, leaving them behind in desperation and abandonment. In the world of HIV/AIDS, prevention means everything to the future of many African, Asian, and European families alike.

Some Constraints Hindering Effective HIV/AIDS Interventions in Africa

Though many conditions and circumstances influence the effectiveness of HIV/AIDS programs, I will look at four main constraints that seem to have a preponderant effect: funding, human and physical infrastructure, political will, and corruption. I use the term "constraints" to refer to the shortcomings within African countries. The lack of funding is often cited as the main problem in instituting programs, yet I question whether this is the most effective way to frame the problem. If this were true, the counterfactual argument would ask, if funding were plentiful throughout the world, would the incidence of HIV be drastically reduced? Would prevention be effective? Is lack of adequate funding the main cause for the rise in new HIV and sexually transmitted disease (STD) infections (Hall et al. 2003) experienced in the United States in 2003?

Funding

Funding for HIV/AIDS services is limited worldwide. The AIDS Drug Assistance Program (ADAP) in the United States has limited funds, and many states currently have waiting lists for program coverage (Southern States AIDS/STD Directors Work Group 2003). This is in a country where health care, funding, and delivery systems are considered among the world's best. Even with all these resources, HIV infection rates continue to increase in the United States. So, while limited funding is an important constraint, there is more that explains consistent increases of HIV transmission and high prevalence. Other important factors must be at play in hindering effective HIV prevention in the United States, Africa, and the rest of the world. Understanding these factors is important in designing more effective prevention strategies.

Many countries in Africa are poor and maintain small health budgets that must address all infectious diseases: the recent polio outbreak in Nigeria, the yearly measles and meningitis outbreaks in Kenya, schistosomiasis in Egypt and Sudan, and malaria and tuberculosis, which are endemic throughout sub-Saharan Africa (Anonymous 2003g; Mwaniki 2003). These diseases put a strain on health budgets of African countries. Additional external funding is necessary to assist efforts to confront the HIV/AIDS issue. Improving funding availability is highly necessary for prevention endeavors to effectively reach rural populations, and for treatment, especially in the purchase and distribution of drugs. However, lessons from Uganda, Senegal, Botswana, and South Africa demonstrate that the availability of funding in and of itself does not necessarily translate into effective HIV intervention or reduction of incidence. Botswana, one of the richest countries in Africa, has also received generous international funding in addition to its own significant national health budget. Yet its HIV rates remain at an all-time high, with poor prevention strategies in place and relatively few individuals receiving treatment.

Uganda, on the other hand, has been able to implement effective prevention strategies from early on in the epidemic with little funding, achieving one of the greatest reductions in infection rates in Africa (Allen 2002; Hogle et al. 2002). According to Low-Beer (2003), Uganda's effective prevention program cost U.S.$21.7 million over a five-year period, because its elements focused on aspects of cultural dynamics in sexual behavior and investing in good public health practices. Having fewer partners, delayed sexual debut, and condoms were the cornerstones of Uganda's prevention strategy. The strategy is currently known as ABC ("Abstinence," "Be faithful," and "Condoms"). Also, Senegal has been able to implement effective prevention strategies, through delaying sexual debut and reducing the number of partners (Anonymous 2003e; USAID 2003).

With careful investment in measures that enhance safety of the blood supply and mobilization of communities through mass education, Senegal has been able to minimize HIV incidence, keeping infection rates at one of the lowest levels on the continent (Anonymous 2003e). Compound the severe lack of funding in Africa with poor political leadership, mediocre infrastructure, conditions of extreme poverty, corruption, and political and economic instability, and it becomes apparent that as much as funding is a critical aspect, solely focusing on its scarcity will not help make progress toward HIV prevention.

Political Will

The national political leaders of Senegal and Uganda took a different view of the HIV/AIDS pandemic to overcome their scarce resource base. Since they did not have abundant resources, financial or otherwise, to pursue treatment or commercialized prevention as the immediate response, they recognized locally based prevention as the best alternative. They saw strong leadership as a central component in the fight against HIV/AIDS. Despite the cultural traditions of polygyny and early marriage in the population, the leadership in these countries built a program based on abstinence, being faithful, and condom usage, but with primary emphasis on A and B, rather than C (Singh et al. 2003). This strategy has resulted in behavior change when compared to countries like Botswana, where financial resources are much more abundant, making commercial prevention of HIV/AIDS through condom promotion possible. The difference between Botswana and Uganda is the end result of prevention efforts. Exclusive promotion of the condom as preventing HIV infection has proved less effective, while condoms linked to abstinence and being faithful have produced demonstrable results (Hearst and Chen 2003; Low-Beer and Stoneburner 2003).

Ugandan and Senegalese political leadership focused their prevention efforts on mobilizing local resources within the public sector, private enterprise, and civil society to build local capacity for prevention through education in schools, churches, and other social organizations in rural communities. This meant all sectors of society were going to have a conversation about HIV/AIDS. In Uganda, President Yoweri Museveni himself led this conversation and instituted an effective social dialogue about prevention strategy by making trips to rural communities and talking to village and church leaders about HIV/AIDS and what they needed to do to prevent it (Anonymous 2003d). Some examples of the mobilization outcomes are depicted through the effective work of the Ministry of Education, faith-based organizations (FBOs), and community-based organizations (CBOs).

A health official in one of the fifteen PEPFAR countries once noted, "My country has an excellent strategy for HIV prevention and treatment.

We are just waiting to get some money to implement it" (Onjoro 2003b). I then asked if they had mobilized the rural communities, churches, and schools, and what role the government was currently playing to work with these groups to take the lead on prevention. What if external funding were not available? Does that mean the government will never do anything? He looked at me as if I were talking about some bizarre strategy. I told him about a national strategy for building local capacities for HIV care. I proceeded to comment that African countries are not taking the necessary responsibility toward HIV prevention by doing simple things like building local capacities (for example, mobilizing local women's groups, traditional healers, local men's groups, youth groups, churches, market gatherings) to talk about HIV/AIDS in contexts that do not necessarily require massive funding. The Ugandan experience demonstrates that building local capacity does not require substantial funding or waiting for foreign aid to support health systems. It takes creativity and resourcefulness to build sustainable programs directed by committed leaders with a strong message to drive behavioral change.

Success in Uganda and Senegal and recent efforts in initial stages in Kenya and Zambia demonstrate that effective and committed political leadership must accompany funding in order to bring about successful prevention programs. The advantage political leadership lends is the ability to unify the country and communities behind local health needs and to align resources, both national and international, in building the infrastructure to address HIV/AIDS. HIV is a highly stigmatized disease, and if government officials speak openly about it, the rest of the country is better able to have public and private discourse about the disease. Political leadership is critical in setting an agenda to fight HIV/AIDS or any health crisis. While the Ugandan experience demonstrates that bold leadership is key to effective prevention and fighting stigma, the poor political leadership in Kenya or South Africa has shown how the lack of such bold leadership can lead to many lives lost to HIV/AIDS. Hopefully, the recent changes in HIV/AIDS policy in both Kenya and South Africa can be maintained and expanded so lives will be spared. Authentic and effective political leadership must be sought, developed, and nurtured to set a platform for effectively fighting HIV/AIDS.

Infrastructure

Of equal importance in stemming the HIV pandemic is the need for an accessible and efficient health infrastructure. The availability of funding and strong political leadership fosters the likelihood of building the necessary infrastructure and network to support HIV/AIDS initiatives. Almost all African countries lack sufficient infrastructure to fully support HIV prevention and treatment. Infrastructure spans the entire public health system, including education and health communications processes. It includes medical facilities—clinics, hospitals, adequate laboratories, and pharmacies—and the necessary personnel—doctors, nurses, nurse practitioners, social workers, lab technicians, health management professionals, counselors, and family support professionals. Infrastructure also includes building local capabilities and systems to support prevention and palliative care initiatives through training and education in rural sectors of society. Even Uganda, a country way ahead of other African nations in its prevention and treatment programs, has yet to provide treatment for half of its patients or to reduce stigma in all sectors of society (Coutinho 2003).

While Uganda has managed to develop effective and simple community HIV care reaching some rural parts of the country, many African countries are far from demonstrating such progress. The competing health demands from regular polio, malaria, measles, or meningitis outbreaks means that HIV care does not receive the attention it requires. Even South Africa, with the best medical facilities on the African continent, still lags behind instituting effective HIV prevention and treatment infrastructure. HIV treatment centers are concentrated in large cities, leaving the rural population with poor and very limited access to voluntary counseling and testing (VCT) or treatment facilities.

Political leadership is necessary to provide coordination of national strategies for responding to HIV/AIDS and to ensure that donor funds and activities adequately address local HIV/AIDS with the requisite effectiveness. Building appropriate infrastructure will also call for coordination and the encouragement of partnerships within and between countries in all HIV care facilities, both private and public. Political leadership is essential to establish and implement a national internal oversight entity for effective provision of care to ensure that all citizens who need HIV care, orphan services, or palliative care receive it. Building infrastructure that caters to HIV and other pressing infectious diseases calls for shifting from reactive care to actively pursuing a preventive primary health care model, as recommended in the 1978 Declaration of Alma Ata (Anonymous 1978). Such an undertaking, however, requires a coordinated effort between donors and countries for the efficient use of both local and foreign aid funding to minimize corruption by instituting administrative platforms to ensure transparency in expenditures and clear accountability.

Corruption

The new infusion of funding for HIV treatment to begin in 2004 from the U.S. government faces serious risks due to weak governance capacities of recipient nations. Their inability to prevent corruption creates important constraints for HIV program delivery. Corruption has made it impossible for many African officials to put the needs of their nations before personal greed and interest. Corruption too often forms part of the fabric of many African political government entities. This is a taboo subject, often dealt with indirectly and timidly in the discourse of international organizations, which has made it very difficult for foreign entities to develop transparent and honest collaborations with the countries they fund.

There is corruption, and then there is what I call organized corruption: multiple layers of donor funding being swindled at various levels of government, often involving top government officials. The British and U.S. ambassadors to Kenya recently sent a strong message to Kenyan authorities regarding endemic corruption within the current government (Teyie and Agina 2004). The Goldenberg scandal (Karanja 2003) in Kenya provides a good example of organized corruption. The scandal, which involved cabinet members, government lawyers, top bank officials, and others, was a compensation scheme ostensibly designed to promote exports of precious metals. The scheme authorized the withdrawal of millions of dollars from the Kenyan Central Bank. With over $720 million missing, the alleged thieves have yet to be charged or funds recovered (Anonymous 2003c). Nigeria and South Africa have also faced these types of scandals. In most cases, the supposed corrupt accountant is fired as a punishment. Meanwhile, the funds simply disappear, perpetrators often continue free with impunity, and none of the planned outcomes are achieved.

Another example involving HIV funding is the scandal recently revealed in Kenya concerning its National AIDS Council (NAC), funded by the Global Fund. While many rural areas went without proper HIV education, and VCT sites and government hospitals were operating with poor equipment, the NAC executive director received a monthly salary of U.S.$29,000 (equivalent to about 2 million Kenyan shillings). Her stipulated salary, however, was supposed to be U.S.$4,000 a month (about 300,000 Kenyan shillings) (Agina 2003; Muriuku 2003). Receiving $29,000 a month for this kind of a position is unheard of in any job market in Kenya. Soon after this discovery and the subsequent firing of the executive director, it was also revealed that NAC was funding fictitious agencies, one of which paid for her inflated salary. Though the executive director was fired, the money she squandered has yet to be recovered, and she has yet to face any charges.

While this is only one example, the question it raises is how it was possible that the Kenyan government and the Global Fund did not have adequate safeguards established to immediately detect such aberrations of trust. It also raises the question of how many other acts of corruption involving HIV funding are going undetected, while people living with AIDS continue to die daily due to lack of basic HIV services. The loss of funding through corruption is a serious constraint to the success of HIV/AIDS funding. Without proper mechanisms to ensure accountability, it will continue to be difficult for Kenya, and many other African countries, to achieve the desired outcomes of HIV/AIDS interventions with or without Western donations. Western nations have been criticized, and often rightly so, for having too many strings attached to foreign aid money. Such strings often create dependency relationships and collusion. On the other hand, in cases where dependency is minimized, program outcomes are often embedded with local corruption. Of these two shortcomings, dependency and corruption, local corruption poses the worst impediment to program outcomes.

It is beyond the scope of this chapter to explore the causes and strategies for dealing with corrupt practices in public programs. The point here is to call attention to corruption and other constraints as common examples adversely affecting HIV/AIDS initiatives. Internal constraints are compounded by problems arising from HIV/AIDS international agencies' policies and practice.

Some Important Reasons behind HIV/AIDS Program Failures

From my viewpoint (Onjoro 2001) and that of many other social scientists, the main reason for HIV/AIDS program failures in Africa is embedded in the direct importation and imposition of a Western health development model as the solution to the health problems of African nations. The main problem lies with the fact that the Western models by design tend to ignore the cultural realities and strengths, history, and philosophical reality of African people (Airhihenbuwa 1995; Green 2003; Janzen and Green 2003; Kwame 1995; Makinde 1988; Masolo 1994; Onjoro 2003a; Purcell and Onjoro 2002). A second problem arises from the fact that Western efforts are poorly coordinated within the country, making it impossible to consolidate resources and avoid duplication and unnecessary overhead expenses.

Most HIV/AIDS foreign aid programs ignore empirical evidence of African philosophical beliefs that drive health behavior and healing practices.

The validity of African philosophy, indigenous knowledge, and worldviews in directing cognitive perception, and the consequent action, has been explored by philosophers such as Alcoff and Potter (1993), Gyekye (1995), Williams and colleagues (1994), and Wiredu (1995), and by social scientists such as Airhihenbuwa (1995) and Antweiler (1998).

For example, Africans' perceptions of health and illness affect their health-seeking behavior. In general, most Africans do not attend health screenings to simply affirm that they are in good health. They rush to hospitals almost exclusively in the face of an emergency or obvious sickness. Thus, it is not surprising that Africans do not flock to VCT centers unless they have reason to suspect HIV infection or the onset of AIDS. The strategy of convincing HIV-infected, but otherwise healthy, Africans to attend HIV testing, learn their status, and ultimately adopt more responsible sexual behavior needs to be formulated based on how they perceive health and healing from their own cultural viewpoint. Health screenings are popular in Western societies, but we should not forget that even there the practice has flourished only recently and after a few decades of investments. Proper understanding of African perceptions concerning health and healing is basic to designing effective HIV prevention strategies.

Lack of interest in attending biomedical screenings does not mean that Africans do not indulge in daily or frequent traditional health maintenance. They do through traditional healing. Use of various preventive herbal treatments is common in many families. I remember when growing up, my grandmother made us drink a bitter herb made from a plant we called *mafua*. In her healing concept, *mafua* cured everything from stomachaches to sniffles. When we got sick or complained of congestion, my grandmother's first action of choice was to make us drink *mafua*, not to take us to the local clinic. You can imagine how many times her grandchildren had to drink it. In fact, at times we denied being sick just to avoid the nasty taste of drinking *mafua*. Oddly enough, the leaves of that same plant are also used as the most popular local toilet tissue paper.

A few times a year, for the sake of prevention and for no other apparent reason, she would cover us with a blanket for about thirty minutes sitting over a hot pot steaming of this herbal medicine. After one of us was done, she would replenish the pot content and move on to the next child. Each one of us dreaded our turn. To this day, I do not know what she had in the pot. However, I do not remember our being sick often or being taken to the doctor for anything serious. My grandmother, like many Africans, employed a prevention strategy without engaging causation or targeting a particular illness. On the contrary, the biological routes of HIV infection are now well understood and can be directly targeted for prevention. The point is: Africans do have their own well-developed strategies of maintaining good health based on their own cultural understanding of health, illness, and healing that does not necessarily include biomedical understanding, explanations, and screenings. It would make sense to build Western program initiatives around culturally appropriate health practices and beliefs (Castro and Marchand-Lucas 2000; Cernea 1991; Dei 1992; Galanti 1991; Hahn 1995; Imperato 1977).

Like many past health development endeavors, most HIV/AIDS programs and policies implemented in Africa are based on Western cultural ideas and assumptions of prevention and sexual behavior. For example, until the beginning of 2003 most of the prevention work by the U.S. Agency for International Development (USAID) and Centers for Disease Control and Prevention (CDC) focused on the abundant distribution of condoms: strategies targeting what were considered to be high-risk groups—in the Western perception. This prevention strategy perceives sex only as a mechanical act and not also as a complex behavioral practice embedded in cultural beliefs, values, and practices. Western prevention strategies hence focused on sex workers, truck drivers, and drug users, reflecting a similar emphasis in Western countries. While I recognize that truck drivers and drug users need to be targeted and should receive attention for prevention, they are not the group most at risk in Africa for HIV infection. Based on Western notions of what constitutes high risk, programs have focused on teaching sex workers to use safer sex, or encouraging them to give up sex work all together. There is no question that safer sex should be promoted among truck drivers and sex workers; however, I see the most at-risk group in Africa as the heterosexual family in both polygynous and monogamous marriages.

Efforts should be made toward understanding the root causes of high rates of HIV infection in Africa. For example, poverty forces the low-income segment of society into temporary migratory patterns to and from sugar factories or mines, where new liaisons are formed and the virus is passed back and forth. Epidemiologic research sets the tone for prevention interventions in early years, with little behavioral research. My concern is that to date, very little effort has been put toward behavioral research to identify effective strategies on how to target the most at-risk group in Africa—the heterosexual couple or polygynous unit.

Health development, like other forms of development, "is caught up in a clash of philosophical ideals. With only limited exceptions, in both the literature and in practice, development has come to mean a replication of the West. . . . The equalization of development with Westernization impeded the construction of an authentic development theory" (Baeck 1988). On the one hand, there is the underlying assumption that poor nations should mimic the path to progress enjoyed by the West. At the other end of the spectrum lies the cultural reality of local communities in the developing world. This conflict between Western and developing nations' ideals provides only a part of the context needed to understand the evolution of an encompassing comprehensive and effective health development model. The remaining contextual information lies with the competing agendas of the key stakeholders in the process—those agencies and governments that control funding, and hence set the agendas for development process and determine the direction of progress, including the role local communities play (Dewalt 1999; Sillitoe 1998).

Another ignored but detrimental factor fueling HIV infection is the "sugar daddy" (Anonymous 2003a; Luke and Kurz 2002). A sugar daddy is an older man who engages in one or more sexual relationships with young girls, some of whom are still in primary or high school, in exchange for gifts and cash. If infected with HIV, the young girl may, in turn, infect her age-mate lover. Targeting the so-called Western high-risk groups, while ignoring the principal modes of HIV infection within the African population, misjudges the role heterosexual practices play in fueling HIV infection.

Like the national HIV prevention strategy of the United States, the massive social-marketing promotion of condom use undertaken by USAID and WHO through the end of 2002 is a good example of cultural incompatibility in HIV prevention policy. Even as ABC prevailed in Uganda and studies substantiated this approach, Western agencies ignored such success and continued on their charted course, focusing on Western notions of risk groups and condoms as the primary means of prevention. There is no doubt that the use of condoms helps to prevent HIV. However, focusing exclusively on condoms as the main prevention strategy has failed miserably in Africa, and continues to be debated, even in the U.S. prevention platform. Condoms were aggressively promoted in Botswana and made available in rural villages, yet the incidence of HIV infection continued to rise at alarming rates.

During a trip to Botswana in 2003, a representative from the Ministry of Health stated to our delegation that the country was once again launching another massive condom promotion strategy in the country, installing 10,000 condom machines in various parts of the country. The condom distribution strategy was not effective the first time. I am not sure why the government thinks it is going to reduce the incidence this time. To me, this was a clear sign how perceiving HIV prevention in the Western sense as a mechanical act fails to generate results in the country. When the Washington, D.C., Health Department recently announced it was planning to have condoms available in every public place, the idea raised heated and interesting debates among parents, teachers, youth, religious, and advocacy groups. The question is, why has U.S. taxpayer money been used for years to promote the same strategy in Africa without any debate whatsoever? For over a decade, I seldom heard or read of anyone calling into question the validity and morality of such a strategy. Many of these programs are still operating, despite their ineffectiveness, sinking taxpayer money with no tangible success, yet nobody is marching in the streets in protest of these wasted resources.

Condoms can be forced on Africans, but expecting condoms to work as they might in other cultural settings is proving to be a different story. There is stigma in African societies attached to the use of condoms, and this is a rare consideration for argument in the HIV/AIDS debates. Condoms, in addition to preventing transmission of HIV, also inhibit procreation, which is highly valued and the main reason for marriage in Africa (Maillu 1988). By way of example, a mother of four in her midthirties who lived in my village became very upset when her husband suggested she should consider using birth control to avoid having more children. Her argument was, "I am still young and my eggs fresh; why should I stop having children?" Having a house full of children and a big family are more important to a majority of Africans than the economic burden raising many children might pose. HIV prevention strategies that hinder the process of procreation should be designed with the local people at the table if a high level of adherence is the ultimate goal. Initiatives that seek strong community participation are often more effective and sustainable (Annis and Hakim 1988; Blanchard 1988; Galtung 1974; Taylor and Mackenzie 1987, 1992).

Despite its vital role in HIV prevention, I see several faults with a condom-focused strategy of prevention. Condom-focused prevention is a narrow and limiting approach. Condoms may be perceived as risk free; they allow the user to have sex with multiple partners and still feel protected. They take away individual responsibility for making hard personal choices, such as being faithful to a partner, delaying sexual debut, or becoming monogamous. Condoms are male centered. A man has to use a condom, and this does not give women any control over HIV prevention. It excludes other forms of prevention, like abstinence and fidelity, to those who prefer these choices. In addition, despite massive promotion, the effectiveness of condoms and the likelihood that they will be used properly 100 percent of the time in order to achieve the desired prevention outcome are still matters of intense debate. Africans have the ability to make their own rational choices if provided with appropriate and correct information and education about a disease and various alternatives choices. They should be presented with an array of prevention options and sufficient education to make informed choice. Decisions affecting their lives should be made with them and not for them.

For two decades, condoms were the main strategy for HIV prevention recommended to many African countries—the C part of ABC. In the United States, many see the A and B parts of the ABC strategy as controversial and rather limiting the natural human need for a broad and diversified enjoyment of safe sexual encounters. Abstinence and being faithful are thus associated with repressive, judgmental, and sex-negative ideologies. Instead, these opponents emphasize the rhetorical aspects of abstinence and being faithful, focusing on morality issues. Abstinence or delaying sexual debut until one is mature enough to make responsible personal choices about sex is and can be beneficial for straights and gay men alike. Equally, faithfulness or partner reduction is healthy and beneficial to relationships, regardless of one's sexual orientation. Rotello (1997) was clear on this message after witnessing many of his gay friends get infected through multipartnering and die. The argument against abstinence or being faithful does not have any scientific substantiation and ignores the few but growing number of strong supporters in the United States. A lot of gay men and lesbians believe in monogamy and abstinence, while many more do not. The issue is making many choices available to everyone. We need broad, culturally appropriate prevention strategies designed and tailored to African cultures, especially in countries where there are financial limitations to purchase condoms.

HIV/AIDS programs also fail because they are adversely affected by poor collaboration among Western donor agencies on the ground. Without proper coordination and focus, programs financed through multiple agencies and organizations may continue to produce very limited results. Most of the work conducted by Western donors, through USAID, CDC, the Global Fund, or WHO, are implemented with little interagency or donor collaboration. This is the case in several countries, such as Kenya, Botswana, and South Africa. For example, in Uganda, where the CDC, the U.S. embassy, and USAID work closely together, one can see different results in program outcomes. In other countries where this is not the case, programs are scattered and poorly coordinated.

During my visit to Kenya in August 2003, it was disappointing to discover that USAID and CDC operate as totally separate and divergent programs in terms of their physical location and efforts on the ground. No one at the U.S. embassy could clearly explain to me what each of the two agencies was doing in Kenya. I had to visit each agency separately to learn of its activities. The CDC's Global AIDS Program (GAP) in the country seemed fairly well organized; however, the USAID office could not provide me with one updated report on its current efforts in Kenya. Nor was it broadly knowledgeable of what GAP was doing. Such fragmentation makes working with foreign agencies quite cumbersome and creates the likelihood of duplication of services and efforts. If donor agencies originating from the same country cannot collaborate among themselves, how do we expect collaboration between donor countries with similar development interests and actions in each country?

Components of Successful HIV/AIDS Prevention Strategies in Africa

Now that I have examined some factors that are not beneficial for HIV/AIDS initiatives in Africa, I want to focus on how such programs might be successful in the future. In addition to securing appropriate funding and committed political leadership, effective HIV/AIDS interventions need to build on the knowledge integration model; focus on preserving the African family; explore beneficial and important cultural aspects that can promote less risky sexual behaviors and integrate them as part of the prevention strategy process; promote poverty reduction strategies to boost family incomes; incorporate traditional healers and national and regional political leadership; and build partnerships between civil, public, and private entities. But ultimately, interventions must be "people driven"; in other words, they must be designed with the local people at the table as part of the planning and implementation decision-making processes (Ayittey 2003; Onjoro 2003a; Purcell and Onjoro 2000).

Effective HIV/AIDS programs should be based on the balanced integration of Western scientific and local knowledge systems. Several authors, including myself, have addressed the issue of knowledge integration as an approach critical for program development and sustainability (Ayittey 2003; Emery 2000; Onjoro 2003a; Purcell and Onjoro 2002). Decades of poor outcomes have demonstrated the need and value for integrating local and foreign knowledge in the development of applied international programs, through allowing communities to get involved and take partial ownership for defining problems and identifying solutions to them. Development of HIV/AIDS interventions is no exception. Uganda's and Senegal's successes demonstrate the validity of local knowledge integration in building sustainable HIV/AIDS programs.

Better success can be achieved if HIV/AIDS prevention is built around strengthening and producing healthy African families. So far, HIV prevention has not focused on making polygyny (a fundamental African custom) a safer sex environment. Instead of building prevention around it, polygyny is perceived as a root cause of HIV transmission that should be stamped out. The question I would like to see asked is what role must polygyny play in HIV prevention? As an African, I strongly believe this inclusion of polygyny as a positive force in HIV prevention must be done, and it can be done more efficiently than by focusing on the elimination of polygynous behavior. Senegal, a Muslim culture with acceptance of up to four wives, has one of the lowest rates of HIV/AIDS infections in Africa. This does not mean that the fundamental cultural beliefs necessarily need to change, though in some cases they may need to evolve for survival. It does imply that cultures must adapt to the reality of AIDS by creating alternative ways to think about sexuality in order to bring about behavioral change.

Cultures always change, and it is people who change them. Making the right personal choices to survive HIV/AIDS will induce important changes in African cultures that will conserve their essence and make a healthy life possible. External change agents should be facilitators and not the decision makers of this self-sustaining process, providing scientific knowledge and relevant information in an appropriate way so that people in local communities can make better decisions about sexual behavior and achieve more understanding about themselves in the context of HIV/AIDS.

Although many African families today are nuclear families (constituted by parents and children only) in structure, sexual interactions and dynamics of adults in them have not been sufficiently researched or understood to provide insight for prevention strategies. HIV programs downplay the role played by extramarital sex between adult women and men and between sugar daddies and young females in the spread of HIV infection in Africa (Epstein 2004; Gisselquist and Potterat 2003). The diversity of cultural norms and customs that shape African sexual practices has not been explored and incorporated as part of HIV prevention programs. These sexual practices need to be understood within the context of the nuclear family and polygyny, and the findings employed in designing prevention programs.

I have seen only anecdotal evidence of prevention programs targeting intergenerational sexual relationships—for instance, in Uganda and Botswana. However, such prevention issues have not been the subject of substantial prevention research efforts. Thus, little is being done to research the dynamics of these behaviors and how they can be addressed to reduce HIV infection among youth, single men and women, and adult married couples. In addition, prevention should seek to address some of the socio-economic needs that foster the spread of HIV/AIDS, while encouraging behavior change toward less risky behaviors where family survival depends on such income. HIV prevention programs must work together with other international organizations like the United Nations Development Program, the World Food Program, the World Bank, and other donors in crafting viable strategies that link economic and health outcomes.

HIV prevention models in Africa must seek to involve the traditional health system and its practitioners as well (Ayittey 2003; Green 2003; Janzen and Green 2003; Onjoro 2003a). With training, traditional healers can expand HIV prevention and treatment efforts, and their health care system can be incorporated as education, information, testing, home health care, and palliative care sites. Traditional healers are the entry point to a health system for many Africans, hence the involvement of traditional healers could mean getting more people tested and referred to HIV care sooner rather than later (Kaiser Daily HIV/AIDS Report 2003; Onjoro 2001).

Any prevention effort should seek to involve public, private, and civic society at the national and local levels. Involving all three sectors means forging the teamwork and a comprehensive approach for building new capacities needed to combat the spread of HIV/AIDS. It also ensures that messages about HIV/AIDS are consistent and widespread throughout all sectors of society. Building effective prevention strategies for Africa will mean Western development agencies must learn to change the way they usually do business, relinquish some control, and accept sharing project control with local communities.

Research Needs for Developing More Effective HIV/AIDS Policies and Intervention in Africa

Considering the nature of the obstacles to effective HIV/AIDS prevention, perhaps it is time to expand investment in social science research to more fully explore the dynamics of HIV/AIDS within different cultural milieus. Key research needs should include: culturally appropriate models of prevention; dynamics of sexual behaviors, including generational sex and sex within polygynous and monogamous marriages; local strengths and resources that can be mobilized and enriched for more effective HIV prevention, treatment, and palliative care—home-based care and hospice care.

The battle against HIV/AIDS must be fought on two fronts simultaneously; treatment and prevention efforts need to go hand in hand. Research on new drugs is crucial and must be supported to keep HIV treatment a viable option for those already infected, especially in the face of increasing drug resistance to ARV therapy. Likewise, it is important to identify ways to reduce new HIV infections through understanding the culturally driven risk behaviors that fuel its spread. The steady increase in new HIV infections all over the world (UNAIDS 2003a) demonstrates that past prevention strategies have lost their zest and that many people at risk for HIV infection are becoming complacent, especially with the promise of effective treatment. We cannot continue to witness the rise in HIV incidence and hope to eradicate this disease without implementing radically different strategies that are effective. We need new and effective models for HIV prevention in Africa. The Ugandan ABC model has had encouraging success with locally based models, especially in comparison to results of alternative strategies that focus on Western perceptions of high-risk behaviors to which massive condom distribution efforts have been directed. However, while some aspects of the Ugandan model are worth replicating, we cannot assume it will have the same level of success in other parts of Africa without local adaptation. Local adaptation for appropriateness is of critical importance. Identifying through substantive local research what combination of preventive strategies, including the ABC model, work best in other parts of Africa provides a scientific foundation for building more sustainable programs.

A one-size-fits-all Western approach to development has proven it can only achieve limited and brief success in program effectiveness and should not be encouraged in HIV/AIDS care, prevention, or treatment. Focused practical research should be conducted in diverse cultural settings on an ongoing basis to identify and test approaches and models that address true needs of different ethnic and language groups, and the varying needs of men, women, and youth within those groups. The research should not only investigate new approaches, messages, and models, but also develop strategies with local people on how the new models can be incorporated as effective prevention strategies in each cultural setting. This is not to suggest dressing the same old models in new clothes, but rather changing the fundamental paradigms on which these models are based (Brewer et al. 2003). A lion in sheep's clothing is still a lion and not a sheep. New paradigms would be based on knowledge integration that fully involves the participation of local people, flexibility that tailors programs to different cultural and socioeconomic settings, and the capacity to nurture program innovations as needed to improve effectiveness.

Besides developing intervention models, it is necessary to launch new studies that bring a fresh understanding of the dynamics governing African sexual behavior. While several anthropologists have studied African sexuality during the mid-twentieth century, new social and economic changes have influenced many aspects of African cultures in significant ways in the twenty-first century. Sexual dynamics have changed dramatically in various geographic regions during the last forty years and will continue to change in the United States, Africa, and other parts of the world. New studies and data are now necessary to better understand the new complexities of African sexual behavior and dynamics and how HIV prevention can be effectively introduced targeting specific desired behavioral changes. Modernization of sexuality, marital relations, economic liberalization, social organization, technology, and communications has played an important role in forcing those changes, and social actors must find new and creative ways to address specific strategies that will inform primary and secondary prevention. The active engagement and involvement of Africans and their leaders in understanding and analyzing these issues should become an essential part of the paradigms used by researchers.

Even though it seems quite obvious, investing in research looking at the dynamics of how HIV is actually transmitted in Africa is urgently needed. Surprisingly, this has been seriously neglected. In the long run, developing strategies to address cultural behaviors promoting the spread of HIV is much more cost efficient and logical than investing in the massive distribution of condoms.

Another area that should receive research attention is understanding and identifying local cultural and noncultural strengths and resources, and how they can be mobilized by the communities themselves to build capacity for HIV prevention, palliative care, and care for orphans. Any research done locally must involve close collaboration with indigenous leadership. There is no question that AIDS has devastated many African communities, and they want it to just go away. Gandhi once said, "You must be the change you wish to see in the world" (Anonymous 2004b). Africans must be part of the change they wish for by actively engaging in the fight against HIV at the grassroots level. Local strengths and resources include: local healers and their specialties, and their current level of knowledge about HIV; local knowledge regarding health and healing; what neighbors know and can do about HIV; social groups and organizations and their institutional capacities; local social and political networks, and their capabilities; and local family networks. African communities must be empowered to exert greater responsibility for the survival of their families, even if it means changing aspects of their cultural norms.

Another crucial area of research is identifying how to reduce the stigma that continues to fuel HIV infection and negatively affects the lives of those already infected (Nyblade et al. 2003). "Breaking the Silence" (Kinyua 2001), a booklet about Kenyan families coping with HIV/AIDS, clearly demonstrates the depth of stigma in communities and the need to determine how to diffuse it. Social stigma generates fear and shame, which inhibits acceptance of HIV-positive status. Under these conditions, denial and ignorance prevail, and those infected do not assume responsibility for their sexual behavior; do not seek testing, care, or treatment; and often continue to infect others. Destigmatization strategies need to be developed through understanding the cultural dynamics behind stigmatization.

Although much is known about the biological causes of HIV infection, such as unprotected sex and blood transfusions, the continued increase in new infection demonstrates that strategies to reduce incidence must be sought through further understanding of behaviors that promote infection. In addition to cultural factors, political, economic, and environmental factors also contribute to the spread of HIV. Anthropological research can be of value in understanding the dynamics of sexual behaviors in these different contexts in order to develop more nuanced strategies.

The Value of Anthropological Research in Policy Making for the Fight against HIV/AIDS in Africa

Social scientists looking at risk factors and routes of transmission of HIV/ AIDS have made significant contributions to HIV research (Aggleton 1996; Bolton and Orozco 1994; Glick-Schiller et al. 1994; Leap and O'Connor 1993; Norr et al. 1996; Preston-White 1995; Sweat and Denison 1995). Others have explored issues surrounding human behavior and cultural environment and how they influence risk behavior (Ajzen and Fishbein 1980; Becker and Joseph 1988; Frankenberg 1995; McGrath et al. 1993; Schoepf 1991, 1995; Streefland 1995; Weeks et al. 1993). At the 2003 Society for Applied Anthropology annual meeting, several research papers were presented related to HIV/AIDS (Anonymous 2004b). Research and reports by several social scientists, including Green (2003) and Hogle and colleagues (2002), have nourished the debate around HIV/AIDS policy in U.S. foreign aid and have played a significant role in a policy shift to prevention based on the ABC model. Designing and promoting effective and comprehensive prevention strategies beyond condom use mean clearly understanding behaviors that lead to infection among the diversity of world cultures.

Anthropological research into HIV/AIDS is critically important to orient policies that affect the lives of millions of people. It is only through the scientific examination of human behavior and aspects of culture that infections through sexually transmitted diseases (STDs), such as HIV, can be adequately contextualized and their transmission understood in order to develop effective interventions. Unfortunately, most anthropological research often ends at conference presentations or journal articles, or as the final product report to a research funding agency. Thus, good informative data is often not geared to reach and inform policy makers and program managers, even when such intention is claimed.

While many anthropologists would like to make their research useful, the desire to do so often ends as good intentions. Wrapped up in our own academic politics and agenda, many anthropologists have yet to reach the policy table in a consistent and tangible way that informs and influences effective change through policy. HIV is a public health issue strongly embedded in human behavior, poverty, and history. Influencing and causing effective prevention will need to involve understanding human behaviors, as well as considering the underlying effects of historical and economic factors affecting various African groups. Such understanding should lead to positive change. Given anthropologists' strong claim of a greater understanding of human culture, I see this as an area where anthropological research should be in the forefront of informing policy. The persistent disconnect between anthropological research and HIV/AIDS policies and program development reveals the need to evaluate research practices and improve their applicability.

Building an effective interface between anthropological research about HIV/AIDS and policy makers is an important and urgent challenge in the public health community. It is often argued that policy makers pay little attention to anthropological research, yet anthropologists often do not strive to write for policy makers. Anthropological research intended for the policy market needs to be free of academic jargon, distributed to appropriate venues, and linked in a cogent fashion to the key issues surrounding the particular policy. In other words, anthropologists should understand the anthropology of policy making in different contexts and conditions. Presenting policy papers at conferences has limited effect on driving policy. We need to design new strategies so the important knowledge gathered by our research reaches the hands of policy makers at the appropriate time to effect change. Timing is crucial, and so are content and format. As grant writers, we learn to write in the terms and tone that catches the interest of the grantors. We also need to educate ourselves about how anthropological work can be applied to affect and promote policy. If we cannot be at the table where key policies are made, we need to learn the language of policy makers and write policy reports that can reach the policy-making table because they address critical policy interests and concerns at hand. Now more than ever, our research can have an important impact on the lives of those who have a limited voice in the policy process.

Anthropologists have conducted tremendously valuable cultural and behavioral research on HIV/AIDS that should be informing prevention and treatment programs, including in Africa (Aggleton 1996; Ajzen and Fishbein 1980; Becker and Joseph 1988; Frankenberg 1995; Gregson et al. 1998; MacPhail and Campbell 2001; McGrath et al. 1993; Moses et al. 1994). Resignation that our voices are not heard because policy makers are not listening is not the best approach and cannot be an option while thousands die from AIDS every day. It takes time to make good voices heard, and the squeaky wheel does get the grease. It took nearly ten years to convince and change U.S. policy abroad on HIV prevention strategies. I applaud Edward Green and his colleagues, who have championed the ABC approach, for not giving up despite many discouraging episodes.

Policy makers are more cognizant and in dire need of good scientific data than ever before, especially if this can readily demonstrate new orientations for designing effective HIV prevention strategies and HIV care. The reward from Green's research was that in the beginning of 2003, the United States adopted the ABC strategy to guide its prevention efforts. However, ABC is not a panacea for HIV prevention, but it is an important place to start because of its success. What followed has been a string of debates that continue to hinder effective outcomes for this prevention approach due to the lack of scientific research available in policy deliberations that demonstrates the advantages of such comprehensive approaches. The Ugandan experience in HIV prevention depicted through social science research serves as a lesson to policy makers that the scientific knowledge presented by anthropologists merits greater consideration in informing, designing, and evaluating programs.

Anthropologists will have to create opportunities to interface with policy makers and ensure that their research can improve policies and HIV programs on the ground. Anthropological research can help identify unique cultural patterns that encourage HIV infection and embed stigma, hindering timely diagnosis and optimum treatment outcomes. Anthropologists work throughout the myriad cultures of the world, and their collective efforts can provide information from diverse cultural environments.

Conclusion

As we continue to fumble with the HIV/AIDS problem, the disease is affecting increasing numbers of young people and more Africans, and unraveling the fabric of African cultures. The future of Africa is at stake, and we must act responsibly and urgently. HIV prevention strategies as promoted by Western donors have not been working effectively. This means rethinking HIV prevention research and introducing new models and strategies. These have to be more focused, grounded in anthropological knowledge, and better integrated into the reality of the African way of life. The new interest and recent adoption of the ABC model by the U.S. government in its foreign aid programs are a welcome change, but the ABC model should not be taken as a panacea, either. The policy-making process for HIV/AIDS should seek sound evidence-based science.

With greater resources available for treatment, there will be a natural tendency to gravitate away from prevention. This would be a serious policy oversight and must be resisted. Treating HIV/AIDS must go hand-in-hand with strong prevention programs. Focus on prevention as the front-line strategy is the only way to control the epidemic, since there will never be enough resources to treat everyone who gets infected. These resources will also accentuate weaknesses in existing programs if these are not dealt with in new programs. It is especially critical that a new partnership between donor nations and African governments be forged in which each party assumes the burdens of its responsibilities and proper measures are established to ensure high levels of coordination efforts and effectiveness in the mobilization, allocation, and use of resources.

Anthropologists have an important and exciting role in the fight against HIV/AIDS. Understanding human behavior, stigma, and sexual practices is the key to preventing HIV transmission. How different people understand their sexuality, and its links to their cultural identity, and the increasing need for everyone to become more aware of these dynamics in order to bring about change mean anthropologists have a newfound responsibility to research, learn, and educate. The special kinds of knowledge that anthropologists generate, document, and disseminate can provide a new platform of hope in HIV prevention. Our task has never been so vitally important.

Notes

The views expressed in this chapter are those of the author, as a public health professional and an applied medical anthropologist, and by no means necessarily represent the views of her current or former employers.

References Cited

Aggleton, Peter. 1996. "Global Priorities for HIV/AIDS Intervention Research." *International Journal of STD AIDS* 7 (Supplement 2): 13–16.

Agina, Ben. 2003. "Ngilu Sacks Drug Supply Chief." *East African Standard*, June 18.

Airhihenbuwa, Collins O. 1995. *Health and Culture Beyond the Western Paradigm.* Thousand Oaks, Calif.: Sage.

Ajzen, Icek, and Martin Fishbein. 1980. *Understanding Attitudes and Predicting Social Behavior.* Englewood Cliffs, N.J.: Prentice Hall.

Alcoff, Linda, and Elizabeth Potter. 1993. *Feminist Epistemologies.* New York: Routledge.

Allen, Arthur. 2002. "Sex Change: Uganda v. Condoms." *New Republic*, May 27, 14.

Annis, Sheldon, and Peter Hakim. 1988. *Direct to the Poor: Grassroots Development in Latin America.* Boulder, Colo.: Lynne Rienner.

Anonymous. 1978. Declaration of Alma-Ata. Statement at the International Conference on Primary Health Care. Geneva, Switzerland: World Health Organization Regional Office for Europe. http: //www.who.dk/AboutWHO/policy/20010827_1.

Anonymous. 2002. *Strategic Plan for the Period 2003–2007.* Kampala, Uganda: The AIDS Support Organization (TASO).

Anonymous. 2003a. *Dangerous Liaisons: People in Cross-Generational Relationships Underestimate Risk.* Research Brief No. 2. Population Services International. February.

Anonymous. 2003b. "Hundreds Resistant to All HIV Drugs." *BBC News.* http: //news.bbc.co.wc/2/hi/health/3208511.stm, accessed October.

Anonymous. 2003c. "Kenya Launches Inquiry into £400 Export Scam." *Guardian*, February 25.

Anonymous. 2003d. "Museveni Denies Condoms Reduced HIV in Uganda." Panafrican News Agency. October 29.

Anonymous. 2003e. "Senegal: Involve Community Networks in Adolescent Reproductive Health Operations Research Summary No. 35. www.carefacts.com.

Anonymous. 2003f. "Teenager Searching for a Wife and Mother." *Daily Nation* (Nairobi), November 5.

Anonymous. 2003g. "WHO: Polio Outbreak Spreads in West Africa." *New York Times*, January 27. www.nytimes.com/aponline/international/AP-UN-Polio.html.

Anonymous. 2004a. "AIDS Drugs Selling in City Streets." Horizon Correspondent. *Daily Nation Supplements*, January 22. www.nationaudio.com.

Anonymous. 2004b. The Society for Applied Anthropology Web site. http: //www.sfaa.net/am.html.

Anonymous. 2004c. "TASO Services: Medical Care." http://www.tasouganda.org/.

Antweiler, Christoph. 1998. "Local Knowledge and Local Knowing: An Anthropological Analysis of Contested 'Cultural Products' in the Context of Development." *Anthropos* 93: 469–494.

Ayittey, George B. N. 2003. "Leadership in the Campaign to Fight AIDS in Africa." Presentation to the Presidential Advisory Council on HIV/AIDS, July 18.

Baeck, Louis, 1988. "Shifts in Concepts and Goals of Development." In *Goals of Development*, 37–53. Paris: UNESCO.

Becker, Melvin H., and Jill G. Joseph. 1988. "AIDS and Behavioral Change to Reduce Risk: A Review." *American Journal of Public Health* 78 (4): 394–410.

Blanchard, David. 1988. "Empirical Strategies of Bottom-Up Development." In *Approaches That Work in Rural Development*, ed. John Burbidge, 318–338. New York: Institute of Cultural Affairs International.

Bolton, Ralph, and Gail Orozco. 1994. *The AIDS Bibliography: Studies in Anthropology and Related Fields*. Arlington, Va.: American Anthropological Association. http://www.aaanet.org/committees/commissions/aids/aids2.htm, accessed October.

Brewer, Devon D., Stuart Brody, Ernest Drucker, David Gisselquist, Stephen Minkin, John Potterat, Richard Roltienberg, and Francois Vachon. 2003. "Mounting Anomalies in the Epidemiology of HIV in Africa: Cry the Beloved Paradigm." *International Journal of STD and AIDS* 14: 144–147.

Camillo, Emmanuel. 2003. "Children Dropping Out of School Because of AIDS, Officials Warn." *Associated Press*, November 6.

Castro, Arucha, and Laure Marchand-Lucas. 2000. "Does Authoritative Knowledge in Infant Nutrition Lead to Successful Breastfeeding? A Critical Perspective." In *Global Health Policy, Local Realities: The Fallacy of the Level Playing Field*, ed. Linda M. Whiteford and Lenore Manderson, 233–264. Boulder, Colo.: Lynne Rienner.

Cernea, Michael. 1991. "Knowledge from Social Science for Development Policies and Projects." In *Putting People First*, ed. Michael Cernea, 1–37. New York: Oxford University Press.

Coutinho, Alex. 2003. "A Situation Analysis of HIV/AIDS in Uganda and the Role of VCT." Speech given at the First Annual General Meeting of the AIDS Information Center (AIC). Kampala, Uganda, February 21.

Dei, George. 1992. "The Indigenous Responses of a Ghanaian Rural Community to Seasonal Food Supply Cycles and Socio-Environmental Stress of the 1980s." In *Development from Within: Survival in Rural Africa*, ed. D. R. F. Taylor and Fiona Mackenzie, 58–81. New York: Routledge.

Dewalt, Billie. 1999. "Using Indigenous Knowledge to Improve Agriculture and Natural Resource Management in Latin America." In *Traditional and Modern Natural Resources Management in Latin America*, ed. Francisco Pichon, Jorge Uquillas, and John Frechione, 101–121. Pittsburgh: University of Pittsburgh Press.

Emery, Alan. 2000. *Integrating Indigenous Knowledge in Project Planning and Implementation*. Ontario: KIVU Nature.

Epstein, Helen. 2004. "Why Is AIDS Worse in Africa?" *Discover* 25 (2): 68–75.

Floyd, Kolbe. 2003. "Can We Become More Effective in Preventing HIV Infection among Young People?" Presentation to the Presidential Advisory Council on HIV/AIDS, August.

Frankenberg, Ronald. 1995. "Learning from AIDS: The Future of Anthropology." In *The Future of Anthropology: Its Relevance to the Contemporary World*, ed. A. S. Ahmed and C. Shore, 110–133. London: Athlone Press.

Galanti, Geri-Ann. 1991. *Caring for Patients from Different Cultures: Case Studies from American Hospitals*. Philadelphia: University of Pennsylvania Press.

Galtung, Johan. 1974. "Technology and Dependence." *Ceres* (September–October): 45–50.

Gisselquist, David, and John J. Potterat. 2003. "Heterosexual Transmission of HIV in Africa: An Empirical Estimate." *International Journal of STD and AIDS* 14: 162–173.

Glick-Schiller, Nina, S. Crystal, and D. Lewellen. 1994. "Risky Business: The Cultural Construction of AIDS Risk Groups." *Social Science and Medicine* 38 (19): 1337–1346.

Green, Edward C. 2003. *Rethinking AIDS Prevention*. Westport, Conn.: Praeger.

Gregson, Simon, Tom Zhuwau, Roy M. Anderson, and Stephen K. Chandiwana. 1998. "Is There Evidence for Behaviour Change in Response to AIDS in Rural Zimbabwe?" *Social Science and Medicine* 46 (3): 321–330.

Gyekye, Kwame. 1995. "The Concept of the Mind." In *Readings in African Philosophy*, ed. Safro Kwame, 69–84. New York: University of America Press.

Hahn, Robert A. 1995. *Sickness and Healing: An Anthropological Perspective*. New Haven, Conn.: Yale University Press.

Hall, Hi, R. Song, and M. T. McKenna. 2003. "Increase in HIV Diagnosis—29 States, 1999–2002." *Mortality and Morbidity Weekly Report* 52 (47): 1145–1148.

Hearst, Norman, and Sanny Chen. 2003. "Condoms for AIDS Prevention in the Developing World: A Review of the Scientific Literature." Paper presented to the Presidential Advisory Council on HIV/AIDS.

Hogle, Janice, Edward C. Green, V. Nantulya, R. Stoneburner, and J. Stover. 2002. *What Happened in Uganda? Declining HIV Prevalence, Behavior Change, and the National Response*. Washington, D.C.: U.S. Agency for International Development and the Synergy Project, September.

Imperato, Pascal James. 1977. *African Folk Medicine*. Baltimore: York Press.

Janzen, John, and Edward C. Green. 2003. "Continuity, Change, and Challenge in African Healing." In *Medicine Across Cultures*, ed. Helaine Selin and Hugh Shapiro, 1–26. Dordecht: Kluwer Academic.

Kaiser Daily HIV/AIDS Report. 2003. "HIV/AIDS Is 'Disease of Young People': One Youth Infected Every 14 Seconds Worldwide, UNFPA Report Says." Kaiser Foundation, October.

Karanja, William. 2003. "Kenya: Corruption Scandal." *World Press Review* 50 (10): 28.

Kinyua, Muriithi. 2001. *Breaking the Silence: Kenyan Families Coping With HIV/AIDS*. Nairobi, Kenya: Nairobi Family Planning Private Sector.

Kwame, Safro. 1995. *Readings in African Philosophy*. New York: University Press of America.

Leap, William, and K. O'Connor. 1993. "Introduction: Applying Anthropology in HIV/AIDS Research." *Practicing Anthropology* 15 (4): 3–4.

Low-Beer, Daniel. 2003. "Personal View: This Is a Routinely Avoidable Disease." *Financial Times*, November.

Low-Beer, Daniel, and Rand L. Stoneburner. 2003. "Behavior and Communication Change in Reducing HIV: Is Uganda Unique?" *African Journal of AIDS Research* 2 (1): 9–21.

Luke, Nancy, and Kathleen M. Kurz. 2002. *Cross-Generational and Transactional Sexual Relations in Sub-Saharan Africa: Prevalence of Behavior and Implications for Negotiating Safer Sexual Practices*. Washington, D.C.: International Council for Research on Women and Population Services International. September.

MacPhail, Catherine, and Catherine Campbell. 2001. "'I Think Condoms Are Good but, Aai, I Hate Those Things': Condom Use among Adolescents and Young People in a Southern African Township." *Social Science and Medicine* 52 (11): 1613–1627.

Maillu, David. 1988. *Our Kind of Polygamy*. Nairobi, Kenya: Heinemann Kenya.

Makinde, M. Akin. 1988. *African Philosophy, Culture and Traditional Medicine*. Monographs in International Studies, African Series, No. 53. Athens, Ohio: Ohio University Center for International Studies.

Masolo, A. D. 1994. *African Philosophy in Search of Identity*. Bloomington: Indiana University Press.

McGrath, Janet W., Charles B. Rwabukwali, Debra A. Schumann, Johnny Pearson-Marks, Sylvia Nakayiwa, Barbara Namande, Lucy Nakyobe, and Rebecca Mukasa. 1993. "Anthropology and AIDS: The Cultural Context of Sexual Risk Behaviour among Urban Baganda Women in Kampala, Uganda." *Social Science and Medicine* 36 (4): 424–439.

Moses, Stephen, E. N. Ngugi, Janet E. Bradley, E. K. Njeru, G. Eldridge, E. Muia, J. Olenje, and F. A. Plummer. 1994. "Health Care Seeking Behavior Related to the Transmission of Sexually Transmitted Diseases in Kenya." *American Journal of Public Health* 84: 1947–51.

Muriuku, Muriithi. 2003. "MP's Furious Over Misuse of AIDS Funds." *Daily Nation*, November 7.

Mwaniki, Mike. 2003. "TB Epidemic Looms Large Over Kenya." *Horizon*, June 12.

Norr, F. Kathleen, B. J. McElmurry, M. Moeti, and S. D. Tlou. 1996. "AIDS Prevention for Women: A Community-Based Approach." *Nursing Outlook* 40 (6): 250–256.

Nyblade, Laura, Rotini Pande, Sanyukta Malhur, Kerry MacQuarrie, and Ross Kidd. 2003. *Disentangling HIV and AIDS Stigma in Ethiopia, Tanzania, and Zambia*. Washington, D.C.: International Center for Research on Women.

Onjoro, Elizabeth A. 2001. "Knowledge Integration in Development: The Relative Authority of Western and Indigenous Knowledge in Traditional Birth Attendants Health Practice in Rural Kenya." Ph.D. diss., University of South Florida.

———. 2003a. Cultural Integration for Effective AIDS Prevention. *Anthropology News* http: //www.aaanet.org/press/an/infocus/0310_onjoroaids.htm, accessed November.

———. 2003b. Personal conversation with a health official.

Porco, Travis C., Jeffrey N. Martin, Kimberly A. Page-Shafer, Amber Cheng, Edwin Charlebois, Robert M. Grant, and Dennis H. Osmond. 2004. "Decline in HIV Infectivity Following the Introduction of Highly Active Antiretroviral Therapy." *AIDS* 18 (1): 81–88.

Preston-White, Elizabeth M. 1995. "Half-Way There: Anthropology and Intervention-Oriented AIDS Research in Kwazulu/Natal, South Africa." In *Culture and Sexual Risk: Anthropological Perspectives on AIDS*, ed. Han Brummelhuis and Gilbert Herdt, 315–338. Amsterdam: Gordon and Breach.

Purcell, Trevor, and Elizabeth Akinyi Onjoro. 2000. "Toward Epistemological Equitability: A Proposed Model of Knowledge Integration in Planned Social Change." Paper presented at Association of Social Anthropologists Conference, the School of Oriental and Asian Studies, London, April 3.

———. 2002. "Indigenous Knowledge, Power and Parity: Models of Knowledge Integration." In *Practicing Development: Approaches to Indigenous Knowledge*, ed. Paul Sillitoe, Alan Bicker, and Johan Pottier. New York: Routledge.

Redfern, Paul. 2003. "Drug Resistant Strains of HIV Start to Develop." *Daily Nation*, June 26.

Rotello, Gabriel. 1997. *Sexual Ecology: AIDS and the Destiny of Gay Men*. New York: Dutton.

Schoepf, Brooke G. 1991. "Ethical, Methodological and Political Issues of AIDS Research in Central Africa." *Social Science and Medicine* 33 (7): 749–763.

———. 1995. "Culture, Sex Research and AIDS Prevention in Africa." In *Culture and Sexual Risk: Anthropological Perspectives on AIDS*, ed. Han Brummelhuis and Gilbert Herdt, 29–52. Amsterdam: Gordon and Breach.

Sillitoe, Paul. 1998. "The Development of Indigenous Knowledge: A New Applied Anthropology." *Current Anthropology* 39: 223–252.

Singh, Susheela, Jacqueline Darroch, and Akinrinola Bankole. 2003. "A, B, and C in Uganda: The Roles of Abstinence, Monogamy and Condom Use in HIV Decline." Occasional Report No. 9. New York and Washington, D.C.: Alan Guttmacher Institute.

Southern States AIDS/STD Directors Work Group, in collaboration with the National Alliance of State and Territorial AIDS Directors. 2003. *Southern States Manifesto. HIV/AIDS and STDs in the South: A Call to Action!* http: //www.southernaidscoalition.org/FinalSouthernStatesManifesto.pdf.

Streefland, Peter H. 1995. "Methodological and Management Issues in Applied Interdisciplinary AIDS Research in Developing Countries." *Human Organization* 54 (3): 335–339.

Sweat, Michael, and J. Denison. 1995. "Reducing HIV Incidence in Developing Countries with Structural and Environmental Interventions." *AIDS* 9 (Supplement A): S251–S57.

Taylor, D. R. F., and Fiona Mackenzie. 1987. "Indigenous Autonomy for Grassroots Development." *Cultural Survival Quarterly* 11: 8–12.

———. 1992. *Development from Within: Survival in Rural Africa*. New York: Routledge.

Teyie, Andrew, and Ben Agina. 2004. "British Envoy Tears into Kibaki Government Over Graft." *East African Standard*, July 14. http: //www.eastandard.net/headlines/news14070412.

UNAIDS. 2003a. *AIDS Epidemic Update 2003*. December. Geneva, Switzerland: World Health Organization.

———. 2003b. *Fact Sheet: HIV/AIDS and Food Security.* Geneva, Switzerland: World Health Organization.

———. 2003c. *Treating 3 Million by 2005: Making It Happen.* Geneva, Switzerland: World Health Organization.

USAID (U.S. Agency for International Development). 2003. *Country Profile: Senegal.* June. Washington, D.C.: USAID.

Weeks, Margaret, M. Singer, and J. J. Schensul. 1993. "Anthropology and Culturally Targeted AIDS Prevention." *Practicing Anthropology* 15 (4): 17–20.

Williams, Cicely, Naomi Baumsla, and Derrick Jellife. 1994. *Mother and Child Health.* New York: Oxford University Press.

Wiredu, Kwasi. 1995. "The Concept of the Mind." In *Readings in African Philosophy*, ed. Safro Kwame, 125–151. New York: University of America Press.

Editor's note: While the editor of this volume does not support the ABC approach and de-emphasizing condom use in Africa, this chapter presents an alternative view shared by some anthropologists specializing in HIV/AIDS research.

11

Tugende Uganda

Issues in Defining "Sex" and "Sexual Partners" in Africa

SUSAN MCCOMBIE AND ARIELA ESHEL

Preface by Susan McCombie

This chapter draws on data from AIDS-related research that I was involved with in several countries between 1989 and 1998. Most of the examples are from Uganda, hence the title "Tugende Uganda" (Let's go to Uganda). Uganda was the first country in Africa that I visited, and I will always think of it as a second home. On the first day of my first visit in April 1989, I had the good fortune to be taken to the National Theatre, where Philly Lutaya was addressing a full house. He was the first Ugandan celebrity to publicly announce that he had AIDS and to attempt to turn his misfortune into an opportunity to educate others. His actions had a tremendous impact on attitudes, and many believe it was a turning point for AIDS prevention efforts in Uganda. This chapter is dedicated to Philly Lutaya, Francis Rwakagiri, Kenneth Dunnigan, and all of the people in Uganda who devoted themselves to AIDS prevention while living with HIV.

Introduction

AIDS was first recognized in Uganda in 1982. By the time HIV was identified and prevention efforts initiated, prevalence rates were already very high, with a median prevalence of 24 percent among pregnant women in urban areas (UNAIDS 2003). Uganda was one of the first countries in Africa to recognize and respond to the AIDS epidemic. The median rates among pregnant women in urban areas peaked at 30 percent in 1992 and fell to 11 percent by 2000 (UNAIDS 2003). Unfortunately, many countries in Africa have experienced an opposite trend, with low infection rates in the late

1980s and early 1990s that have mushroomed into explosive epidemics in the twenty-first century. This tragedy, which could have been prevented, is due at least in part to a failure of people to realize that their sexual behavior was putting them at risk. AIDS prevention messages that focused on "risk groups" or "risky partners" may have contributed to losing the opportunity to prevent AIDS in many parts of Africa.

One result of the AIDS epidemic was an increased interest in research surrounding sexual behavior. Many international agencies have conducted large sample surveys in order to determine if changes in reported behavior have occurred as a result of prevention programs. The use of standardized questionnaires to conduct research on sexual behavior has been the topic of considerable discussion centering on concerns about validity. The major focus of concern is that people will refuse to answer, give inaccurate answers, or both. There has been little attention to issues of translating terms for sexual activities and sexual partners.

Sexuality is defined and given meaning in a variety of ways in different sociocultural settings. There are substantial differences in definitions of sex and types of partners both intraculturally and cross-culturally. It is not possible to say "sex" or "wife" and assume a universal understanding of the terms. This chapter problematizes the use of language in sexual behavior surveys and explores its relationship to categorization of sexual partners, lay perceptions of risk for HIV infection, and patterns of condom use with different types of partners.

Language, Sex, and AIDS

Alfred Kinsey's (1948, 1953) studies of sexual behavior, although extensive and revolutionary, began a tradition of surveys based on the mistaken assumption that "sex," "spouse," and "sexual partner" are unambiguous constructs. Hunt and Davies (1991: 43) point out that the notion of a "sexual encounter" is central to studies of sexual behavior in general, and to the epidemiology of sexually transmitted diseases (STDs) in particular, but is rarely defined: "The question 'How many sexual partners have you had?' is asked explicitly or implicitly in all studies of sexual behavior. A moment's thought should, however, suffice to convince that the question, 'who is a partner?' begs the question, 'what counts as sex?'"

For many people, what counts as "sex" includes more than "sexual intercourse" (Bolton 1992; Michaels and Giami 1999; Smith 1999). Cross-culturally, people tend to categorize sex as either physical or affective. But within these two general categories, "sexual acts" may range from kissing to "full sex," where the latter implies vaginal or anal intercourse culminating in orgasm. What counts as sex may be defined not only by type of activity but also by location: "sex in a bathroom," "sex in private" (Hunt and Davies 1991: 48). A "sexual encounter" may imply a strictly physical sexual activity involving particular parts of the body, while a "sexual partner" may imply a relationship between two individuals (Hunt and Davies 1991; Michaels and Giami 1999). As Bolton (1992: 166) states, "Unless greater specificity is provided, 'number of sexual partners' is rather devoid of substance."

Defining Types of Partners

"Sexual partner" is often divided by Westerners into several categories, including "casual partner," "steady partner," "regular partner," "girlfriend/boyfriend," "sex worker," and "wife/husband." The cognitive separation of the sexual act from the sexual partner with whom the act takes place has implications for studies of sexual behavior, risk perception, and condom use. The "risk group" approach, which involves using racial or ethnic categories and sexual orientation as indicators of an individual's risk for HIV, has been a contentious issue for AIDS prevention programs (McCombie 1986; Schiller 1992). Statements proclaiming that "even if condoms are 99 percent effective, they provide less protection than does choosing a low-risk partner" (Anonymous 1988: 147) reinforce misconceptions that infection can be prevented by a social or psychological assessment of one's potential partner.

These culturally constructed categories have been used explicitly or implicitly in prevention messages in a number of educational campaigns in Africa (for example, "Love Carefully" in Uganda in 1989, "Avoid Casual Sex to Prevent AIDS" in Ghana in 1991). Implicit in many of these messages is the notion that sex with a "spouse" is safer than sex with other types of partners, and that risk increases as one moves through this continuum to "prostitute." This notion illustrates the tendency to associate AIDS with what is defined as illicit sex, and a reluctance to accept that heterosexual intercourse that meets legal and moral standards of appropriateness could be risky.

As stated above, sexual terms are not universally understood. A seemingly straightforward survey question asking American respondents to self-identify as homosexual, heterosexual, or bisexual received the following answer from a female respondent: "It's just me and my husband, so bisexual" (Smith 1999). In another survey, respondents who found the terms "vaginal intercourse" and "anal intercourse" difficult to understand were more likely to report "zero" when asked the number of people with whom they had vaginal/anal intercourse (Binson and Catania 1998). While these examples may be anecdotal, they illustrate that possibilities for error are abundant even when the interviewer and interviewee speak the same language. The issue becomes more complicated when it is examined from the perspective of translating a questionnaire.

In 1989, McCombie began preparations for a survey that would provide the baseline data to evaluate a workplace-based peer education project in Uganda. The program was implemented by the Federation of Uganda Employers and the Experiment in International Living, with technical assistance and funding from the U.S. Agency for International Development (USAID). The primary purpose of the program was to facilitate sexual behavior change among workers, their friends, and families. An instrument with a variety of questions concerning knowledge, attitudes, and practices related to AIDS was formulated, pretested in English, and prepared to be translated and back translated.

Luganda, a Bantu language, was chosen as one of the languages to be used in the questionnaire. More than one million people speak Luganda as their first language. Many more Ugandans communicate in Luganda while working, trading, or engaging in social interaction. The questionnaire was also translated into Swahili. Both questionnaires were independently back translated and revised for clarity.

In Luganda, the question "Are you married now?" has a very close translation (*oli mufumbo*). *Oli* means "are you," and *mufumbo* means "married." *Bufumbo* (marriage) is a term related to *kufumba* (to cook), and the question "Who cooks for you?" can imply a sexual relationship. The definition of who is "married" is complex. In the United States, persons are considered married when a couple has obtained a certificate from a government agency and participated in a ceremony presided over by an authorized civil servant or religious official. The distinction between who is married and who is not is relatively clear-cut, and marriage implies a lifelong monogamous relationship.

In Uganda, persons are described as "married" under a number of other circumstances. Among the traditional Baganda, marriage was a contract between a man and the father of a woman. The contract was finalized through the transfer of bridewealth (usually in cattle or currency). In the postcolonial period, a number of changes took place, and there are a number of ways in which a couple may come to be considered by the community as married:

1. A traditional ceremony with transfer of bridewealth or gifts.
2. A civil marriage registered with the government.

3. A ceremony within a religious institution such as the Church of Uganda, Catholic church, or mosque.
4. Two people begin to live together.
5. Two people are recognized as having a long-term sexual relationship.

The traditional practice of polygyny (one husband marries two or more wives) remains common. Polygynous marriages are not recognized in Christian churches and cannot be registered by the national government (Brown 1988). However, polygyny is accepted among Moslems and in traditional settlements. As a result, men living in identical situations might describe their partner relationships differently, depending on their religion, the extent to which they have been affected by Westernization, and the social context in which the relationship is being discussed.

Consider a man who has two female partners with whom he engages in sex and produces children. He may live with one and visit the other, or separate his time between the households, providing economic support for the woman and children in each. When asked the question "How many wives do you have?" one man might say "two" and another might say "one." In fact, if neither relationship was certified by civil registration or religious ceremony (methods 2 and 3 listed above), a conceivably correct answer would be "none." A Christian for whom the first marriage was recognized in church would be likely to say that he had one wife and one girlfriend. Separating "wives" from "girlfriends" in the analysis of survey data becomes problematic.

In Luganda, one word for wife is *omukyala*, which also translates as "lady," distinct from *omukazi* (woman). The concept of steady partner can be translated as *muganzi wo owenkalakalira* (*muganzi* = lover, *wo* = your, *owenkalakalira* = permanent). The concept of a "casual partner" is less easily translated. The closest approximation is *muganzi wo owolumu*, (*muganzi* = lover, *wo* = your, *owolumu* = once). With a high incidence of HIV infection among the general population, one "casual partner" can represent less risk in terms of frequency than a "wife."

Sexual behavior studies typically reduce ambiguity in the definition of partners by allowing respondents to choose their own definitions, imposing a standard definition, or working toward a common definition (Hunt and Davies 1991). All three strategies have limitations, and since different studies use different definitions, comparisons of data can yield misleading results. One step toward solving this problem is to explicitly define what each term means in the context of a particular survey. Although this step does not guarantee respondents' understanding of the question (Binson and Catania 1998), it can increase the validity of the data, especially for comparisons.

In the Uganda survey, since the phrase that achieved the best translation of "casual partner" was not frequently used and possibly subject to misinterpretation, the question used in the interview was a translation of: "In the last two months, have you had sex with anyone besides a spouse or steady partner?" This leads to the question of how to say "sex."

Defining Sex

Sexual intercourse is defined as "genital contact, especially the insertion of the penis into the vagina followed by orgasm" (*Webster's Unabridged Dictionary of the English Language*, 2nd ed., s.v. "sexual intercourse"). The definition of sexual relations is "any sexual activity between individuals." Interestingly, another definition of sexual relations is "sexual intercourse" (Ibid., s.v. "sexual relations"). Sexual relations, then, are either specifically defined as one (presumably heterosexual) activity, or left to one's imagination. In English, the word "sex" itself is ambiguous, because it is also used to describe a person's gender.

In preparing for a survey of sexual behavior in Great Britain, English terms for sexual intercourse were found to range from "the biblical ('couple,' 'copulate,' 'fornicate'), to the vernacular ('screw,' 'fuck'), from the euphemistic ('doing it,' 'having it'), to the romantic ('making love'), and from lay terms ('having sex,' 'sexual intercourse') to the scientific ('coitus')" (Wellings et al. 1994: 18). Misunderstanding of terms was so common that a glossary was included in the self-administered questionnaire (Wellings et al. 1994).

In Luganda, the literal translation of "sex" (as vaginal intercourse) is *okutomba*. This word is considered highly offensive and is used only in certain situations (for example, while joking among very close friends of the same sex and age). The closest analogy in American English would be "fuck." However, "fuck" is a less offensive term that is used in a variety of contexts, while *okutomba* is used only to indicate sexual intercourse.[1]

A euphemistic way to refer to sexual intercourse is *okulola omukazi* (to work a woman). Here okulola, the ordinary word for work ("I work at a bank"), is interpreted in the context of the sentence as referring to sex. It is less rude than *okutomba* (a taboo word), but would not be used in ordinary conversation. It might be used in joking between male friends. A similar reference is found in *bamulide omukazi* (to eat a woman).

The term that was ultimately chosen for the questionnaire was *okwebakaka*, which means "to sleep with." It has a high level of specificity when used in the proper context (two unrelated persons of the opposite sex). It is also the ordinary term for sleep ("a mother sleeps with her baby"). Although it seems closely related to the euphemistic term used in American English, some Luganda speakers consider using *webakako* to refer to sex too rude for polite conversation, especially if speaking to a member of the opposite sex or an elder. Some of the interviewers objected to using the phrase in these contexts. A more polite but less specific phrase that was sometimes substituted was *wegatako nomukazi/nomusaja*. Used in a question, it means "did you join with a woman/man." It is an ordinary expression to ask whether a person has "met with" or "been with" someone, but could be interpreted as indicating a sexual encounter when used in the proper context.

Translation issues can arise even when dealing with different dialects of English. Ugandans who speak English use a variety of phrases to refer to sex. Where Americans might say "have sex," Ugandans would say "play sex." Where Americans might say "he is always fooling around," Ugandans would say "he is always moving around" or "he is always moving up and down." In American English, the phrase "to sleep around" implies someone who has sex with a lot of partners. The meaning of "sleep around" is much different in Ugandan English, where it is interpreted as "Do you live around here?" As a result, it is quite possible to ask a Ugandan man, "Do you still sleep around?" and he will cheerfully reply "yes," meaning simply that his home is nearby. So while *webakako* refers to sleep and can be used to imply sex in Luganda, "sleeping around" and "sleeping with" are much different concepts in English for Ugandans.

The fact that the most direct translation of "sex" that can be feasibly used in a Luganda questionnaire is the same as a polite euphemism used in American English illustrates the complexity of studying seemingly simple concepts of sexual behavior cross-culturally. Obtaining measures of frequency of intercourse or specific acts is even more complicated. After translation, the question "How many times have you 'had sex' with that partner?" would be interpreted as the number of nights spent together rather than the number of acts of intercourse.

In Kenya in 1994, USAID officials were puzzled by the discrepancy between condom distribution numbers and reports of use from the 1993 Demographic and Health Surveys (DHS). There seemed to be many more condoms disappearing than could have been used based on reported use and sexual frequency found in the survey. However, the question used in the DHS was, "In the last four weeks, on how many days did you have sexual intercourse?" Research involving in-depth interviews with male condom users found that having more than one "round" a night was common, and some were using more than one condom per "round" (McCombie 1994). This information, which was not ascertained in the DHS, helped account for the discrepancies in estimates of the numbers of condoms per individual.

Partner Type, Risk Perception, and Patterns of Condom Use

A review of the literature uncovered a virtually endless number of terms used for types of partners in sexual behavior surveys in Africa. Often the terms were not defined in English, and issues of translation into a variety of languages were never discussed. Table 11.1 is a partial list of terms found in studies cited in this chapter. Comparison across studies is rendered virtually impossible, and the attempt leads one to ponder whether a "new partner" can be a "faithful partner." A "new partner" may be a subcategory of "casual partner," a "potential wife/husband," or a "one-night stand." A "casual partner" may become a "regular partner" if the relationship continues. Spouses or regular partners might refrain from sex for a period of time or be separated because of labor migration. If someone has not had sex with their regular partner in a month, is the person still a regular partner?

An equally diverse set of terms is evident when one considers types of partnerships (Table 11.2). Types of partnerships are often defined in terms of what they are not (for example, nonmarital, noncommitted sexual relationships). "Non" seems to be used to describe partnerships that are less acceptable. One does not find "noncasual partners," only "nonregular partners." Uncertainty about partnerships is revealed in terms such as "possibly committed sexual relationship." If the diversity in types of partnerships were a result of using locally defined categories of partners, it would be interesting from an ethnographic standpoint to know more about the classifications. However, the terms used seem to reflect the attempt of the researchers to impose order on sexual behavior and divide it into what is risky and what is not.

"Prostitute" is an especially problematic term, with no exact translation in the Luganda language. In 1989, one respondent stated, "There is really no such thing as a traditional prostitute in Uganda. A prostitute is a woman who is over twenty-five and unmarried." Second, "wives" who were visited by the fathers of their children and given money would be classified as "prostitutes" by Western AIDS researchers. Pickering and colleagues (1997) also noted that the role of a woman engaged in a relationship with a "casual partner" may include domestic duties and caring for the partner's children, not unlike a wife. In Tanzania, sex workers were found to have

Table 11.1. Terms for Types of Partners Found in Studies of Sexual Behavior in Africa

Anonymous partners	Nonmarital, noncohabiting partner
Casual girlfriend	Partner of high frequency/partner of low frequency
Casual partner	Penetrative sexual partner
Casual paying partner	Potential sex partner
Casual, non-sex worker partner	Prostitute
Commercial sex partner	Recent partner
Current sex partner	Regular/nonregular partner
Faithful partner	Regular nonmarital partner
Friend	Risky partner
Future partner (fiancé/fiancée)	Sex worker
Girlfriend/boyfriend	Sexual contact
Heterosexual/homosexual partner	Sexual partner
Last partner	Sexual partner of an IDU
Low-risk/high-risk partner	Spousal/nonspousal partner
Marital/nonmarital partner	Spouse
Mistress	Steady partner
New partner	Unmarried, sexually active partner
Nonanonymous partner	Wife/husband

Table 11.2. Terms for Types of Partnerships Found in Studies of Sexual Behavior in Africa

Concurrent relationships
Concurrent short relationships
Formerly married
High-risk sexual partnerships
High-risk sexual relationships
Marital (legal, religious, consensual)
Married committed relationships
Monogamous regular partnership
Multiple sexual partnerships
Nonmarital, noncommercial sexual relationships
One-night stands
Ongoing sexual relationship
Partners who also have sex with other people
Possibly committed sexual relationships
Primary sexual relationship
Regular nonmarital relationship
Risky and less risky sexual relationships
Serial short relationships
Sexual partnerships outside of marriage or regular relationships
Simultaneous, relatively long-lasting partnerships outside of marriage
Steady and casual premarital/extramarital sexual relationships
Uncommitted sexual relationships
Visiting union

several categories of partners, ranging from single-time contacts to long-term relationships (Outwater et al. 2000).

A report on attempts to standardize definitions for use in World Health Organization (WHO)/UNAIDS surveys illustrates the difficulties involved in trying to define "risky partners" (Anonymous 2001). Initially, WHO and UNAIDS defined "regular partner" as "a partner to whom you are married or with whom you are living." "Nonregular partners" were partners with whom one had a sexual relationship that lasted or was expected to last for less than a year.

> As experience with the WHO questionnaire grew, it became clear that many people were confused by the definition [of] "non-regular part-ner." Even more problematic was the finding that the definition was not capturing all high-risk partnerships, as it was intended to do. This is because, in some cultures, people have several simultaneous, but relatively long-lasting partnerships outside marriage. This is clearly a risk for HIV, since these partners are likely also to have other partners, but this situation was not included as risky under the WHO definition (Anonymous 2001: 10).

The solution was to define "regular partner" as a partner one was married to or living with, and define all other partners as "nonregular" and at higher risk (Anonymous 2001). These definitions are problematic. As illustrated above, "marriage" is not as easily defined as one might assume. In addition, with labor migration and economic difficulties the norm in much of Africa, a woman may define a regular partner as a man with whom she has had a longstanding economic relationship (Pickering et al. 1997). A regular partner, then, might be someone with whom a woman or man engages in sexual activities, but is neither married to nor living with. Likewise, using the corresponding definitions, "nonmarital" and "noncohabiting," to lump together partnerships ranging from a person with whom one has children, a person with whom one has had a sexual relationship of more than one week, a person with whom one exchanges money for sex, and a "one-night stand" is clearly erroneous.

Although there is considerable cross-cultural variation in ways of classifying partners and talking about sex, there is remarkable consistency in attitudes toward condoms and patterns of condom use. Between 1991 and 1992, McCombie and colleagues (2001) conducted an evaluation of an AIDS prevention campaign in Ghana. At the time, AIDS was very rare in Ghana, and most people thought the disease was not a problem in the country.

In both Ghana and Uganda, condom use was much less frequent with

Table 11.3. Reasons for Not Using Condoms among Sexually Active 15–30-Year-Olds in Ghana and Uganda Who Have Never Used a Condom

	Ghana 1991 Percent	Uganda 1990–1991 Percent
Not familiar	24.9	34.2
Using other forms of birth control	14.3	0.0
Don't like	22.1	8.6
Trust partner	16.1	47.7
Want children	7.1	2.8
Not around at time	2.4	0.0
Partner objects	5.2	0.0
Not safe	2.8	5.2
Can't get/expense	1.7	4.3
N =	539	465

Note: The data from Uganda are from three surveys (n = 1,599) conducted between March 1990 and October 1991 in workplaces in Kampala and Jinja. The data from Ghana are from one survey (n = 1,553) conducted in July 1991 in Cape Coast and Techiman.

partners who were defined by respondents as "spouses" or "steady partners" than it was with "casual partners." The pattern was consistent even though overall condom use was higher in Ghana, and the structure and order of question about types of partners were much different in the two surveys. In both surveys, "casual partners" were reported by a small percentage of all sexually active individuals aged fifteen to thirty years (6 percent in Uganda, 10 percent in Ghana). A possible explanation for this is found in Bolton's (1992: 187) critique of the concept of "promiscuity": "Casual sex is another term easily misinterpreted. For most people, sex is not 'casual,' no matter how many partners they have."

A number of common themes emerged when people in the two countries were asked their reasons for not using condoms. Dislike of condoms and trusting one's partner were common responses. However, there was a significant difference in attitudes toward condoms in the two countries in the early 1990s. In Uganda, many people were unfamiliar with condoms, and they had rarely been used for contraception. According to the DHS of 1988, fewer than 1 percent of women in Uganda had ever used condoms for contraception, compared to 5 percent in Ghana. At the time that AIDS awareness was growing in Uganda, many people had never heard of a condom. Condoms came to be associated with AIDS, and many people were concerned that condoms would actually spread AIDS.

Table 11.3 shows the reasons young people in the two countries gave in the baseline surveys for not using condoms. Note that in Uganda, no one mentioned use of another form of birth control as a reason for not using condoms. Almost half said they did not use a condom because they trusted their partner, compared to only 16 percent in Ghana. This reflects the fact that condoms were not as stigmatized in Ghana, where more people were using them for contraception prior to becoming aware of AIDS.

Although there were differences in the overall pattern, statements from respondents in both countries also reveal similarities in reasons for dislike of condoms:

> Woman in Ghana: "Condom takes enjoyment from sex. You won't feel the taste of the thing."
> Man in Uganda: "You can't eat sweets in a wrapper."

The connection of condoms with issues of lack of trust and respect in a sexual union emerges repeatedly, and it is not only men who raise objections:

> Woman in Ghana: "Using it means I have a disease. It's a disgrace."
> Woman in Uganda: "Condoms are casual sex. When a man uses it, he is not respecting you. He is treating you like a prostitute."

Although attention often focuses on men's objections and women's lack of power in negotiating condom use, in these studies women had similar objections. Women in Uganda were just as likely as men to say it was difficult to ask a partner to use a condom.

In spite of the similarity, there were a number of fears about the use of condoms in Uganda that were not expressed by respondents in Ghana. These included concern that men would poke holes in the condoms so they could make a woman pregnant, that men would reuse a condom with another woman, that condoms themselves carried the AIDS virus, and that they were too small. Some of those who believed that condom use would aid in prevention still expressed concerns that the virus would go through or around the condom. One man in 1989 repeatedly asked about the risk from female fluids that would touch his body even when using a condom. He was perfectly sincere when he stated: "They should make a condom for men that is like underwear."

Studies elsewhere in Africa in the 1990s reveal a similar pattern of fears about using condoms and highlight the relationship between partner categorization, risk perception, and patterns of condom use. Messersmith and colleagues (2000: 213) state: "Sexual activity and condom use are determined by a complex assessment of each relationship and vary greatly depending on the nature of the relationship, the meaning and level of trust in that relationship, the relative power and ability to assess and control the sexual behavior of the partner, the perceived risk of unwanted pregnancy and of contracting an STD, and the future prospects of the relationship."

In Nigeria, condom use was highest in commercial sex, inconsistent in casual relationships, and lowest in marriage (Messersmith et al. 2000). Men perceived themselves as being at high risk for STDs if they reported having five or more sex partners, or if they visited a sex worker in the year prior to the survey. "Sex worker" was defined as a woman engaging in sex in exchange for money at bars and hotels as a means of making a living. Reasons for using condoms varied according to how partners were categorized. Protection from STDs and AIDS was a reason to use condoms with a sex worker, but not a casual partner or wife. Condoms were used with casual partners and wives primarily to prevent pregnancy. Although more than half of the men sampled reported contracting an STD from casual partners who were not sex workers, condom use was rare in casual and committed relationships. The authors concluded that "men and women are vulnerable in casual and in some marital relationships because they rarely use condoms" (Messersmith et al. 2000: 213).

Innocent and colleagues (2003) found that in Ghana and Zambia, condom use was significantly associated with risk perception. Sex with a non-regular partner was perceived as more risky than sex with a regular partner, and condom use generally increased with an increased number of casual sexual partners. People defined themselves as not at risk for HIV if they were not sick, were abstinent, had one sexual partner, or were involved in protected sex. Respondents involved in "gainful sex" were more likely to use condoms than those involved in "sex for pleasure" (Innocent et al. 2003: 11).

In another study in Zambia, condom use was significantly associated with nonmarital sexual activity (Agha 1998). Men and women whose last sexual intercourse was with a regular or casual partner rather than a marital partner were significantly more likely to have used a condom. Age and education level were also important determinants for condom use for men. Many believed that one-night stands, rapid intercourse, or intercourse followed by a shower was risk free. Condom use was lowest in marriage (Agha 1998). Similarly, in Zimbabwe, pills were reported as the preferred contraceptive in marriage. Men generally reserved condom use for nonmarital relationships (Adetunji 2000).

In Uganda, Pickering and colleagues (1997) found that women claimed that their male partners used condoms in 93 percent of contacts with casual partners, but never with regular partners. In a review of the variety of fac-

Table 11.4. Percent of Currently Married Women Who Have Ever Used a Condom for Contraception

	Percent	n
Benin 1996	5.2	4,198
Benin 2001	7.6	4,563
Burkina Faso 1992/93	4.8	5,326
Burkina Faso 1998/99	5.1	5,181
Cameroon 1991	7.7	2,868
Cameroon 1998	18.7	3,676
Côte d'Ivoire 1994	9.6	5,271
Côte d'Ivoire 1998/99	15.4	1,863
Ghana 1988	4.5	3,156
Ghana 1993	12.6	3,204
Ghana 1998	14.2	3,131
Kenya 1989	4.3	4,765
Kenya 1993	7.3	4,629
Kenya 1998	9.7	4,834
Madagascar 1992	3.8	3,736
Madagascar 1997	4.9	4,435
Malawi 1992	8.5	3,492
Malawi 2000	8.4	9,452
Mali 1987	0.4	2,948
Mali 1995/96	2.4	8,222
Mali 2001	2.2	10,723
Niger 1992	0.3	5,561
Niger 1998	0.5	6,382
Nigeria 1990	2.0	6,880
Nigeria 1999	5.6	5,757
Rwanda 1992	1.5	3,785
Rwanda 2000	2.0	5,052
Senegal 1986	1.4	3,365
Senegal 1992/93	3.0	4,450
Senegal 1997	5.0	5,851
Tanzania 1992	3.6	6,038
Tanzania 1996	6.5	5,411
Tanzania 1999	9.5	2,653
Togo 1988	3.3	2,454
Togo 1998	11.7	5,819
Uganda 1988	0.7	3,180
Uganda 1995	4.1	5,136
Uganda 2000/01	10.4	4,881
Zambia 1992	10.5	4,457
Zambia 1996	18.6	4,902
Zimbabwe 1988	17.0	2,643
Zimbabwe 1994	24.4	3,788
Zimbabwe 1999	19.6	3,609

Source: Macro International Demographic and Health Surveys.

tors that may have contributed to the decline in HIV rates in Uganda, Hogle and colleagues state, "Most HIV transmission now occurs within monogamous regular partnerships, where bacterial STIs [sexually transmitted infections] tend to be rare" (Hogle et al. 2002: 9).

In a study of four cities in Benin, Cameroon, Kenya, and Zambia, Lagarde and colleagues (2001) found that condom use with spouses ranged from 2.4 to 7.4 percent, while condom use with nonspouses ranged from 10.8 to 24.8 percent. They concluded that "rates of condom use may not have been sufficient to impact on aggregate HIV/STI levels in the four cities even though some individual impact could be found on men's self-reported history of STI symptoms" (Lagarde et al. 2001: S77). This study was unfortunately cited as an example of evidence that shows that condom use rates do not correlate with HIV rates. This is a serious misrepresentation, since the authors appropriately noted the limitations of their cross-sectional ecological study. It is possible that condom use was higher in cities where HIV rates were higher, because people were more aware of the need for safer sex. In any case, the real problem is that the condom use rates were relatively low in all of the cities (with all types of partners).

Condom use has risen in many African countries over the last ten years. Table 11.4 shows the percent of married women who have ever used condoms as a means of contraception for the eighteen countries that have had at least two sequential DHS. Sixteen countries showed an increase, one showed a decrease, and one showed an increase followed by a decrease. However, levels still remain relatively low, and consistent use is rare. This measure ("ever using a condom") is the bottom of an iceberg whose tip barely reaches the surface. Levels of "current use" were so much lower than "ever use" that creating a table did not seem worthwhile, since so many of the percentages were below one. In most African countries, the majority of women marry at a young age and do not use any form of contraception. When they do use contraception, condoms are rarely the method of choice. This unfortunate situation contributes to the growing health emergency facing the continent.

Discussion

There are substantial differences in definitions of sex and types of partners in different cultures. However, patterns of condom use and reasons for lack of use with different types of partners show predictable patterns. On the one hand, there is variation in how sexual relationships are discussed and defined. On the other hand, there is consistency in how condom use is reported and perceived with respect to sexual relationships.

There are striking similarities in patterns of condom use and reasons for lack of use in different cultures. Condoms are less frequently used with "spouses" than with "casual partners." Trusting one's partner is a common reason for not using condoms in many parts of the world. The underlying misconception is that partners of high frequency (such as "spouses") are equated with safety from HIV, while partners of low frequency are assumed to pose an increased risk of HIV. However, from the viewpoint of HIV, a steady partner represents more opportunities for transmission. Many laypeople and public health officials have failed to realize that a retrovirus cannot distinguish between sexual acts that are defined as illicit and those that satisfy cultural norms of appropriateness.

Reluctance to promote condom use for people in "committed," "marital," or "regular" partnerships has been an obstacle to HIV prevention since the mid-1980s. The resistance comes from two sides of the behavior change coin—the target population (the "other") and those who want the "other" to change (the HIV prevention program implementers). Many HIV prevention specialists retain negative attitudes about condom use and have never used a condom with their "regular partner." A suitable cliché is "they talk the talk, but don't walk the walk." When faced with obstacles to condom use from "the target population," the negative attitudes public health communicators have about condom use allow them to create loopholes in the attack on HIV ("Well if you must . . . do that . . . use a condom"). Of course, few individuals ever imagine they are doing "that."

If the topic were washing one's hands after defecation, the prevention message would be very clear and consistent, and few could rationalize their behavior around it.[2] It is hard to imagine health officials abandoning logic and creating educational messages like, "Wash your hands if you think you are somewhere you might get a disease." Yet that is what they have done with HIV, by promoting messages that encourage selecting partners "carefully" and using condoms only "when all else fails."

Most sex occurs between people who "trust" one another, at least at a particular moment. Positioning condoms as a last resort for those who cannot abstain or be faithful does little to change prevailing misconceptions about partner selection as a prevention strategy. In addition, messages that emphasize fidelity or having only one partner have little salience for adolescents who have never had a sexual partner. In Malawi in 1989, an AIDS prevention poster advised people to "Maintain regular sexual partner." For young people coming of age in Africa, the challenge will be to find that partner. We hope they do not undertake that challenge without using a condom.

Unfortunately, HIV is only the tip of the iceberg. Those who continually voice their hope for a cure or a vaccine that will allow these inconveniences to be abandoned are apparently unaware of a simple fact: every encounter, sexual or otherwise, between two humans creates an opportunity for the transmission of pathogens, both new and old. It is not possible to chase every one of these pathogens with specific programs and messages. Human medical technologies are unlikely to stop the evolution of biological agents such as bacteria and viruses and send them to the list of extinct species. Rather, our best technological interventions (drugs and vaccines) actually speed up the evolution of these biological entities. In the meantime, we must promote behaviors that reduce their chances of being transmitted all of the time. Condom use is one of those behaviors. Please don't forget to use one with your favorite partner.

Acknowledgments

The list of people whose thoughts and experiences informed the authors in writing this chapter is long enough to become an entire book. Hence our acknowledgments emphasize key institutions rather than individuals.

The evaluation research in Uganda was conducted in collaboration with the Federation of Uganda Employers (FUE) and the Experiment in International Living (EIL). The research in Ghana was conducted in collaboration with John K. Anarfi, of the Institute of Statistical, Social and Economic Research, University of Ghana, and with the Ministry of Health of Ghana. Both projects were funded by the U.S. Agency for International Development Contract No. DPE 5972-Z-00-7070-00 (AIDSCOM) to the Academy for Educational Development. The evaluation of this project's programs in Africa was performed under a subcontract to the Annenberg School of Communications at the University of Pennsylvania. Most important, Peter K. Ssebbanja, of The AIDS Support Organization (TASO), translated the questionnaire into Luganda and provided invaluable information on terminology.

Notes

1. However, even *Anthropology News* edited the word "fuck" out of a brief report on the Uganda research.

2. The word "defecation" is used because of the need for specificity. In Uganda, McCombie found that "going to the bathroom" could be misinterpreted as meaning washing hands after using the toilet.

References Cited

Adetunji, Jacob. 2000. "Condom Use in Marital and Nonmarital Relationships in Zimbabwe." *International Family Planning Perspectives* 26 (4): 196–200.

Agha, Sohail. 1998. "Sexual Activity and Condom Use in Lusaka, Zambia." *International Family Planning Perspectives* 24 (1): 32–37.

Anonymous. 1988. "Choose Sexual Partners Very Carefully, AIDS Researchers Caution." *Family Planning Perspectives* 20 (3): 146–147.

Anonymous. 2001. "Measuring Risky Sex and Condom Use." *Measure Evaluation Bulletin* 2: 9–12.

Binson, Diane, and Joseph A. Catania. 1998. "Respondents' Understanding of the Words Used in Sexual Behavior Questions." *Public Opinion Quarterly* 62 (2): 190–208.

Bolton, Ralph. 1992. "AIDS and Promiscuity: Muddles in the Models of HIV Prevention." *Medical Anthropology* 14 (2–4): 145–223.

Brown, Winifred. 1988. *Marriage, Divorce, and Inheritance: The Uganda Council of Women's Movement for Legislative Reform*. Cambridge African Monographs 10. Cambridge: University of Cambridge.

Hogle, Janice A., Edward Green, Vinand Nantulya, Rand Stoneburner, and John Stover. 2002. *What Happened in Uganda? Declining HIV Prevalence, Behavior Change, and the National Response*. Washington, D.C.: U.S. Agency for International Development and the Synergy Project.

Hunt Andrew, and Peter Davies. 1991. "What Is a Sexual Encounter?" In *AIDS: Responses, Interventions and Care*, ed. Peter Aggleton, Peter Davies, and Graham Hart, 43–52. Bristol, Pa.: Falmer Press.

Innocent, Najjumba Mulindwa, James Ntozi, Fred E. Ahimbisibwe, Jonathan Odwee, and Nata Agiya. 2003. "Risk Perception and Condom Use in Uganda." *Union for African Population Studies* 18 (1): 68–79.

Kinsey, Alfred. 1948. *Sexual Behavior in the Human Male*. Philadelphia: W. B. Saunders.

———. 1953. *Sexual Behavior in the Human Female*. Philadelphia: W. B. Saunders.

Lagarde, E., B. Auvert, J. Chege, T. Sukwa, J. R. Glynn, H. A. Weiss, E. Akam, M. Laourou, M. Carael, A. Buve, and the Study Group on the Heterogeneity of HIV Epidemics in African Cities. 2001. "Condom Use and Its Association with HIV/Sexually Transmitted Disease in Four Urban Communities of Sub-Saharan Africa." *AIDS* 15 (Supplement 4): S71–S78.

McCombie, Susan C. 1986. "The Cultural Impact of the 'AIDS' Test: The American Experience. *Social Science and Medicine* 23: 455–459.

———. 1994. *Frequency of Sex and Condom Use in Kenya: Results from Preliminary Qualitative Research*. Report to the Futures Group International for USAID.

McCombie, Susan C., Robert Hornik, and John K. Anarfi. 2001. "Effects of a Mass Media Campaign to Prevent AIDS among Young People in Ghana." In *Public Health Communication: Evidence for Behavior Change*, ed. R. Hornik, 147–161. Mahwah, N.J.: Lawrence Erlbaum Associates.

Messersmith, Lisa J., Thomas T. Kane, Adetanwa I. Odebiyi, and Alfred A. Adewuyi. 2000. "Who's at Risk? Men's STD Experience and Condom Use in Southwest Nigeria." *Studies in Family Planning* 31 (3): 203–216.

Michaels, Stuart, and Alain Giami. 1999. "Review: Sexual Acts and Sexual Relationships: Asking About Sex in Surveys." *Public Opinion Quarterly* 63 (3): 401–420.

Outwater, Anne, Lucy Nkya, George Lwihula, Patricia O'Connor, Melzideck Leshabari, Justin Nguma, Blastus Mwizarubi, Ulrich Laukamm-Josten, Edward C. Green, and Susan E. Hassig. 2000. "Patterns of Partnership and Condom Use in Two Communities of Female Sex Workers in Tanzania." *Journal of the Association of Nurses in AIDS Care* 11 (4): 46–54.

Pickering, H., M. Okongo, K. Bwanika, B. Nnalusiba, and J. Whitworth. 1997. "Sexual Behavior in a Fishing Community on Lake Victoria, Uganda." *Health Transition Review* 7: 13–20.

Schiller, Nancy Glick. 1992. "What's Wrong with This Picture? The Hegemonic Construction of Culture in AIDS Research in the United States." *Medical Anthropology Quarterly* 6 (3): 237–254.

Smith, Tom W. 1999. "Review: The JAMA Controversy and the Meaning of Sex." *Public Opinion Quarterly* 63 (3): 385–400.

UNAIDS. 2003. *Epidemiological Fact Sheets on HIV/AIDS and Sexually Transmitted Infections: Uganda.* www.unaids.org.

Wellings, Kaye, Julia Field, Anne Johnson, and Jane Wadsworth. 1994. *Sexual Behaviour in Britain.* London: Penguin Books.

12

HIV/AIDS and the Context of Polygyny and Other Marital and Sexual Unions in Africa

Implications for Risk Assessment and Interventions

TERESA SWEZEY AND MICHELE TEITELBAUM

Introduction

Some attention has been paid to the impact AIDS has had on the African family with respect to widows and orphans. Orphans and vulnerable children have especially been the target of funding and multiple interventions to address their needs. Limited observations have been made about the impact of AIDS on formal marital arrangements, but little has been done to incorporate a realistic view of African marriage into policy, funding, and interventions. Some policies and funding decisions appear to be based on an idealized, prescriptive concept of marriage. Most notably, the "ABC" approach to HIV/AIDS prevention—abstain, be faithful, and condom use—promotes abstinence before marriage, fidelity to one partner within marriage, and targeted use of condoms by high-risk groups.

This chapter explores a less idealized concept of marriage, one that shows that African marriage can be a relatively fluid concept that includes polygyny, several other arrangements that can be called "de facto polygyny," and serial monogamy. This broader concept of marriage, interacting with gender dynamics and current economic reality in Africa, has implications for assessment of risk for HIV/AIDS. Household-level data collected from Basoga Muslims in Uganda also suggest that gender stereotypes of women as either virtuous wives or commercial sex workers have obscured the wider range of roles that women may have in contributing to risk within marriage.

A broad view of marriage in Uganda and a wide perspective on women's sexual behavior can be seen as a positive development, in much the same way that many see the "sexual revolution" in Western society, which has led to acceptance of sex without marriage and serial monogamy in many segments of society. Similarly, Western society has frankly acknowledged a wide range of sexual behavior among heterosexuals and gay men and lesbians, and a less prescriptive view of marriage, as prerequisite to effective mitigation of the risk of HIV/AIDS. We argue for comparable frankness in risk mitigation in Africa, which would include a more realistic approach to risk assessment than one focused on monogamous sexual dyads, or "couples." We also point to the need to address underlying socioeconomic factors that may lead to an increase of risky behavior. For example, in Western society, AIDS programs address sex-for-drugs exchanges; in developing countries of Africa, we may need to address situations of economic vulnerability that lead some women to increase the number of their sexual partners.

Marriage Does Not Mitigate Risk

Irrespective of the need for a broader approach, for many women in sub-Saharan Africa, a commitment to monogamy within a marital union or steady partnership is no guarantee against HIV infection. An estimated 60 to 80 percent of women infected with HIV in the region have had only one lifetime sexual partner (Rivers and Aggleton 1999; see also Whelan 1999). Most women living with HIV/AIDS in sub-Saharan Africa, as well as globally, were infected by their "primary partner" (O'Leary 2000).[1] The results of a ten-year longitudinal study in the Masaka District in Uganda found, for example, that "in married couples where both partners are not infected, men bring HIV infection into the marriage at twice the rate of women. This is probably owing to extramarital sexual behaviour" (Whitworth 1999: 181).[2]

The idea that women who remain "faithful" will be at less risk, or that women are in a position to effectively negotiate condom use with their husbands or steady male partners, is belied by gender power differentials within marital relations and other unions. These gender power differentials in control over sexuality within and outside of marriage mean that many women have little control over their husbands' or steady male partners' sexual behavior (Blanc 2001; McGrath et al. 1993; Gupta et al. 1996; Schoepf 1998; Simmons et al. 1996; Ulin 1992). Given this, de Bruyn and colleagues (1998: 14) argue that "marriage should be squarely acknowledged as a major risk factor for women in many societies." If monogamous marriage has so little impact on risk mitigation, an understanding of the dynamics of a broader range of marital arrangements and sexual unions in sub-Saharan Africa is a critical precursor to understanding social risk factors of the HIV/AIDS epidemic in the region.

African Marital Relations and Other Unions

Marriage in sub-Saharan Africa is changing as economic decline, geographic mobility (especially migration to urban areas in search of work, resulting in the separation of spouses), and rapid urbanization contribute to new forms of unions. The burden on men and their families to generate the costs of bridewealth and other wedding-related costs is also increasing the number of informal unions. These unions are variously referred to as "concubinage," "outside marriages," "second office," "sugar daddy relationships," "visiting unions," and "serial monogamy" (Aryee 1997; Bledsoe 1990; Bledsoe and Pison 1994; Karanja 1994; Locoh 1994; McGrath et al. 1993; Meekers and Nadra 1995; Obbo 1987; Ocholla-Ayayo 1987; Van de Walle and Meekers 1994). While these unions are known by a variety of names, Bledsoe (1990: 120) argues that they are "de facto polygynous templates."

These changes in relationship patterns have a number of consequences for women (Adepoju 1997; Ahlberg 1991; Caldwell et al. 1994; Caraël 1994). Commenting upon the Kikuyu in Kenya, Ahlberg (1991) notes that in the past, the decision to add another wife to the family was made jointly by both the husband and wife. Currently, many women learn that they have co-wives, or that their husband has mistresses, through other sources. Thus, husbands are now shared with unknown women. This also means that the husband's resources are stretched even more thinly among many women and their families. Teenage pregnancies and pregnancies outside of marriage have increased, as has fertility among married women and related complications. Such unions expand the sexual network for all involved and increase the risk of sexually transmitted diseases (STDs), including HIV/AIDS. On the one hand, if men use condoms with their extramarital partners, then the expanding sexual networks created by new forms of unions pose little risk to existing wives. Even if condoms are available and used with all extramarital partners, however, "the wives of husbands already infected prior to condom use would nevertheless remain unprotected" (Ahlberg 1991: 220).

Marriage—in whatever form—is nearly universal in sub-Saharan Africa (Adepoju 1997; Adepoju and Mbugua 1997; Bledsoe 1990; Garenne and

Van de Walle 1989; Mbugua 1997). "Most African men are involved in long-term relationships with more than one woman at any given moment, a situation that for the majority of African women has led to the inevitability of being in a polygynous consensual or formal union" (Adepoju and Mbugua 1997: 42). While there is a wide diversity of marriage practices and rates of different forms of marriage, some common patterns emerge. In polygynous societies, women generally marry at an earlier age than men, and there is often a significant age gap between husbands and wives. This is especially true of junior wives, who may be many years younger than their husbands (Adepoju and Mbugua 1997; Bledsoe 1990; Bledsoe and Pison 1994; Lesthaeghe et al. 1989).

Divorce and widowhood are more common in polygynous societies; women often remarry quickly after becoming widowed or divorced. Women who remarry because of divorce or widowhood frequently remarry into already polygynous unions as junior wives. A woman who has not produced children with a man may either leave or be divorced by him and remarry someone else (again, often as a junior wife in a polygynous union) in the hopes of fulfilling her socially sanctioned roles and statuses as wife and mother. Women are thus usually in some form of union for most of their lives (Adepoju and Mbugua 1997; Bledsoe 1990; Bledsoe and Pison 1994; Lesthaeghe et al. 1989). Many women in monogamous unions are those who are younger and have been married for a shorter duration (Pebley and Mbugua 1989). "The institution that maximizes the time women spend in union, despite wide age gaps between spouses and often high rates of divorces, is polygyny" (Bledsoe 1990: 117).

The rate of polygyny is usually framed in terms of two measures: incidence and intensity. Incidence, in general, refers to the number of new cases during a specified time period. The incidence of polygyny provides a measure of the number of men married to more than one wife. Intensity is discussed either as the average number of wives per polygynous man or as the number of men who are married to more than two wives (Clignet 1970; Van de Walle 1968). Given the flexibility of marriage forms and the likelihood that many currently monogamous marriages may become polygynous, an alternative conceptualization of intensity is "not only whether a man is married but how married he is. In this view, polygyny is not a state distinct from monogamy but simply farther along a continuum that ranges from 'not at all married' to 'intensely married'" (Blanc and Gage 2000: 165).

The incidence of polygyny varies widely by region and by ethnic group. The rates are generally highest in West and central Africa and lower in East and southern Africa. About 40 percent of women in West Africa and 30 to

39 percent of women in much of central Africa are in polygynous unions, compared to a rate of between 20 and 30 percent in East Africa. The percentage of women in polygynous marriages is 20 percent or less in southern Africa (Lesthaeghe et al. 1989). The high incidence of polygyny has persisted despite efforts on the part of both colonial and contemporary states and religious institutions to decrease or eliminate it through the enactment of legal and religious codes (Bledsoe 1990; Bledsoe and Pison 1994).

Data from a series of Demographic and Health Surveys (DHS) conducted from 1990 to 1993 in nine sub-Saharan African countries (Burkina Faso, Cameroon, Ghana, Kenya, Malawi, Niger, Rwanda, Senegal, and Tanzania) among men ages twenty to fifty-four years show a low of about 9 percent polygyny in Rwanda and Malawi to a high of approximately 28 percent in Senegal and Burkina Faso. The rates for Kenya and Tanzania were 11.6 percent and 14.9 percent, respectively. Calculations of the intensity of polygyny show that most polygynous men in the nine-country study are married to two wives. The number of wives that a man is married to increases, however, over his lifetime (Blanc and Gage 2000).

In ethnographic studies conducted by one of the authors in Liberia in the mid-1970s, in traditional villages in one region, the rate of polygyny was consistently under 10 percent. Most polygynous men had only two wives, and often the second was an inherited widow. Men with more than two wives had acquired additional wives after becoming wealthy, and those men were usually chiefs. Inconsistencies and time lags in data collection limit our capacity to generalize, but clearly there has been great variation in the rate of polygyny in sub-Saharan Africa, and it is possible that de facto polygynous unions have increased in response to economic decline and sociopolitical change in Africa.

Beyond Dyads to Risk Clusters

Irrespective of the ambiguities, it is clear that HIV/AIDS research in sub-Saharan Africa too often focuses on "couples" as though they exist in isolation and are not embedded in larger units that may be relevant to HIV/AIDS transmission. In the case of either formal or informal polygynous unions, each dyadic "couple" is linked to the others, and to the past and current sexual partners of all of them. Interventions intended to mitigate risk of HIV/AIDS often consider that a man may infect more than one wife and/or women who are not his wives. The man is viewed as the center of a constellation from which risk emanates to its satellite components. This view assumes that women are either virtuous wives or wanton single women, most likely commercial sex workers. A realistic model needs to acknowledge that currently monogamous unions may become polygynous and may have been polygynous in the past, and that the past and current behavior of married women may contribute to the risk of their husbands and co-wives, and other partners of the husbands and co-wives.

Instead of dyadic or constellation models, we use the concept of "risk cluster," which moves beyond individual and dyadic levels, and male-focused views, to address the risk of both husbands and wives within the same or linked households. Teresa Swezey developed this concept to analyze data from surveys, focus groups, and interviews conducted among polygynous households of Basoga Muslims in Uganda. A consistent theme of these data was that the behavior of all partners within the marital union affects one's HIV/AIDS risk and ability to reduce that risk. Wives were concerned about their co-wives' behavior, as well as their husband's behavior, and husbands were concerned about their wives' behavior.

Morris and Kretzschmar (2000) identify concurrent sexual partnerships (that is, partnerships "that overlap in time") as one way that the HIV/AIDS epidemic has spread rapidly in sub-Saharan Africa. For analytical purposes, they identify two types of concurrent partnerships: long-term (marriages) and short-term (all other sexual relationships). Having more than one partner at a time contributes to the spread of the epidemic because

first, from the virus-eye view, there is less time lost after transmission occurs waiting for that partnership to dissolve, or between the end of one partnership and the beginning of another. Second, the effect of partner sequence on exposure risk is reduced. Under serial monogamy, each partner increases the risk of infection to a subject, so earlier partners are less likely to be exposed to an infected subject than later ones. If partnerships are concurrent, much of the protective effect of sequence is lost. Earlier partners remain connected to the subject, and are exposed when the subject becomes infected by a later concurrent partner. And finally, concurrency has a critical effect on the "connected component," the number of persons in the population that are directly or indirectly connected at any point in time. Under sequential monogamy, the maximum size of the connected component cannot exceed [two]. Under concurrency, by contrast, the maximum size of a connected component can become quite large: individuals have partners who are themselves connected to others, these others are again connected to additional persons, and so on. Concurrency creates a large, loosely structured, constantly shifting web of connected persons in a network, enabling an infectious agent to spread rapidly and pervasively.[3] (Morris and Kretzschmar 2000: 4)

The network aspect of polygynous, and de facto polygynous, unions means that all partners are linked to each other through a complex web of sexual, economic, and social relationships. Polygynous unions thus consist of these linkages between two or more "dyads." These dyads do not exist in isolation from each other, yet more often than not they are analyzed in this manner in the existing "couples" research on reproductive health and, to a much lesser extent, in HIV/AIDS research in sub-Saharan Africa. Analyses of "couples" data that include people in both monogamous and polygynous unions may be restricted to only monogamous "couples" because of the difficulties inherent in analyzing data from a husband and more than one of his wives. Alternately, if people in polygynous unions are included in the study, researchers may restrict the analysis to husbands and only one of their interviewed wives, or they may count a husband and each of his interviewed wives as a "couple" (Dodoo 1998). Co-wives and their husband, and all of their partners, are rarely considered as a "unit."

While sexual behavior occurs at the dyadic level, the limited research on women's views of polygyny in sub-Saharan Africa shows that women in polygynous unions may consider their co-wives' reproductive behavior when deciding on whether to have another child (Bledsoe 1993; Meekers and Nadra 1995; Ware 1979; Wittrup 1990). It seems reasonable to also analyze assessments of HIV/AIDS risk within marital unions to include the question of whether concerns about co-wives' behavior influences the HIV risk assessments of individuals in polygynous unions.

Perceptions of Polygyny as a Risk Factor

Polygyny as a risk factor for AIDS emerged as a consistent theme in focus groups and interviews during two periods of research (1994–1995 and 1997) with Basoga Muslims in Uganda. Many of the reasons articulated for polygyny being considered a risk factor are linked to an imbalance of power within marital unions and its consequences for the embodiment—or lived experience—of risk for women. Both women and men framed polygyny as a potential risk factor in terms of "trust/mistrust" (concern about the behavior of their spouse/spouses and/or co-wife/co-wives), the possibility that a new wife added to the union might be infected, and challenges for men in treating all their wives equally, which might lead to one or more of the wives seeking outside partners. Many women also expressed concerns about the possibility that even if they remained "faithful" within their po-lygynous union, their co-wife/co-wives might have outside partners, which would increase their risk.

The focus on polygyny and risk in this chapter is not intended to im-ply that Muslims are at greater risk for AIDS because polygyny is officially sanctioned in Islam. Indeed, a multiyear study (Carpenter et al. 1999: 1087) on HIV transmission within marriages in the rural district of Masaka, with serodiscordant partners (one partner HIV positive, the other HIV negative) found that the rates of new infection (incidence rate) "for non-Muslims were significantly higher than those of Muslims for men (age-adjusted RR = 3.5 percent . . .) and women (age-adjusted RR = 2.7 percent . . .)."[4] Another study in Uganda (Mcintyre et al. 2001) found that Muslims were more likely to report behavior change than were members of other religious groups. Moreover, the practice of polygyny is not limited to Muslims in Uganda. While Muslims accounted for only about 11 percent of the country's popu-lation in the 1991 census, an estimated 30 percent of all women were in cur-rently polygynous unions.[5] Polygyny is not, in and of itself, necessarily a risk factor for AIDS on the individual level. It becomes a potential risk factor for all spouses if any one of them has extramarital partners, or had premarital partners, with whom they have had unprotected sex (Berkley 1994; Morris and Kretzschmar 1995).

Women in sub-Saharan Africa identify one of the major disadvantages of polygyny as creating tensions within polygynous families—between not only husbands and wives but between or among co-wives. Women com-pete for resources from shared husbands for themselves and their children. Husbands may show favoritism toward a new wife, which results in a lack of support for the other wife or wives and their children (Kilbride and Kilbride 1990; Meekers and Nadra 1995; Ware 1979; Wittrup 1990). An additional challenge is the expectation of husbands treating all wives equally (emo-tionally, materially, and sexually). While this is especially the ideal in Islamic societies, the way it is played out at the local level among the Basoga Mus-lims reveals a gap between ideal and practice. The likelihood that adding another wife to the union will result in some wives being neglected sexually is summarized in this comment from an educated male survey respondent: "Men like [sexual] variety, so they have many wives along with outside part-ners. . . . In the end, they forget or neglect some of their wives as far as sex is concerned."

Among this population, there is also a fairly high rate of "wife leaving" (that is, wives leaving their marital unions). Wives who are unhappy about the addition of another wife to the union may choose to leave. Wives' re-

sponses showed that as many as 40 percent of partners in currently monogamous unions may have been in polygynous unions in the past. This
highlights the fluidity of marital unions along a shifting continuum of currently monogamous, currently polygynous, intending to become polygynous (Speizer 1995), and a possible fourth category that should be added to
Speizer's marriage trichotomy—formerly polygynous. The high percentage
of currently monogamous marital unions that were likely polygynous at
some point in the past introduces additional concern for HIV risk because
of the past additional partners.

Basoga Muslim survey respondents who stated that polygyny is a risk
factor for HIV infection were asked a follow-up question about their reasons for this judgment. The most frequent response (by 51 percent of 140
respondents) was "can't trust co-wives," which was stated almost exclusively
by women, 87 percent of whom (out of seventy-nine women) identified this
as a reason for considering polygyny a risk factor.

Wives in polygynous unions were more likely than wives in monogamous unions to mention mistrust of co-wives as a reason for polygyny being a risk factor (63 percent and 39 percent, respectively.) Men (62 percent
of sixty-one men) often gave "can't trust all your wives" as a reason. Only
three respondents—all men—identified "can't trust husband" as a reason
for considering polygyny a risk factor. About equal percentages of women
and men (35 percent and 30 percent, respectively) stated that it is "difficult
to treat all wives equally," which was the second most frequently cited reason for polygyny being a risk factor for AIDS.

The emphasis on co-wife infidelity in the survey data may be a somewhat
paradoxical finding, given the concerns about husbands' behavior that were
raised by women in focus groups, in-depth interviews, and informal conversations during both periods of research. These concerns are summarized
in the following comment from a women's focus group: "As married women
in the man's home, we do not move out [travel outside the home], but men
move out and women find themselves infected." Further, "Generally women
have no power over their risk, because they can stay home and be faithful,
but they cannot rule their husbands and force them to stay home." Additionally, slightly more than a quarter (28 percent) of the wives who ranked
their HIV risk as "moderate/great" gave responses indicating that they mistrusted their husband as one of their reasons.

The group discussions also included a fair amount of wife blaming on
the part of both women and men regarding why women have extramarital
partners. While the husbands' inability or unwillingness to meet all of their
wives' emotional, sexual, and material needs was cited as a reason for wives

to have outside partners, the men who are those outside partners were curiously absent from the discourse on blame. In short, while the respondents did associate polygynous men with sexual behavior that increased the risk of HIV infection for themselves and their wives, they clearly recognized the risk introduced by the sexual behavior of wives in polygynous unions. The view from within these polygynous Basoga Muslim unions supports the need for the analytic concept of a risk cluster, as opposed to dyadic or constellation models.

Basoga Muslims in polygynous risk clusters were significantly more likely to assess their AIDS risk as "moderate/great" than those in monogamous risk clusters. Sixty percent of wives and 49 percent of husbands in polygynous risk clusters considered themselves at "moderate/great" risk compared to 33 percent of wives and 31 percent of husbands in monogamous risk clusters. Wives in polygynous risk clusters were 2.4 times more likely to assess their risk of getting AIDS as "great" than wives in monogamous risk clusters. Similarly, husbands in polygynous risk clusters were 3.2 times more likely than husbands in monogamous risk clusters to report that they were at "great" risk of HIV infection. Both women and men identified poverty as a major reason for women choosing to have outside partners.

Economic Vulnerability and Women's Risk

What is the basis for suspicion of infidelity among Basoga Muslim co-wives? Is it simply an aspect of co-wife jealousy or sexual competition? Is co-wife suspicion related to dispersed living arrangements and lack of cooperative work obligations among this population? If so, the phenomenon of co-wife infidelity and suspicions of infidelity might vary greatly among African polygynous societies, to the extent that co-wife relationships and co-wife living and farming arrangements vary throughout the continent. However, when Basoga Muslim respondents refer to the difficulty of meeting material needs of co-wives and their children, they address an underlying theme that is becoming pervasive throughout sub-Saharan Africa.

The 2002 UNAIDS report on the global AIDS epidemic identified gender inequality with respect to access to valued societal resources, worsening of economic conditions, and younger women marrying older men as some of the reasons that a higher percentage of younger women are infected with HIV in sub-Saharan Africa:

Women and girls are commonly discriminated against in terms of access to education, employment, credit, health care, land, and inheritance. With the downward trend of many African economies increasing the ranks of people in poverty, relationships with men (casual or formalized through marriage) can serve as vital opportunities for financial and social security, or for satisfying material aspirations. Generally, older men are more likely to be able to offer such security. But, in areas where HIV/AIDS is widespread, they are also more likely to become infected with HIV. The combination of dependence and subordination can make it very difficult for girls and women to demand safer sex (even from their husbands) or to end relationships that carry the threat of infection.[6] (UNAIDS/WHO 2002: 18)

In developing economies, the practice of women exchanging sex for financial security and/or sociocultural security should not be assumed to be limited to adolescents or to sex workers, although studies and policies related to HIV prevention have often made this assumption. Under conditions of economic scarcity, married women also make risky choices. In polygynous households, if resources are strained and all wives and their children are not supported equally—even when custom or religion dictates that they should be—economic need, or perceived need, may be the root cause of decision making about behavior that increases women's risk for HIV/AIDS.

The cordoning off of "risk groups" from the "general population" in the social and epidemiological literature, which has been customary, is therefore an unrealistic approach and comes with a number of negative consequences. Other authors have noted that as increasing numbers of women are trading sex for money or material goods in order to survive during economic crises, the "boundary" encircling the "general population," separating it from acknowledged populations at risk, becomes increasingly blurred (Farmer 1996a, 1996b; Schoepf 2001; Schoepf, Engundu, et al. 1991;, Schoepf, Wa Nkera, et al. 1991; Simmons et al. 1996; Standing 1992). Most notably, when "prostitutes," or "commercial sex workers," are set in opposition to "wives and mothers," this "dichotomization . . . [makes invisible] most women at risk. . . . Some women may at times exchange sex for financial security, material goods, or specific services—including support for their children. Many women who sell sex do not identify themselves as prostitutes" (Booth 1998: 130; see also Carovano 1991).

This issue of how women are sexually defined, first, reflects a bias that may impact on risk assessment: dichotomizing women as either virtuous wives or "prostitutes" fails to acknowledge the extent to which a wide range of women are at risk, including women who are living culturally appro-

priate and meritorious lives in their own societies. Whether the dichotomous view emerges out of ignorance, lack of good research, or prescriptive
ideology, interventions based on this view will ultimately fail to address
the tremendous risk mitigation needs of the AIDS epidemic in Africa. Additionally, ignoring the wide range of sexual partnering that is motivated
by economic necessity fails to recognize the need for policies and interventions to increase the economic autonomy and viability of women as a
means of mitigating their risk of HIV/AIDS. Currently, funding agencies
most often earmark funds separately, in unconnected programs; there are
funds for HIV/AIDS care, prevention, and for interventions that might have
an impact on women's financial viability, such as skill building and micro-
credit.

Faith-Based Prevention Approaches in Africa

A number of assessments of U.S. global AIDS policy, such as the recent
evidence-based analysis by the Center for Health and Gender Equity
(CHANGE 2004), have suggested that U.S. AIDS policy is influenced by
fundamentalist religious ideology. That view is certainly consistent with the
circumscribed notions of risk and marriage that we cite as limiting and
characteristic of approaches such as "ABC." However, while we agree that
ideological biases should not be imposed on African cultures, we have seen
evidence that ideology consistent with African views and cultural practices
can be advantageous in AIDS prevention.

The Basoga Muslim study cited in this chapter was conducted among
a largely Muslim population, in cooperation with the Islamic Medical Society of Uganda's Family AIDS Education and Prevention Through Imams
(FAEPTI) project. The FAEPTI project trains imams (religious leaders) and
laypeople to be AIDS educators. The imams incorporate prevention messages into their sermons, and both imams and lay educators address gender and economic power relations as influences on risk and risk reduction
within the Muslim community. As Islam permits polygyny, this faith-based
project was able to be supportive of a practice that is widespread among
both Muslim and non-Muslim populations in Africa. The "be faithful" message of the "ABC" approach to AIDS prevention was framed in terms of
all partners staying within the union. In reminding Muslim men of their
religious obligations, FAEPTI was able to discourage men from taking
on more wives if they could not support all wives equally and adequately.
Drawing on Islamic teachings emphasizing women's rights to earn and
control their own income, the FAEPTI project addressed the link between

women's economic vulnerability and AIDS by encouraging men to support their wife's/wives' efforts regarding earning and controlling income. The latter two strategies could lead to a reduction of risky sexual behavior that is motivated by women's economic needs. Indeed, both women and men reported that the initiation of income-generating projects for women had contributed to a reduction in women's economic vulnerability and their AIDS risk.

Thus, the imposition of alien ideology may be of no value or have negative consequences, particularly if it prevents a realistic assessment of risk and the development of appropriate risk-mitigating interventions. On the other hand, a compatible ideology can be supportive of indigenous practices and also advocate risk mitigation.

Conclusion

The findings discussed in this chapter and other research suggest that AIDS prevention in Africa is not as easy as "ABC." Women in marital relations and other unions face many challenges in trying to control their risk. We have emphasized the need for a more fluid and realistic view of marriage and sexual unions, one that is not prescriptive and that acknowledges many challenges for AIDS prevention. As a tool to assess these relationships for epidemiologic and other analyses, the concept of "risk cluster" is suggested as more appropriate than models that are couple focused or male focused.

A more realistic view of sexual partnering in developing countries, and reasons for women's decisions about sexual partnering, leads to the conclusion that economic need exposes a wide range of women to greater risk of AIDS. Some attention has been paid to the general need for empowering women, particularly with respect to negotiating sexual relationships, but we need to pay more attention to the bottom-line issue of financial empowerment. Interventions designed to encourage women to "abstain" or "be faithful" and negotiate the use of condoms are useless without interventions that give women the skills and resources to support themselves and their children and to make independent choices.

Faith-based initiatives that are compatible with and supportive of indigenous views can be effective agents for change. However, policies or intervention strategies that are based on alien ideologies can seriously bias and impede AIDS prevention efforts in Africa. Researchers need to support evidenced-based, culturally appropriate strategies for more effective mitigation of the AIDS epidemic in Africa.

Acknowledgments

Teresa Swezey gratefully acknowledges funding assistance from the Social Science Research Council International Pre-dissertation Fellowship Program, the Fulbright Institute of International Education for Research Abroad, and the U.S. Department of Education's Title VI Foreign Language Areas Studies Fellowships administered through Michigan State University's Center for the Advanced Study of International Development. She also thanks the Basoga communities who participated in the field research and members of the Islamic Medical Association of Uganda's Family AIDS Education and Prevention through Imams Project for their invaluable collaboration and assistance.

Notes

1. The phrase "living with HIV/AIDS" refers to all individuals who are HIV positive, regardless of whether they have developed symptoms associated with AIDS (UNAIDS/ WHO 2002). For further examples of the risks posed to women by their steady male partners in sub-Saharan Africa, see Allen and colleagues (1991) and Carpenter and colleagues (1999).

2. The largely rural Masaka and Rakai districts in southwestern Uganda have been especially affected by the HIV/AIDS epidemic.

3. See Robinson and colleagues (1999) and Ssengonzi and colleagues (1999) for further discussion of the role of concurrent partnerships in HIV transmission. As noted by Robinson and colleagues, short-term concurrent partnerships play an important role in the rapid spread of HIV during the early stages of an HIV epidemic. In the latter stages of an HIV epidemic, however, long-term concurrent partnerships between serodiscordant partners also play an important role.

4. This longitudinal project (the Medical Research Council General Population Cohort) has followed 10,000 people residing in fifteen neighboring villages in rural Masaka District, Uganda, since 1989. It, along with the Rakai Project conducted in a neighboring district of Uganda, is one of the few research studies in sub-Saharan Africa able to provide incidence as well as prevalence (number of total cases) HIV/AIDS data over an extended period of time. The authors observe that the lower incidence rates in Muslim men may be linked, in part, to male circumcision, which has been hypothesized as a protective factor for HIV transmission. All of the Muslim men in the study were circumcised, compared to about 10 percent of the non-Muslim men. The authors do not—at least in this article—extend the discussion of what accounts for the significantly lower rates of new infections among Muslim women and men in their study beyond this finding (Carpenter et al. 1999).

Another group of researchers who have conducted a long-term longitudinal study in the neighboring Rakai District (Gray et al. 2000; Gray et al. 2002) suggest that several factors related to being Muslim (in addition to nearly universal circumcision) may contribute to lower HIV incidence rates among Muslims. Other researchers dispute the potentially confounding influence of religion on the effect of male circumcision on lower HIV prevalence and incidence.

5. The most recently available Uganda DHS provides a slightly higher figure of 33 percent of all currently married women in polygynous unions.

6. This gendered difference in the percentage of young women and men living with HIV/AIDS in sub-Saharan Africa is also linked to women's lower level of knowledge about HIV/AIDS (as many as 80 percent of women in the fifteen-to-twenty-four-year-old cohort are estimated to lack adequate knowledge) and to physiological factors (immature cervical cells) that increase the risk of girls and young women for being infected with HIV (UNAIDS/WHO 2002).

References Cited

Adepoju, Aderanti. 1997. "Introduction." In *Family, Population, and Development in Africa*, ed. Aderanti Adepoju, 1–24. Atlantic Highlands, N.J.: Zed Books.

Adepoju, Aderanti, and Warira Mbugua. 1997. "The African Family: An Overview of Changing Forms." In *Family, Population, and Development in Africa*, ed. Aderanti Adepoju, 41–59. Atlantic Highlands, N.J.: Zed Books.

Ahlberg, Beth Maina. 1991. *Women, Sexuality and the Changing Social Order: The Impact of Government Policies on Reproductive Behavior in Kenya*. Vol. 1, International Studies in Global Change Series. Yverdon, Switzerland: Gordan and Breach.

Allen, Susan, Christina Lindan, Antoine Serufilira, Phillipe Van de Perre, Amy Chen Rundie, Francois Nsengumuremyi, Michel Caraël, Joan Schwalbe, and Stephen Hulley. 1991. "Human Immunodeficiency Virus Infection in Urban Rwanda: Demographic and Behavioral Correlates in a Representative Sample of Childbearing Women." *Journal of the American Medical Association* 266 (12): 1657–1663.

Aryee, A. F. 1997. "The African Family and Changing Nuptuality Patterns." In *Family, Population, and Development in Africa*, ed. Aderanti Adepoju, 78–96. Atlantic Highlands, N.J.: Zed Books.

Berkley, Seth F. 1994. "Public Health Measures to Prevent HIV Spread in Africa." In *AIDS in Africa*, ed. Max Essex, Souleymane Mboup, Phyllis J. Kanki, and Mbowa R. Kalengayi, 473–496. New York: Raven Press.

Blanc, Ann K. 2001. "The Effect of Power in Sexual Relationships on Sexual and Reproductive Health: An Examination of the Evidence." *Studies in Family Planning* 32 (3): 189–213.

Blanc, Ann K., and Anastasia J. Gage. 2000. "Men, Polygyny, and Fertility Over the Life-Course in Sub-Saharan Africa." In *Fertility and the Male Life-Cycle in the Era of Fertility Decline*, ed. Caroline Bledsoe, Susana Lerner, and Jane I. Guyer, 163–187. Oxford: Oxford University Press.

Bledsoe, Caroline. 1990. "Transformations in Sub-Saharan African Marriages and Fertility." *ANNALS, AAPSS* 510: 115–123.

———. 1993. "The Politics of Polygyny in Mende Education and Child Fosterage Transactions." In *Sex and Gender Hierarchies*, ed. Barbara Diane Miller, 170–192. Cambridge: Cambridge University Press.

Bledsoe, Caroline, and Gilles Pison. 1994. Introduction. In *Nuptuality in Sub-Saharan Africa: Contemporary Anthropological and Demographic Perspectives*, ed. Caroline Bledsoe and Gilles Pison, 1–22. Oxford: Clarendon Press.

Booth, Karen M. 1998. "National Mother, Global Whore, and Transnational Femocrats: The Politics of AIDS and the Construction of Women at the World Health Organization." *Feminist Studies* 24 (1): 115–139.

Caldwell, John C., Pat Caldwell, E. Maxine Ankrah, John K. Anarfi, Dominic K. Agyeman, Kofi Awusabo-Asare, and I. O. Oruboloye. 1994. "African Families and AIDS: Context, Reactions, and Potential Interventions." In *Sexual Networking and AIDS in Sub-Saharan Africa: Behavioural Research and the Social Context*, ed. I. O. Oruboloye, John C. Caldwell, Pat Caldwell, and Gigi Santow, 235–247. Canberra, Australia: Health Transition Centre, Australian National University.

Caraël, Michel. 1994. "The Impact of Marriage Change on the Risks of Exposure to Sexually Transmitted Diseases in Africa." In *Nuptuality in Sub-Saharan Africa: Contemporary Anthropological and Demographic Perspectives*, ed. Caroline Bledsoe and Giles Pison, 255–273. Oxford: Clarendon Press.

Carovano, Kathryn. 1991. "More Than Mothers and Whores: Redefining the AIDS Prevention Needs of Women." *International Journal of Health Services* 21 (1): 131–142.

Carpenter, Lucy M., Anatoli Kamal, Anthony Ruberantwiri, Samuel S. Malamba, and James A.G. Whitworth. 1999. "Rates of HIV-1 Transmission within Marriage in Rural Uganda in Relation to the HIV Sero-Status of The Partners." *AIDS* 13 (9): 1083–1089.

CHANGE. 2004. *Debunking the Myths in the U.S. Global AIDS Strategy: An Evidence-Based Analysis*. Takoma Park, Md.: Center for Health and Gender Equity, March.

Clignet, Remi. 1970. *Many Wives, Many Powers: Authority and Power in Polygynous Families*. Evanston, Ill.: Northwestern University Press.

de Bruyn, Maria, Helen Jackson, Marianne Wijermars, Virginia Curtin Knight, and Riet Berkvens. 1998. *Facing the Challenges of HIV/AIDS/STDs: A Gender-Based Response*. Amsterdam, The Netherlands, and Harare, Zimbabwe: Royal Tropical Institute (KIT) and the Southern Africa AIDS Information Dissemination Service (SAfAIDS).

Dodoo, F. Nii-Amoo. 1998. "Men Matter: Additive and Interactive Gendered Preferences and Reproductive Behavior in Kenya." *Demography* 35 (2): 229–242.

Farmer, Paul. 1996a. "On Suffering and Structural Violence: A View from Below." *Daedalus* 125 (1): 261–270.

———. 1996b. "Women, Poverty, and AIDS." In *Women, Poverty, and AIDS: Sex, Drugs, and Structural Violence*, ed. Paul Farmer, Margaret Connors, and Janie Simmons, 3–38. Monroe, Me.: Common Courage Press.

Garenne, Michel, and Etienne Van de Walle. 1989. "Polygyny and Fertility among the Sereer of Senegal." *Population Studies* 43 (2): 267–283.

Gray, Ronald H., Noah Kiwanuka, Thomas C. Quinn, Nelson K. Sewankambo, David Serwadda, Fred Wabwire Mangen, Tom Lutalo, Fred Nalugonda, Robert Kelly, Mary Meehan, Michael Z. Chen, Chuanjun Li, and Maria J. Wawer, for the Rakai Project Team. 2000. "Male Circumcision and HIV Acquisition and Transmission: Cohort Studies in Rakai, Uganda." *AIDS* 15 (5): 2371–2381.

Gray, Ronald H., Maria J. Wawer, Noah Kiwanuka, David Serwadda, Nelson K. Se-wankambo, and Fred Wawbire Mangen. 2002. "Male Circumcision and HIV Acquisition and Transmission: Rakai, Uganda" [correspondence]. *AIDS* 16 (5): 809–810.

Gupta, Geeta Rao, Ellen Weiss, and Daniel Whelan. 1996. "Gender and the Global HIV/AIDS Pandemic." In *The Gendered New World Order: Militarism, Development, and the Environment*, ed. Jennifer Turpin and Lois Ann Lorentzen, 147–161. New York: Routledge.

Karanja, Wambui Wa. 1994. "The Phenomenon of 'Outside Wives': Some Reflections on Its Possible Influence on Fertility." In *Nuptuality in Sub-Saharan Africa: Contemporary Anthropological and Demographic Perspectives*, ed. Caroline Bledsoe and Gilles Pison, 194–214. Oxford: Clarendon Press.

Kilbride Philip Leroy, and Janet Capriotti Kilbride. 1990. *Changing Family Life in East Africa: Women and Children at Risk*. University Park: Pennsylvania State University Press.

Lesthaeghe, Ron, Georgia Kaufmann, and Dominique Meekers. 1989. "The Nuptuality Regimes in Africa." In *Reproduction and Social Organization in Sub-Saharan Africa*, ed. Ron J. Lesthaeghe, 238–337. Berkley: University of California Press.

Locoh, Thérèse. 1994. "Social Change and Marriage Arrangements: New Types of Unions in Lomé, Togo." In *Nuptuality in Sub-Saharan Africa: Contemporary Anthropological and Demographic Perspectives*, ed. Caroline Bledsoe and Gilles Pison, 215–230. Oxford: Clarendon Press.

Mbugua, Wairiara. 1997. "The African Family and the Status of Women's Health." In *Family, Population, and Development in Africa*, ed. Aderanti Adepoju, 139–157. Atlantic Highlands, N.J.: Zed Books.

McGrath, Janet W., Charles B. Rwabukwali, Debra A. Schumann, Jonnie Pearson-Marks, Sylvia Nakaywia, Barbara Namande, Lucy Nakobye, and Rebecca Mukasa. 1993. "Anthropology and AIDS: The Cultural Context of Sexual Risk Behavior among Urban Baganda Women in Kampala, Uganda." *Social Science and Medicine* 36 (4): 429–439.

Macintyre, Kate, Lissanne Brown, and Stephen Sosler. 2001. "'It's Not What You Know, But Who You Knew': Examining the Relationship between Behavior Change and AIDS Mortality in Africa." *AIDS Education and Prevention* 13 (2): 160–174.

Meekers, Dominique, and Franklin Nadra. 1995. "Women's Perceptions of Polygyny among the Kaguru of Tanzania." *Ethnology* 34 (4): 315–325.

Morris, Martina, and Mirjam Kretzschmar. 1995. "Concurrent Partnerships and Transmission Dynamics in Networks." *Social Networks* 17: 299–318.

———. 2000. *A Microsimulation Study of the Effect of Concurrent Partnerships on the Spread of HIV in Uganda*. Population Research Institute Working Paper 00–07. University Park: Population Research Institute, Pennsylvania State University.

Obbo, Christine. 1987. "The Old and the New in East African Elite Marriages." In *Transformations of African Marriage*, ed. David Parkin and David Nyamwaya, 263–282. Manchester: Manchester University Press for the International African Institute.

Ocholla-Ayayo, A. B. C. 1987. "The African Family between Tradition and Modernity." In *Family, Population, and Development in Africa*, ed. Aderanti Adepoju, 60–77. Atlantic Highlands, N.J.: Zed Books.

O'Leary, A. 2000. "Women at Risk for HIV from a Primary Partner: Balancing Risk and Intimacy." *Annual Review of Sex Research* 11: 191–234.

Pebley, Anne, and Wariara Mbugua. 1989. "Polygyny and Fertility in Sub-Saharan Africa." In *Reproduction and Social Organization in Sub-Saharan Africa*, ed. Ron J. Lesthaeghe, 338–364. Berkley: University of California Press.

Rivers, Kim, and Peter Aggleton. 1999. *Men and the HIV Epidemic.* Geneva: UNDP HIV and Development Programme.

Robinson, N. J., D. Mulder, B. Auvert, J. Whitworth, and R. Hayes. 1999. "Type of Partnership and Heterosexual Spread of HIV Infection in Rural Uganda: Results from Simulation Modeling." *International Journal of STD and AIDS* 10 (11): 718–725.

Schoepf, Brooke Grundfest. 1998. "Inscribing the Body Politic: Women and AIDS in Africa." In *Pragmatic Women and Body Politics*, ed. Margaret Lock and Patricia A. Kaufert, 98–126. Cambridge: Cambridge University Press.

———. 2001. "International AIDS Research in Anthropology: Taking a Critical Perspective on the Crisis." *Annual Review of Anthropology* 30: 335–361.

Schoepf, Brooke Grundfest, Walu Engundu, Rukarangira Wa Nkera, Payanzo Ntsomo, and Claude Schoepf. 1991. "Gender, Power, and Risk of AIDS in Zaire." In *Women and Health in Africa*, ed. Meredith Turshen, 187–203. Trenton, N.J.: Africa World Press.

Schoepf, Brooke Grundfest, Rukarangira Wa Nkera, Claude Schoepf, Walu Engundu, and Payanzo Ntsomo. 1991. "AIDS and Society in Central Africa: A View from Zaire." In *AIDS in Africa: The Social and Policy Impact*, ed. Norman Miller and Richard C. Rockwell, 211–225. Lewiston, N.Y.: Edwin Mellon Press.

Simmons, Janie, Paul Farmer, and Brooke G. Schoepf. 1996. "A Global Perspective." In *Women, Poverty, and AIDS: Sex, Drugs, and Structural Violence*, ed. Paul Farmer, Margaret Connors, and Janie Simmons, 39–90. Monroe, Me: Common Courage Press.

Speizer, Ilene. 1995. "A Marriage Trichotomy and Its Application." *Demography* 32 (4): 533–542.

Ssengonzi, Robert, Martina Morris, Maria Wawer, and Nelson Sewankambo. 1999. *Spatial Networks of Sexual Partnerships in a Rural Ugandan Population: Implications for HIV Transmission.* Population Research Institute Working Paper 99-08. University Park: Population Research Institute, Pennsylvania State University.

Standing, Hilary. 1992. "AIDS: Conceptual and Methodological Issues in Researching Sexual Behavior in Sub-Saharan Africa." *Social Science and Medicine* 34 (5): 475–483.

Ulin, Pricilla R. 1992. "African Women and AIDS: Negotiating Behavioral Change." *Social Science and Medicine* 34 (1): 63–73.

UNAIDS/WHO. 2002. *AIDS Epidemic Update, December 2001.* Geneva: Joint United Nations Programme on HIV/AIDS (UNAIDS) and World Health Organization (WHO).

Van de Walle, Étienne. 1968. "Marriage in African Censuses and Inquiries." In *The Demography of Tropical Africa*, 183–238. Princeton, N.J.: Princeton University Press.

Van de Walle, Étienne, and Dominique Meekers. 1994. "Marriage Drinks and Kola Nuts." In *Nuptuality in Sub-Saharan Africa: Contemporary Anthropological and*

Demographic Perspectives, ed. Caroline Bledsoe and Gilles Pison, 57–73. Oxford: Clarendon Press.

Ware, Helen. 1979. "Polygyny: Women's Views in a Traditional Society, Nigeria 1975." *Journal of Marriage and the Family* 41 (1): 185–195.

Whelan, Daniel. 1999. *Gender and HIV/AIDS: Taking Stock of Research and Programmes*. UNAIDS Best Practice Collection. Geneva: UNAIDS.

Whitworth, J. A. G. 1999. "Medical Research Council Programme on AIDS in Uganda—The First 10 Years." *Interdisciplinary Science Reviews* 24 (3): 179–184.

Wittrup, Inge. 1990. "Me and My Husband's Wife: An Analysis of Polygyny among Mandinka in the Gambia." *Folk* 32: 117–141.

13

Gender, Poverty, and AIDS Risk

Case Studies from Rural Uganda

CHARLES B. RWABUKWALI

Introduction

AIDS currently affects all African countries, especially those in eastern, southern, and central Africa (WHO 2002). HIV/AIDS is transmitted there primarily by heterosexual contact (Mann and Tarantola 1996; UN-AIDS 2002). In several African countries, such as Uganda, available data demonstrates that increasingly more women than men are infected with HIV (Berkley et al. 1990; STD/AIDS Control Programme 2002). The rapid spread of HIV/AIDS among women is only now beginning to be fully understood. There is growing awareness that women generally, and women in developing countries in particular, are more vulnerable both biologically and socially to HIV infection than heterosexual men (Esu-Williams 2000; Figuera 2002).

From a purely biological point of view, women seem to be at greater risk of acquiring HIV/AIDS and other sexually transmitted diseases (STDs) than men. First, the volume of male ejaculate, which is deposited directly onto the vulnerable cervical tissue, is often much greater than the cervical and vaginal secretions (Alexander 1990; Susskind 2001). Second, once an infection has been established, the anatomy of the female does not allow ready visualization of the damaged tissue. In developed countries, this is not such a big problem, since modern medical procedures are available for infected women. However, in the developing world, such medical procedures are not readily available, due to scarcity of resources. Last, in most cases when women are infected with STDs, such infections cause no symptoms or such mild ones that many women fail to seek treatment. In effect, even if diagnostic procedures and treatment were available, there is no guarantee that all women would use them (Alexander 1990; Nagy-Agren 2001).

But biological and physiological factors only partially explain gender differences regarding vulnerability to risk of HIV infection. In reality, as Mann and colleagues (1992: 578) observe, "It is people and their behavior that constitute the key dimension in the HIV equation." Therefore, a comprehensive understanding of gender differences in HIV risk must go beyond biological factors to analyze male and female behavior and the ways in which behavior is influenced by gender roles and relationships (Gupta 2001; Gupta and Weiss 1993).

The heart of the problem with regard to female vulnerability to HIV infection, it has been argued, is the unequal role and status of women worldwide (Figuera 2002; Gupta et al. 1996; Whitehead 2001). Often this is subsumed under the rubric of gender relations. It is argued further that these unequal gender relations lead to greater economic and social dependence of women on men, hence increasing their vulnerability both to poverty and risk of HIV infection (Bianco 2001; Gupta 2001; Gupta and Weiss 1993; Henderson 2000). However, the notion that the unequal role and status of women compared to men increases women's vulnerability to AIDS is often based on much generalization. There is a dearth of carefully conducted studies that show—empirically—the link between unequal gender relations and increased vulnerability to HIV/AIDS.

The worldwide recession of the 1980s affected many developing countries negatively, with several of them experiencing a decline in their gross domestic product (GDP). In several countries, those most affected by the decline in GDP tend to be women, who have seen an increase in their poverty levels (Mann and Tarantola 1996). This poverty is compounded by the fact that in several countries, women have no access to education or training and often find it difficult to start small businesses, because they find it hard to get credit since they have no collateral (Cohen 2001; Henderson 2000; Lycette 1984). Many women in the developing world are engaged in agriculture, but female farmers find it almost impossible to get agricultural credit to purchase quality seed and machinery (Esu-Williams 2000; Ramkin and Wilson 2000). In addition, in Africa, very few women are in salaried or in wage employment, and yet increasingly more women are becoming the sole providers for their households in several African countries (Gupta and Weiss 1993; Lycette 1984).

Women's poverty has implications for their increased vulnerability to HIV infection. First, for many women, especially those in developing countries, sexual networking whether by married or unmarried women becomes an important survival strategy (Bianco 2001; Obbo 1993). In India, for example, it has been reported that poor widows, divorced women, and other marginalized women will often have sex with landlords in order to have their rent waived and to have access to other scarce commodities (George and Jaswal 1994). In Uganda, young girls are enticed into sex by rich older males (commonly known as "sugar daddies") by a promise of money and other gifts (Standing 1992).

It has further been shown that poverty influences women's vulnerability to HIV infection to the extent that a poor woman is more likely than a more affluent woman to be "stuck" with a cheating husband (Cohen 2001; Gupta 2001; Mann and Tatantola 1996; Whitehead 2001). To this end, studies show that despite being married and remaining faithful to her husband, a woman can often be at risk of infection with HIV. For example, in Rwanda 20 percent of HIV-infected women had only one lifetime sexual partner, and in Morocco 45 percent of HIV-infected women had been infected by their husbands (Mann and Tarantola 1996). However, it should be noted that it seems these reports are referring to the "monogamy" of the woman, not the man. In countries like Uganda, polygyny (where a man marries two or more women) is still practiced, so even if a woman is being sexually faithful to her husband, she can still be put at risk by the husband if she is in a polygynous union where one of the wives is not faithful, or if the husband engages in extramarital sex. Moreover, as has been pointed out, in many societies married women have few legal rights in marriage, and often have no choice but to accept sex with their spouse, even if their spouse has AIDS (Berkley et al. 1990).

Beyond the above-discussed economic determinants of women's vulnerability to HIV infection, there are important sociocultural factors that are believed to place women at increased risk of HIV infection, hence making it difficult for them to prevent themselves from getting infected. In some cultures, women's modesty is greatly valued, and as such, women are not supposed to know "too much" about their own sexuality (Ankomah 1992). This lack of knowledge about their own physiology leads many women to have unfounded fears about preventive methods, such as condoms. Studies among women in Uganda found that many women believed that a condom could fall off inside the vagina, leading to serious medical complications (Rwabukwali et al. 1994).

In many societies, cultural norms demand sexual fidelity and docile sexual behavior from women while permitting and even encouraging early sexual experimentation, multiple sex partnership, and aggressive, dominating behavior for men (Gupta and Weiss 1993). Therefore, to understand both women's vulnerability and options for prevention, it is important to look critically at cultural norms about men's sexual behavior. For example, in many societies, variety in sexual partners is perceived to be an essential part of men's culture (Goldstein 1994), and in some cultures polygyny is a preferred form of marriage, being a symbol of material wealth and high status (McGrath et al. 1993). Such cultural norms, together with social economic dependency, limit women's ability to negotiate safer sex, and make women more vulnerable to infection with STDs, including AIDS (Gupta and Weiss 1993; Gupta et al. 1996).

In sum, it appears from the research literature that poverty is seen as a risk factor for HIV infection among women, because women may resort to multiple sexual practices or stay with husbands who do. However, not all poor women resort to sex work or risky sexual practices. It is important to examine empirically how poor women react to poverty and not to make sweeping generalizations that they will automatically engage in multiple sexual practices. Second, much of the research literature present women as "stuck" in monogamous relationships and exposed to HIV by their husbands. There may be some element of truth in this, but not all women accept being "stuck" with cheating husbands. Therefore, there is a need to empirically document the circumstances under which one woman may agree to stay with a cheating husband, while another may leave. Last, there is a need for more studies to corroborate findings (such as those by McGrath et al. 1993) that report a strong association between poverty and HIV among some Ugandan cultures. In my view, the important point is to stress the need to understand in empirical terms what it is about poverty specifically that increases women's vulnerability to the risk of infection with HIV. This chapter, therefore, will examine the role that gender and poverty play in one's vulnerability to increased HIV risk among a group of rural Ugandan women.

The Batoro

The data on which this chapter is based are from the Batoro of western Uganda.[1] It is important to understand the sociocultural variables that have an impact on gender relations among the Batoro and how this affects Batoro women's vulnerability to HIV/AIDS. The Batoro are a patrilineal (descent through the male line) Bantu society, and in the past clans and lineages tended to be powerful corporate groups that occupied particular hills, ridges, or villages. Today, however, clans and lineages are not corporate groups, although they still have important economic, cultural, and religious functions. For example, in several instances, clans have been involved in arrangements for succession in the event of a death of a clan member. Clans also help in solving local disputes. However, it is fair to say that currently, clans do not play a crucial and integrative role as in the past.

Toro is a male-dominated society, and in the past the superiority of the male Mutoro (the singular of Batoro) over a woman was regarded as the basic foundation of a Mutoro man's whole way of life. Today, Batoro women continue to do most of the housework in addition to working in the gardens. However, through modern education, new ideas about relationships between men and women are beginning to emerge. For example, while women are still expected to be deferential, respectful, and obedient to their husbands, their status has improved. These days, women enjoy a number of freedoms and privileges. Batoro women can now take up employment outside of the home, and a daughter can inherit her father's property.

Marriage in Toro traditionally took place, and still continues to occur, at an early age, especially for girls. In most cases, the primary purpose of marriage is procreation. In the past, strong value was attached to female virginity, and at the same time there were strong sanctions against an unmarried female bearing a child (Perlman 1975). Some of these values still exist, but they are not held as strongly as before. In the past, most of the marriages were arranged by parents for their children. These days, only a small fraction of marriages are arranged. However, as in the past, payment of bridewealth is required to express transfer of rights in marriage to the husband by the wife's father. Polygyny was, and is, an important conjugal institution, although only a few wealthy and powerful men can afford it. In Toro society, both in the past and today, there is great value attached to children, and a man with many children is regarded as "wealthy."

This study was carried out in Mugoma village, Kabarole District (formerly Toro Kingdom), western Uganda, about 200 miles west of Kampala, Uganda's capital city. This site was selected for two reasons. First, it is a rural community. Despite the fact that the majority of Ugandans live in rural areas, most studies on HIV/AIDS in Uganda have been urban based. This study in rural Kabarole district is an attempt to collect data in a rural setting. A second reason for choosing to study Kabarole is that I was born in the district and belong to the Toro tribe. I speak the local dialect (Rutoro) fluently. Although I have not lived in Kabarole all my life, I grew up in a rural village, and I understand most of the local culture at a personal level. However, I anticipated that some of the rituals, ceremonies, and behaviors would be completely new to me.

Before going to the field, I was aware that being an indigenous researcher has its problems. For example, I might appear to blunder if I asked about matters that people regarded as obvious and expected me to know (Narayan 1993). However, it turned out that being an indigenous researcher was advantageous for me. The villagers as a whole, and the informants in particular, were cooperative, and made it easy for me to establish rapport. Before going into the field, I was aware that my status as an elite male, studying village women, might influence the types of information that I would collect. In general, however, I learned that my "elite" status as a university "professor" made it easy for me to get access to the villagers and made it unlikely that many women would refuse an interview. Instead, I learned that most people in the village were intrigued and also amused that a "big" man like myself could spend a whole year in their village merely talking to people.

I was also aware that being a male interviewer studying village women and asking about several issues, including sexual values and sexual norms, might embarrass some of the respondents and make it hard for them to give truthful answers. In practice, the interviews generally went smoothly. Most of the questions were bland and factual and did not cause embarrassment to the women. Even questions concerning cultural values about sex did not cause much trouble. In any case, most of these questions did not refer to the woman in particular, but rather to Toro culture in general. A few questions on sex values were personal and caused some embarrassment to a few women, but this did cause much discomfort, and only one elderly woman in the entire sample terminated an interview because she thought the questions on cultural values about sex were inappropriate.

Methodology

Interviews with 120 village women aged fifteen years and above, residing in the study area (Mugoma village), were conducted over a period of twelve months. The aim of these interviews was to identify sociocultural and sexual behavioral patterns that influence the vulnerability to HIV/AIDS risk among Batoro women, and to identify sociocultural factors influencing Batoro women's choices of preventive strategies against HIV. Two interviews were held with each woman. The first interview collected sociodemographic data such as age, marital status, economic status, and religion. The second interview collected information concerning such issues as the role of sexuality in Toro society, awareness and knowledge about HIV/AIDS, cultural norms and values that might predispose Batoro women to AIDS, and relative power and prestige between men and women in Toro society. I conducted two separate interviews to avoid taking too much of the respondents' time. Many of these women were very busy, cultivating their gardens and looking after their families. They were unlikely to sit down for very long interviews. Plus, the first interview enabled me to establish rapport with the respondents before asking the more personal questions in the second interview. I did not lose any of the 120 women when I tried to interview them for the second time.

In order to gain a deeper understanding of the intersection of cultural factors, gender relations, and poverty in influencing Batoro women's vulnerability to HIV, in-depth interviews were also done with a subsample of thirty women ("key informants") who were selected using snowball/networking procedures. That is, once a woman was identified as particularly knowledgeable about cultural issues such as sex customs or gender relations, she was recruited and then asked to name two or three other women whom she thought would be a useful resource to interview. The investigator visited each of the thirty "key informants" twice a week for a period of twelve weeks. During this time, informants were asked to describe their "critical life events"—that is, events that were regarded as most formative in their lives socially, economically, and politically. Additional interviews were held with these women to cover neighborhood social settings in which informants spend their time, the informants' social networks, their views on sexual behavior, household economics, and gender relations in the context of poverty and the AIDS epidemic. Participant observation in the community permitted additional observation regarding gender relations.

The 120 semistructured interviews were conducted by me (the principal investigator) and one field assistant. All interviews were tape recorded, with consent. I conducted all "key informant" interviews. To ensure dependability and confirmability of the data collected, both the research assistant and I kept field notes that were written during or soon after an interview or observation. These field notes were later expanded and comments added.

After transcription, data from the semistructured interviews was entered on a laptop computer using the ethnographic software Ethnograph v4.0. This resulted in coded qualitative data, which was then transformed into quantitative information using the EpiInfo 5.0 program to generate frequencies. The data set from the in-depth interviews was analyzed using content analysis. Each of the thirty cases was reviewed in total as a case study, to obtain an understanding of the "whole picture" as it affects HIV risk, and AIDS risk reduction behavior. This chapter presents data arising from the "key informant" interviews.

Women and AIDS: A Portrait of Vulnerability

The following three case studies from the village of Mugoma in Kabarole district of western Uganda are presented to test the thesis that poverty and female powerlessness in rural African society are associated with increased vulnerability to risk of infection with HIV.[2]

Case 1

Atwoki is twenty years old, married for the second time, and Catholic.[3] Atwoki and her husband are desperately poor. They live in one of the most poorly constructed houses in the village. The house is made of grass, which severely leaks during the rainy season. Atwoki informed me that they lost their more permanent house during the earthquake of 1994. But unfortunately, they have not saved or borrowed enough money to buy materials to put up a decent house. As Atwoki puts it: "As you can see, things are not good for us. We are living in a temporary shelter which leaks whenever it rains. My children are now constantly sick because of the poor accommodation. We are trying our best to build a new house, but where is the money? We are so poor."

I asked Atwoki to tell me briefly about her life when growing up as a young girl. She informed me that she was born in the village of Mugoma. Both her parents are alive. Her father had two wives, with her mother being the legally married wife, which made the stepmother a mistress. The stepmother died some time back. Atwoki was the only child of her mother. I asked her if she had ever been to school. She replied: "I went to Kagote primary school up to primary four, but had to leave because my father claimed that he had no money to pay school fees. I think this was not true, because my brothers continued to go to school. I think the main reason he did not pay school fees for me is because I am a girl, and he thought it was a waste of his money to educate girls."

When asked what were the most important social events in her life, she mentioned her two marriages.

After school, when I was about fifteen years old, I got married to my first husband. The man was a driver of a bus that worked on the Fort Portal–Kampala route. He had a lot of money, and at first I was excited by the marriage. Within a short period we had three children. Then the man began to mistreat me. He would disappear for months, and I heard rumors that he had several girlfriends in Kampala. I felt deserted and had to leave after seven years of marriage. I have been with my current husband for about eight years. He is a loving husband, but very poor. He works as a casual laborer. As you can see, my eldest son is out of school because we cannot afford school fees.

On my visits to Atwoki's home, I noticed that she and her family are, even by village standards, extremely poor. They have very few personal possessions in their temporary house, and their compound is so small that when Atwoki washes her laundry, she takes it to a neighbor's compound for drying. As noted above, her eldest son is not in school, and her small daughter walks around naked most of the time. Atwoki has no money to buy clothing for the children. In one of the interviews, I asked her what she saw as the main problem facing households in Mugoma, and she replied:

Two of the biggest problems facing women in the village are scarcity of land and firewood. For example, I cultivate land belonging to a rich man, and it is three kilometers away. I pay rent of 4,000 shillings per season for using the land; at times, the landlord takes part of the produce.[4] This reduces any profit that I might get from the crops. Also scarcity of land means I cannot keep a cow or two, which could provide milk for my children. The situation with regard to firewood is even worse. In the past, we used to collect wood from the nearby swamps, but most of the swamps have been drained and turned into dairy farms by the richer families in the village. It is now very difficult to get firewood.

When I asked Atwoki to describe life in her household, she replied that until recently, relations with her husband were good, despite his poverty. But in recent times, he comes home very late, and rumors reaching her indicate that he is befriending a barmaid in the next village. This has made Atwoki very bitter. "Imagine, this man is poor and now I hear he befriends a barmaid. Where does he get the money? Our son is out of school because he can't pay school fees, we live in the worst house in the village, and the stupid man is having affairs. I think he is mad. If I confirm the rumor, I am going to fight him and the barmaid."

I asked her if she would consider leaving her husband if the rumor proved correct. She replied that she would not, because she has nowhere to go. Her father would not accept her back in his home. He has enough problems of his own. As for relations between men and women in the community, she had this to say: "Mostly they are cordial and warm, but there are some couples who quarrel a lot. Mostly, these are families where the man is a womanizer. When the wife finds out, there are all sorts of trouble. Also some couples quarrel if the man is unable to provide basic necessities for the wife."

On the question of politics, she said that she and her husband are shy about politics. They believe that Resistance Committee level 1 (RC1) has little power, and they are also completely fed up with the behavior of the local politician who represents their district in parliament.[5]

> The politician is terrible. For example, he brought two boreholes [a borehole is a well that has a manual device for pumping water to the surface] to the village, but one of them is located in his courtyard and is guarded by hostile dogs so that we cannot use it. What logic is there for one man to keep a whole borehole to himself? Also, whenever materials come for the benefit of the poor people in the village, the parliamentarian grabs them for himself and his friends. Recently, when this politician won elections, he killed a big cow to celebrate, but few of the villagers were invited. Definitely, he is not popular in the village.

Overall, Atwoki thinks that life is hard socially, economically, and politically. She thinks things may improve under President Museveni's continuing rule.

Case 2

Akiiki is twenty-eight years old, married, and Muslim. She and her husband have two small children. The oldest girl is four years old, and the younger boy is two. Akiiki lives in a fairly nice home, with her house surrounded by many decorative trees and flowering plants. Inside her house, it is equally neat and pleasant. The walls of her living room are covered with all sorts of family photographs, as well as photos from magazines.

I asked Akiiki to tell me about some of the most important events that have shaped her life. She had this to say:

> I was brought up by my father and grandmother, my mother having died shortly after I was born. I attended one of the best secondary schools in the district, but I got expelled after I became pregnant when I was in senior three [tenth year of study].[6] The boy who made me pregnant was my classmate. While I was expelled, he was allowed to continue with his studies. He has now completed technical college and is a successful businessman and builder, while I am nothing. Life is unfair. I should have been given the same treatment as the boy, but

instead, I was blamed for the pregnancy, while the boy was left to go free. Anyway, unfortunately, I had a miscarriage and lost the baby. I could not go back to school, so I was forced to look for a job. I began to work as a shop attendant. While working as a shop attendant, I met my current husband, a fellow shop attendant.

Akiiki continued to inform me that her husband is a Muslim, so when they got married, Akiiki was forced to convert from Catholicism to Islam. I asked her if she converted willingly, and she replied: "I really did not want to convert to Islam, but you know among Muslims, it is [up to] the woman to convert and not the man. Also, in Toro society, women have little power. It is the man who has the power, so the woman should change her religion, but not the man. I had wanted to keep my Catholic religion and had hoped one of my children would take up my faith. But this has been denied to me, and I feel angry and helpless."

Later on, I asked her to describe her marriage currently, and how she gets along with her in-laws. She said:

I am really not happy in my marriage. I am better educated and come from a better home than my husband. I don't really like it. My husband is really poor and many of the things in this house have been provided by my parents who feel sorry for me. My husband works extremely long hours, usually from eight in the morning to eight in the evening. However, I think he lies to me. I think he spends some of the time womanizing. I have heard rumors that he has a girlfriend. He has also hinted to me that as a Muslim he needs to marry a second wife. I think this is a stupid idea, since he cannot even look after one wife properly. I am also worried that if he marries a second wife, the woman may be infected with AIDS and all of us will die. I am seriously thinking of leaving this man. A few men have proposed love affairs with me. So far I have refused, but if my husband brings a second wife, I will have a few affairs of my own or divorce completely.

In general, Akiiki is critical of men in the village. She said men could do more to help their wives with some of the domestic chores. Instead, she pointed out that most men spend time loitering in the village and getting drunk. To her, this was one reason why Mugoma was so underdeveloped.

Case 3

Amooti is forty years old, divorced twice, and Protestant (Church of Uganda). She told me that she studied up to primary five (the fifth year of primary school), but had to leave school because her father claimed to have no money. The little money that was available was used to pay for her brother's school fees. This is not entirely unusual in Toro society. Many parents, if forced to make a choice, will pay for the boys' education over the girls' education, since it is thought that girls do not have a bright future except to get married. But boys can get "good" jobs upon completion of school.

I asked Amooti to describe some of the most important social events in her life, and she responded:

> The most important social events in my life have been my two previous marriages. I contracted my first marriage when I was very young, soon after school. The marriage lasted fifteen years. The husband was a businessman. We produced three children, all boys. The eldest is now working in Kampala. I left the first husband because he became mentally sick and increasingly violent. He blamed his sickness on me, saying that I was bewitching him. This was not true of course, but still the man mistreated me. To make matters worse, he continued to drink alcohol, even after the doctors told him not to. The alcohol made his condition worse. I had no choice but to leave him. Then I married my second husband. The marriage lasted five years, and we had three children, all girls. Again, I was forced to leave this man because he also became abusive and a womanizer. I feared he would give me AIDS. Even now I am not sure I am safe. He may have infected me already.

Amooti is extremely poor. She has no house of her own, and currently lives with her unmarried young brother. After several visits to her home, I learned that she sells alcohol and snacks to get money for survival. This activity is illegal, as it was banned by the RC1 Council, but she does it anyway in order to survive. In her words: "I sell 'tonto' and 'waragi' [two popular drinks], in order to get some money to buy food. I know it is wrong, but what can I do? If I don't get some money, either I will steal or starve to death."

Her extreme poverty and her sale of alcohol could make her vulnerable to sexual advances from men who come to drink at her place, thus putting her at risk of getting HIV/AIDS. I noticed that she is extremely popular in the village, and several young men keep coming to her house either to chat with her or to buy some alcohol. I asked her if she had any "boyfriends" among her customers. She did not give a straight reply, but told me that she might sleep with some of them if "her body got attracted" to them. Whenever I visited Amooti, I was reminded of studies like that of Seeley and colleagues (1994) in rural Masaka District that have found that women who sell alcohol in their homes are more vulnerable to risk of infection with HIV than women in the general population.

I asked Amooti what she thinks of the current political situation, and she was full of praise for President Museveni and the National Resistance Movement (NRM) administration:

> Although I am not very active in politics, I am thankful that Museveni is in power. He has brought peace to our homes. In the past, things were very bad. Former dictator Idi Amin's soldiers and Obote's soldiers used to roam around the village stealing chickens and goats from people. They raped many women, both young and old. They were like animals. They destroyed our houses, and many young men had to run away from the village for fear of those bad soldiers. But those bad days are over. Now soldiers come around, but they pay for whatever they want. We don't fear them anymore. I shall vote for Museveni whether he campaigns or not.

Gender, Poverty, and AIDS Reconsidered

Several studies attribute women's vulnerability to HIV infection to their poverty and unequal status in society compared to men (Gupta and Weiss 1993; Henderson 2000). The prevailing notion from these studies is that poverty increases women's vulnerability to HIV risk. It is argued that poor women will turn to sex work or to multiple sex partners to make ends meet, or that because women have little power, they will quietly endure a husband or boyfriend who is having love affairs, hence increasing their risk of HIV.

The three case histories of Atwoki, Akiiki, and Amooti provide mixed evidence of the assertion that African rural women tend to be poor, marginalized, and powerless, and that this makes them vulnerable to infection with HIV/AIDS. It is true that the three women in the case studies are poor, and it is tempting to conclude that since these women are poor, and since they have less power than men, they are automatically at increased risk of HIV/AIDS. The situation is more complicated than that. For example, not all of the women were completely dependent on men. Akiiki and Amooti have found a way to reduce their poverty and dependence on men. Akiiki gets financial assistance from her well-to-do parents, while Amooti gets money through the sale of alcohol and snacks. Therefore, while some women who are completely dependent on their husbands for sustenance may be said to be vulnerable to the risk of HIV/AIDS because they would be unable to leave a philandering husband, since this would cut them off from the man's support, many women find some way to overcome or minimize their poverty and risk by engaging in trade. Amooti is a case in point.

In effect, it is not poverty as such that creates vulnerability to HIV infection among rural women such as those in Mugoma, but rather it is the combination of poverty and other social, cultural, and structural factors that put women at increased risk of HIV infection (Cohen 2001). For example, the situation of Akiiki and Atwoki, who suspect that their husbands are having extramarital affairs, serves to boost the argument that cultural values that permit men to have multiple sexual relations while insisting on strict female fidelity tend to put women at increased risk of HIV/AIDS.

In conclusion, the three case studies presented here provide mixed results with respect to the notion that women's vulnerability to HIV/AIDS is due to their poverty and lack of power in society compared to men. True, many poor women are vulnerable to HIV, but not all poor women are equally vulnerable. Some have found ways of reducing their poverty and vulnerability, and not necessarily by "selling" sex.

Acknowledgments

Data on which this chapter is based was collected during twelve months of fieldwork in Kabarole district, western Uganda, during 1996 and 1997.

Notes

1. "Mutoro" (singular), "Batoro" (plural), are the people who inhabit the Kingdom of Toro in western Uganda. Their language is Rutoro.

2. Kabarole district is populated by the Batoro, a Bantu ethnic group.

3. All names in these case profiles are pseudonyms.

4. One U.S. dollar is worth approximately 2,000 Uganda shillings.

5. In 1986, when the National Resistance Movement (NRM) came into power in Uganda, it established a system of Resistance Committees (RCs) for the smooth administration of the country. There are five levels of elected representative committees. RC1 is the village level, representing between thirty to fifty households; RC2 is the parish level; RC3 is the subcounty level; RC4 is the county level; and RC5 is the district level. RCs are mandated to identify local problems and to mobilize the people to solve these problems. The RC system allows citizens to participate at all levels of representation without discrimination. Under the new Uganda Constitution enacted in October 1995, Resistance Committees and Resistance Councils have been renamed Local Councils and Committee (LCs).

6. In Uganda, the formal education system runs from primary school to universities and other tertiary institutions. Primary school is for seven years. Secondary school has

two levels: Ordinary "O" level, which is four years (Senior 1–Senior 4), and Advanced "A" level, which is two years beyond O level (Senior 5–Senior 6). When a student completes the thirteenth year of school, Senior 6, the student may enter a university based upon his or her performance on the A-level exams. At the end of either O or A level, students may choose to enter teachers' college or technical school for three years for those who have completed O level, or for two years for those who have completed A level.

References Cited

Alexander, H. J. 1990. "Sexual Transmission of Human Immunodeficiency Virus: Virus Entry into the Male and Female Genital Tract." *Fertility and Sterility* 54 (1): 1–18.

Ankomah, A. 1992. "Premarital Sexual Relationships in Ghana in the Era of AIDS." *Health Policy and Planning* 7: 135–143.

Berkley, S. F., W. Naamara, S. I. Okware, R. Downing, J. Konde- Lule, M. Wawer, M. Musagaara, and S. Musgrave. 1990. "AIDS and HIV Infection in Uganda: Are More Women Infected Than Men?" *AIDS* 4 (12): 1237–1242.

Bianco, M. 2001. "Women, Girls and HIV/AIDS." *Women's Health Journal* 1: 7–11.

Cohen, Desmond. 2001. "Joint Epidemics: Poverty and AIDS in Sub-Saharan Africa." *Harvard International Review* 23 (3): 54–58.

Esu-Williams, Eka. 2000. "Gender and HIV/AIDS in Africa—Our Hope Lies in the Future." *Journal of Health Communication* 5 (Supplement): 123–126.

Figuera, Michaela. 2002. "Gender Inequalities Render Women Particularly Vulnerable." www.communitylawcentre.org.za/ser/docs-2002.

George, A., and S. Jaswal. 1994. *Understanding Sexuality: Ethnographic Study of Poor Women in Bombay*. Women and AIDS Research Report Series. Washington, D.C.: International Center for Research on Women.

Goldstein, D. 1994. *Culture, Class, and Gender Politics of a Modern Disease: Women and AIDS in Brazil*. Washington, D.C.: International Center for Research on Women.

Gupta, G. R. 2001. "'It's Not Fair': AIDS, Gender and Human Rights." In *Reproductive Health, Gender and Human Rights: A Dialogue*, ed. Elaine Murphy and Karin Ringheim, 33–39. Washington, D.C.: Program for Appropriate Technology in Health (PATH).

Gupta, Geeta Rao, and Ellen Weiss. 1993. "Women's Lives and Sex: Implications for AIDS Prevention." *Culture, Medicine and Psychiatry* 17 (4): 399–412.

Gupta, G. R., Ellen Weiss, and Daniel Whelan. 1996. "Women and AIDS: Building a New HIV Prevention Strategy." In *AIDS in the World II: Global Dimensions, Social Roots, and Responses*, ed. Jonathan Mann and Daniel Tarantola, 215–228. New York: Oxford University Press.

Henderson, C. W. 2000. "Breaking the Silence on Abuse of Women and HIV." *Women's Health Weekly*, August 31, 9–10.

Lycette, M. 1984. *Improving Women's Access to Credit in the Third World: Policy and Program Recommendations:* Washington, D.C.: International Center for Research on Women.

Mann, Jonathan, and Daniel Tarantola, eds. 1996. *AIDS in the World II: Global Dimensions, Social Roots, and Responses*. New York: Oxford University Press.

Mann, Jonathan, Daniel J. M. Tarantola, and Thomas W. Netter, eds. 1992. *AIDS in the World*. Cambridge, Mass.: Harvard University Press.

McGrath, Janet W., C. B. Rwabukwali, D. A. Schumann, J. Pearson-Marks, S. Nakayima, B. Namande, L. Nakyobe, and R. Mukasa. 1993. "Anthropology and AIDS: The Cultural Context of Sexual Risk Behavior among Urban Baganda Women in Kampala, Uganda." *Social Science and Medicine* 36: 429–439.

Nagy-Agren, S. 2001. "Infectious Diseases and Women's Health: Link to Social and Economic Development." *Journal of the Medical American Women Association* 56 (3): 92–93.

Narayan. Kirin. 1993. "How Native Is a 'Native' Anthropologist?" *American Anthropologist* 95: 671–686.

Obbo, Christine. 1993. "HIV Transmission through Social and Geographical Networks in Uganda." *Social Science and Medicine* 36 (7): 949–955.

Perlman, Melvin L. 1975. "Children Born Out of Wedlock and the Status of Women in Toro, Uganda." *Rural Africa* 29: 95–119.

Ramkin, William, and Charles Wilson. 2000. "African Women with HIV." *British Medical Journal* 321 (7276): 1543–1544.

Rwabukwali, C. B., Debra A. Schumann, Janet W. McGrath, Cindie Carrol-Pankhurst, Rebecca Mukasa, Sylvia Nakayiwa, Lucy Nakyobe, and Barbara Namande. 1994. "Culture, Sexual Behavior and Attitudes towards Condom Use among Baganda Women." In *Global AIDS Policy*, ed. Douglas A. Feldman, 70–89. Westport, Conn.: Bergin and Garvey.

Seeley, Janet, A. Sam, S. Malamba, Andrew J. Nun, Daan W. Mulder, Jane F. Kengeya-Kayondo, and Thomas G. Barton. 1994. "Socioeconomic Status, Gender, and the Risk of HIV-1 Infection in a Rural Community in South West Uganda." *Medical Anthropology Quarterly* 8 (1): 78–89.

Standing, Hilary. 1992. "AIDS: Conceptual and Methodological Issues in Researching Sexual Behavior in Sub-Saharan Africa." *Social Science and Medicine* 34 (5): 475–483.

STD/AIDS Control Programme. 2002. *HIV/AIDS Surveillance Report*. Entebbe, Uganda: Ministry of Health.

Susskind, Y. 2001. *Women's Health in a Sick World*. www.madre.org.

UNAIDS. 2002. *Report on the Global HIV/AIDS Epidemic*. Geneva: World Health Organization.

Whitehead, A. 2001. "AIDS and Poverty: The Links." *AIDS Analysis Africa* 12 (2): 1–5.

WHO (World Health Organization). 2002. *Epidemiological Fact Sheets on HIV/AIDS and Sexually Transmitted Infections 2002 Update*. Geneva: World Health Organization.

14

Culture in Action

Reactions to Social Responses to HIV/AIDS in Africa

ELEANOR PRESTON-WHYTE

Culture and Tradition in Africa

Discourses around HIV/AIDS in Africa are permeated with references to "culture" or "cultural practice." This is as true of the spoken word as it is of popular and academic texts that emanate both from Africans themselves and from outside observers. Indeed, referring to "culture" often provides a handy cover for arenas of human behavior that are not fully understood by either the speaker, the writer, or possibly the potential audience. For all concerned, however, "culture" is a useful vehicle for indicating what is at once both familiar and understood, in general terms. When used by outsiders, scant sympathy may be expressed for "culture" if this is thought to inhibit successful HIV/AIDS interventions.

Similarly, in much of the early medical literature, "culture" was uncritically assumed to be essentially static and the cause of the vulnerability to infection of particular individuals and groups. This often led to negative stereotyping, marginalization, and possibly even the victimization of those concerned. At the same time, however, in the groundswell of calls for an African renaissance, "African culture" has assumed a revived and iconic importance on the continent (Makgoba 1999). Even this terrain is not uncontroversial or uncontested, particularly in the light of evidence that culture in the form of "tradition" may serve to justify and entrench long standing power and gender inequalities, some of which have been shown to be inimical to attempts to curb the spread of HIV (Leclerc-Madlala 2001, 2002a, 2002b, 2002c; Scorgie 2002).

The end result of either a denigration of the culture of the African "other" or the valorization of African tradition is much the same. Discussion is closed, and there appears to be no pressing need, or justification, for further critical reflection on the nature of the role that culture may or may not play in generating high-risk behavior. Pertinent examples of this occur when men justify the expectation of having multiple sex partners by reference to polygyny in "traditional African culture," or justify violence against women who refuse them sex in terms of traditional male rights over women. It is argued here that it is this closing off of questioning, rather than culture per se, that creates barriers to the development of effective interventions designed to quell the spread and course of the AIDS epidemic in Africa. In itself, the closure of discussion represents a culture of silence that, whether it is the result of ignorance of appropriate methodological tools for understanding culture or of political sensitivity to criticisms of cultural tradition, serves to intensify the growing AIDS crisis on the continent. This silence, although different in origin, adds to the everyday silence engendered by the near universal stigma that surrounds the epidemic in all parts of the world.

As in the case of all generalizations, there are exceptions to the above strictures on the use of the notion of culture within the context of the AIDS epidemic. The exceptions indicate how notions of culture and tradition are used by ordinary people, first to understand how culture operates in the epidemic, and second to map how African peoples' common understandings of culture are sometimes being used to fight the AIDS epidemic. Interpreting and understanding culture have long been the terrain of anthropology, and it is essentially an anthropological perspective that is presented here.

It is one, however, that seeks to speak to a multidisciplinary audience, and particularly an audience that includes biomedical and health scientists working in the AIDS terrain, in research, in clinical practice, or in public health. It seeks also to address laypeople, and especially those infected and affected by the epidemic, whose voices continue to be silenced by fear and stigma and who, in a desperate attempt to understand the epidemic and its spread, themselves resort to explanations couched in terms of "our culture" or "our tradition." In following this route, I will attempt to interpret what people on the continent believe they are doing when they invoke "culture" as an explanation of their beliefs and actions in the face of the crises and emotional turmoil created by HIV/AIDS (Geertz 1983; Reynolds Whyte 2002).

After some introductory remarks about the nature of culture and the closely associated notion of local context, I give a brief indication of some of the lessons that may be learned from the global AIDS epidemic. Pertinent examples are drawn from a number of recent southern African studies based on in-depth qualitative, and predominantly ethnographic, research in order to illustrate how culture operates in the field of HIV/AIDS. These studies offer a nuanced interpretation of the complex perceptions people in Africa have of the epidemic and of the different situations in which it touches their lives. All of these studies go well beyond simplistic, undifferentiated, and monocausal models of culture. Because the African continent is large and diverse, and the AIDS epidemic is moving at different paces across it, it is impossible to do justice geographically, historically, or politically to its complexities.

The choice of material for discussion in this chapter has been dictated by the development of the argument, rather than by an attempt to be exhaustive in spatial coverage, and I have primarily chosen southern African ethnographies for detailed contextual examination. The major reasons for this are that my own fieldwork in the field of HIV/AIDS has been undertaken within southern Africa, and I feel most confident in interpreting the wider literature of that region. That said, it must be noted that in reading the continually growing literature on HIV/AIDS in the rest of Africa, I am forcibly struck by the similarities in the way culture and tradition are interpreted and used (and often consciously manipulated) across the continent. In terms of a working definition of this chapter's primary subject matter, I offer Keesing's (1981) well-worn but still useful characterization of culture as a set of models or "blueprints" for action. Implicit in this formulation is the understanding that culture provides individuals with a set of explanatory concepts, and also options or alternative templates, for future behavior.

Geertz's (1983) concept of "local knowledge" is also useful here. In radically changed circumstances, some blueprints may be abandoned as inappropriate, or reformulated to suit the situation or context within which action must be taken. Although not always perceived clearly by those involved, precedent (or perceived precedent) is relatively seldom followed slavishly, however, and agency and innovation often take precedence over culture, custom, and tradition. In this way, social change is initiated and sustained. Thus, although laypeople often think of culture as unchanging and fixed, and as a set of traditions that are handed down in pristine form from one generation to the next, this is not necessarily the case. Over time, and in practice, action invariably molds and changes culture to a greater or lesser degree as adaptations are made by social actors to fit the context, moment, and circumstances of their actions.

From Culture to Local Context: What's In a Name?

Recently, a competing refrain to "culture" can be detected in the social science literature on HIV/AIDS in the guise of "context," or sometimes "social" or, more often, "local context" (Varga 1997). At worst, this may be merely a substitute for "culture," and adds little to our understanding. In other cases, however, and particularly where it emanates from detailed fieldwork that explores the interface of what people might want to do, and what they do in response to HIV/AIDS, it may suggest possible interventions (Susser and Stein 2004). Here the emphasis is on human agency, although in much of the literature on HIV/AIDS, it is the lack or situational curtailment of agency that appears to dominate behavior.

The gendered position of African women relative to men, and the paucity of alternative support to that provided by men, renders many women unable to say no to unprotected sex (Preston-Whyte et al. 2000; Varga 1997). Similar situations are constantly reported from elsewhere in the developing world, and it is here that the experiences of the global epidemic prove informative. Recently, as we will see, certain categories of heterosexual African men and young boys have also been shown to have little choice in the matter of risky penetrative sex on the streets, or with other men in male migrant hostels and prisons (Lockhart 2002; Niehaus 2002). Meanwhile, mothers who are HIV positive and have not disclosed this to their families hesitate to put their newborn babies on formula feed for fear that by not breast-feeding, they will reveal their HIV-positive status (Preston-Whyte 2003). These are but some of the local contexts that make both women and men, as well as adolescents and newborn babies, vulnerable to HIV infection.

In some cases, culture and local context prove difficult to isolate from each other in practice. A woman who tests HIV positive believes that, despite endangering the life of the infant, "culture" demands that she breast-feed her baby, and not to do so would be heavily criticized by older female kin. For poor women, the cost of formula feeding is not an insignificant consideration: culture and circumstance—or context—join to shape and constrain her choice of action. The question arises not only of where "culture" ends and "local context" begins, but of when and how the local context itself generates new sets of cultural practice and expectations in respect to sexuality and HIV. For this reason, it is sensible to view the complex and multifaceted field we are dealing with as a continuous one.

In many cases, contemporary studies of local context add the detailed situational analysis implicit in the use of Clifford Geertz's (1983) thick description. Intrinsic to this type of analysis is the sketching of pertinent recent and often long-term changes in the local circumstances of everyday life and the concomitant understandings of cultural behavior that characterize different situations and historical periods. Historical perspectives on similar changes in other spheres of social life have long shown tradition to be frequently malleable as well as constraining (Boonzaier and Sharp 1988; Hobsbawm and Ranger 1981).

While cultural meanings and symbols tend to be very different across societies, cultures, and even subcultures, a comparative reading of the literature on the local contexts in which HIV/AIDS is prevalent in Africa (and elsewhere in the world) suggests a number of important commonalities (Farmer 1999, 2003). Although useful to list, it must be stressed that these features do not operate in isolation from each other. They are intimately related to, and feed on, each other and together contribute to the local parameters and magnitude of the epidemic in each context. Two sets of factors may be distinguished. The first is characteristic of the wider social situation or environment, and the second is characteristic of the structures of personal interaction, including those, such as sexual relationships, that render the individual susceptible to HIV infection.

Widespread poverty and economic underdevelopment, exacerbated by global restructuring, appear as the bedrock in almost all cases where the epidemic has gained a stranglehold in Africa. Population mobility also appears consistently, and has been characteristic for well over a century in the continent in the form of long-term labor migration and shorter seasonal movements in search of employment. In today's world made small by the spread of modern transportation, the ubiquitous African truck driver adds to the flow of goods and people, and now very probably HIV, across the continent.

Similarly, sizable population movements occasioned by political instability, forced resettlement, and war appear as regular features in the life histories and experiences of both the infected and affected. It seems that spatial dislocation, and particularly life in refugee camps, provides a fertile breeding ground for the epidemic. Ethnic oppression and discrimination, now fueled by growing xenophobia, are often a precipitating factor in population and individual movements that, in turn, facilitate the spread of HIV.

The second set of contextual factors that appear regularly in association with the spread and impact of the epidemic across the continent are gender inequality and situations of individual and group gender oppression. Both are often bolstered by recourse to the value of past culture and practice and are closely related to differentials in power and access to scarce resources.

In the contemporary situation, these factors focus on access to employment, wealth, or a secure income. They render women, and young women in particular, vulnerable to infection. In some cases, such inequalities may be exacerbated by established and culturally based differentials in age and social status.

Changing Lessons from the Global AIDS Experience

The frontiers of sociological and behavioral understandings and interventions in the AIDS epidemic have changed over time. The tendency in early reports of the epidemic associated risks with certain patterns of sexual behavior. The answer appeared to be clear—avoid high-risk behavior. This, however, proved to be far from simple to achieve, and increasing infection rates threw doubt on the efficacy of informational and educational campaigns to change behavior. It was largely at this point that "culture" surfaced as a convenient explanation for the common barriers to both individual and group behavior change. In the absence of any strong alternative, culture soon became a popular whipping horse among academicians (particularly those from the biomedical domain), laypeople, and the popular press.

Soon social scientists were drawn to the field of behavior change. A major contribution of anthropologists was to use qualitative, and particularly ethnographic, research methods to explore the complexities of culture in the context of HIV. They also brought the fruit of earlier anthropological understandings of cultural processes and thick description to bear on the apparently inexorable trajectory of the epidemic (Parker and Ehrhardt 2001). Many of these studies were either of systems of cultural meaning or local social contexts (Parker 2004; Setel 2000; Susser and Stein 2004).

As the epidemic began to take on a global character, it became clear that if it was to be contained, and the socioeconomic repercussions of AIDS adequately understood, global mobilization and leadership would be necessary. Clearly also, resources on a massive scale would be required for the care and treatment of the infected and affected. These could only come from the rich countries of the developed world (Barnett and Whiteside 2002). At the same time, the refrain of the universality of human rights (Beyrer and Kass 2002), including those of universal access to health care and treatment, was brought to bear forcibly in relation to HIV/AIDS.

When looked at globally, notable regularities were discernable in the trajectory and impact of even the most diverse of local epidemics. HIV/AIDS bit hardest in poor countries (and especially those of the developing world). Women were more at risk of HIV infection than men, and the most severe impact was upon the young, with women between fifteen and twenty-four years of age being particularly vulnerable in Africa. Where access to antiretroviral treatment is minimal, the number of children both infected and affected by AIDS morbidity and the death of their parents is growing steadily. Following Parker (2004), these features may be summarized as pauperization, feminization, and juvenilization. Seen in a global perspective, these now appear to define the coinage of AIDS risk, rather than the minutiae of culture. What then is left to say about "culture" in Africa? To begin to answer this question, we need to listen to what people in Africa say about their culture or tradition in explaining the epidemic to each other, and also how they are dealing with the crises it presents to them.

Culture in Action: Explaining HIV and AIDS, and Dealing with Uncertainty

According to Susan Reynolds Whyte (2002: 170), "As ethnographers, an important part of our job must be to inquire about what people as subjects are trying to do—what they are hoping for, how they deal with their life conditions, and how things unfold for them over time." She introduces the paper in which these words appear with the arresting image of a British Broadcasting Company (BBC) report on a large international conference recently held in Africa. The opening ceremony featured a local traditional healer performing a divination ritual for an AIDS patient. Amid the drumming and general excitement, the commentator explained that most Ugandans believe that AIDS is caused by witchcraft. Reynolds Whyte remarks that this is a vast oversimplification, but is one often heard from Ugandans themselves. The following statements, which she quotes directly from her research participants, could have been uttered in almost any country in sub-Saharan Africa. "'You know those people in the village always blame sickness on spirits.'" Or, "'The traditional people say AIDS is witchcraft. . . . They think it is caused by a curse." Later she quotes a local AIDS counselor as saying that "'most (people here) believe in traditions. We need to make them aware that it's not witchcraft. Instead of wasting money on traditions, they should come for counseling'" (Reynolds Whyte 2002: 171).

Juxtaposing these statements encapsulates the twin crises presented to most people by HIV/AIDS in Africa: how to explain the occurrence and spread of a new and fatal disease, and in the event that it strikes someone close, such as a member of one's family, how to choose among a number of options open for handling the disease. Clearly, the two are connected, and the choice of the course of action follows to a large extent from the answer to the first question.

However, it is not as simple as that. As in most matters of securing health in Africa, there are a number of alternatives and options available, both for explaining the cause of the disease and in dealing with it. In terms of explanation, Western notions of a virus vie with widespread beliefs in the power of spirits or witches, or a curse to cause illness. Similarly, Western medical remedies compete with those of widely respected and trusted traditional healers for attention and allegiance. In the case of AIDS, as Reynolds Whyte and other researchers have shown, the increasing gravity of the symptoms and the near certainty of the tragic end precipitate both fear and emotional crisis. Action is urgently demanded. This, however, may involve simultaneously seeking and following different types of medical treatment, and also taking spiritual advice (Leclerc-Madlala 2002c; Xaba 2002).

In Uganda, illness is often first suspected to be caused by spirits punishing the living for having neglected or annoyed them. Alternatively, it may be blamed on a witch, who in a fit of anger or jealously has cursed the afflicted person. However, a person never knows which is the case until a diviner is consulted. Besides proclaiming the cause of the illness, the diviner invariably suggests a course of remedial action. Until this is followed, Reynolds Whyte observes that people live in a state of intense anxiety, and often after the divination it is judged advisable to try to speedily follow the proffered advice. But alternative advice is also offered by kin or neighbors, and in order not to take chances, this may also be followed. Thus, the different explanations and their remedies provide alternative cultural models for action, which are then often followed at the same time. This was the context in which the AIDS counselor's strictures quoted above were offered, and his remarks epitomize the lack of sympathy of many Western-trained medical personnel for traditional explanations and recourse to indigenous forms of treatment.

On the streets of African towns and in rural villages where there has been little hope of accessing treatments developed and increasingly widely available in the North, an undivided faith in Western medicine is hard, if not impossible, to sustain. As of 2003, UNAIDS (2004) estimates that of the 40 to 42 million adults and children infected by HIV/AIDS worldwide, 26.6 to 29.4 million live in sub-Saharan Africa. Of the 5 million new infections occurring each year, 3.2 million are also in sub-Saharan Africa. More immediately apparent, 2.3 million estimated AIDS deaths occur annually in the region. Although there are marked differences in the numbers and distribution of infections and the epidemic appears to be progressing at different rates across the continent as a whole, few areas remain unaffected. Uncertainty, fear, and stigma prevail and must be handled as best one can.

Maintaining Good Social Relations

Reynolds Whyte further points out that in Africa, individuals do not usually face illness alone. They do so in the company of family members and neighbors, many of whom may have very definite opinions on the matter. This is especially true of those who are senior in the kinship group or are influential in community affairs. To ignore the advice, concern, and beliefs of those who are senior or influential would be lacking in respect and what she refers to as "civility." Health seeking and, in this instance, coping with AIDS morbidity are thus seldom purely personal matters, as they often are in the West. They are shared with others who are both emotionally important to the patient and influential in his or her life. "Civility is a recognition of your involvement with other social actors" (Reynolds Whyte 2002: 182). In the tragic situations engendered by AIDS, it is important to have and keep friends and supporters.

Lockhart (2002) makes the same point in relation to various forms of sexual encounters entered into by "street boys" who struggle to survive on the streets of Mwanza, Tanzania. Ranging in age from about eleven to eighteen years, the youngest of these boys have not previously experienced heterosexual or homosexual sex, and some are largely unaware of the existence of either. Their first sexual experience may be when they wake up in the night to find older boys attempting to have anal intercourse with them. They are formally initiated into street life by an episode of group rape, or are "pizzed on" (the local expression to describe the essentially passive role of the nonpenetrating partner in male-to-male sexual encounters) by older and more powerful boys. They acquiesce largely because they need the continued tolerance and protection of the older boys as they struggle to survive amid the dangers of life on the streets.

Thus, although these sexual encounters were described by the boys in terms of violence and domination of younger boys by the more powerful older boys, they represent also an attempt to ensure the support of the older boys in potentially hazardous encounters outside the group. Lockhart (2002) stresses the importance of the social networks built up and maintained by younger boys as they seek to establish themselves safely on the streets, and both she and previous observers Ranjani and Kudrati (1996) describe what is a local subculture referred to by the boys as *kunyenga*. This unites and distinguishes them from older youths and men, but is characteristic of a stage in their lives rather than as a form of lasting sexual orientation. In addition to penetration, she found that younger boys often engaged in nonpenetrative touching and rubbing, which they described as "play" and did not think of as either sexual or as *kunyenga*.

Cross-Cultural and Contextual Differences in Perceptions of Sexuality and HIV Risk

Not surprisingly, some observers feared that the sexual activities characteristic of *kunyenga* might be potentially dangerous for contracting HIV. Such activities might, moreover, constitute a threat to the wider spread of the disease outside the group if boys engaged in *kunyenga* sex activities and also engage in sex with girlfriends. One of the reasons for Lockhart's study was to assess the reality and magnitude of this danger. Although most of the boys she talked to in Tanzania were aware of AIDS and its routes of transmission, they, like Ugandans, mentioned witchcraft or a curse as an alternative causal possibility. More fundamentally, they did not perceive *kunyenga* sex to carry a risk of HIV. This was because they did not classify it as real sex comparable to what they saw as "normal" heterosexual intercourse.

Some of the boys, when faced with the possibility that *kunyenga* sex might constitute a high level of HIV risk for them, responded fatalistically that this was "no big deal." The lifestyle that they were forced to adopt in order to survive and be independent was, in itself, more dangerous than an illness that was likely to kill them sometime in the distant future (Lockhart 2002). With this, their opinion echoes that of many people living under dangerous circumstances elsewhere in the world. Perhaps the most often cited example of this fatalism is that of commercial sex workers to whom sex with clients without condoms constitutes a major and acknowledged risk of infection, but one that many accept as necessary for economic survival. Hence the rubric of "survival sex," which has been coined to describe such situations, is a useful concept (Preston-Whyte et al. 2000; Varga 1997).

Lockhart (2002) points out that in the case of her respondents, it was not so much the need for making money that led to "survival sex" with other boys as the search for physical protection and emotional support. In the case of South Africa, Preston-Whyte and colleagues (2000) have commented that long-term relationships with a number of men may also be part of an informal and possibly unconscious strategy for survival among women unable and unlikely to find paid employment. Apart from money and gifts, however, these men may also provide the women with physical protection amid the dangers of the urban milieu. Despite the fact that they, too, are open to the risk of HIV infection, these women do not consider themselves to be "prostitutes" (in the sense of women who regularly provide casual sex on the streets), nor do the people living around these women view them as "prostitutes." Context is clearly important to the definition people have of their sexual activities, but also of the risks they accept as part of the job.

Before leaving the streets of Mwanza to look at other situations of male-to-male sexual relationships that may involve risk of HIV infection, it needs to be noted that the Tanzanian boys studied by Lockhart do not classify *kunyenga* sex as "homosexual" in nature. In fact, they characterize a man who had sex with other men derogatively as *mhanisi*, or a "girl-man." Self-masturbation was also classified as *mhanisi*, and to quote Lockhart (2002: 304), this "added further legitimacy to *kunyenga* activities." Such activities were not carried outside or beyond the terms of the boy's participation in *kunyenga* groupings and its associated subculture. By the age of about nineteen, these street boys had moved out of the groups of younger boys to join gangs consisting of young men. At this stage, they gave up *kunyenga* sex in favor of heterosexual relations with women. Something of the same male-to-male forms of sexuality was characteristic of a stage in the lives of many long-term male migrants in Africa. In this case, some of the cultural expectations of heterosexual marriage were temporarily built amid the soulless and emotionally starved environment of the mining compounds.

Using historical and also oral evidence collected from retired miners in South Africa, Niehaus (2002) writes informatively of an arena that has been somewhat unclear in the official record of life in mine compounds, but which includes a high risk of contracting sexually transmitted diseases (STDs). During their years working in the mines when men returned home only infrequently, some older men formed strong relationships with younger men that mimicked the duties, rights, and obligations—and often something of the emotional content—of heterosexual marriages. The younger mine "wives" cooked and performed domestic duties for their mine "husbands," and in return were given gifts and protection. These relationships also involved penetrative anal sex, but more commonly, it appears, sex between the thighs. However, a potential transmission route for STDs was provided. These same-sex "marriages" were public and, within that context, accepted as part of mining life. When the men returned home, they resumed heterosexual relations with their wives or girlfriends. Indeed, many had married before they left for the mines. Cultural patterns were adopted to fill a void created by social and political circumstance. This example is indicative of the flexibility, diversity, and creativity of human cultural behavior.

AIDS, Witches, Local Gossip, and New Moral Scripts in the South African Lowveld

Focusing on southern Africa in the remaining case studies discussed in this chapter, we find further echoes of the themes and concerns around HIV touched on in the cases of Bankole and Mwanza. What really causes AIDS? How should the symptoms of the new disease be interpreted? How should the disease be managed? The same kinds of explanations of HIV/AIDS appear, although in keeping with local histories and social contexts, in slightly different guises.

In South Africa, local gossip and reports in the popular press draw attention to the widespread belief that witches are causing harm to their neighbors. Incidents occur in which people suspected of being witches are chased from local communities and even killed (Niehaus 1997). Stadler (2003b) shows graphically how in the fast-developing epidemic in the northern Lowveld region of South Africa, rumor, fueled by gossip, continuously presents these competing theories to the standard health messages propagated by Western health professionals. People draw conclusions from the sight of returning migrants who present wasting symptoms whispered to be indicative of the new disease. He argues that Western explanations fail to answer the fundamental question of why certain individuals become infected and die, while others (despite their very risky behavior) continue to live. Witchcraft, he argues, successfully explains this contradiction.

Ashforth (2002, 2005) emphasizes the same point, and both analyses recall the seminal work of Evans-Pritchard (1937), who studied witchcraft beliefs and practices in Africa. Among the Azande (with whom Evans-Pritchard lived and studied), witchcraft was used to explain all manner of unfortunate events, including unexpected illnesses and death, and divination provided the answer to where and upon whom the blame might logically fall. In the same way, Stadler, Reynolds Whyte, and numerous other researchers indicate clearly why and how witchcraft provides a satisfying explanation for AIDS. While the existence of witchcraft may be denied by the church or by local clinic staff, rumor and gossip continually suggest that other people take it seriously, and many are convinced that they or their neighbors have evidence to substantiate their belief. The growing number of funerals for the relatively young provides final and conclusive evidence of the possible jealousy of other people. In southern Africa, the ancestors— who may vent their anger for neglect on the living by causing illness—are not usually thought of as going so far as to cause a death within the lineage (Ngubane 1977).

Stadler (2003a) further describes a casual chat with a man after the funeral of a young local woman. Stadler notes that although the man's friends shied away from naming the new disease, from their comments it was clear that all were thinking the same thing. This was confirmed on a later occasion when one of his research participants commented that the woman had been known to have a number of sexual partners who showed her "a good time" and gave her many gifts, including a cell phone. Implicitly, the end result had been inevitable. Listening to casual conversations, Stadler noted further that men and women are characterized as open to risk for different reasons. These scripts sound a warning to others, but also clearly reflect gendered access to local opportunities for employment, and to the status and relative freedom that employment brings. Men are portrayed as powerful, but also as incorrigible womanizers who prey on young women, many of whom have little option but to rely on sexual relations with men for survival, as well as for highly desirable luxury goods.

But women are not always depicted as victims. They are frequently portrayed as very beautiful and out to exploit men. In having many lovers, it is commented that such women are "buying their own coffins." The message of the scripts is clear. In order to survive, both men and women should refrain at all costs from having multiple sex partners. In a subtle and roundabout way, one of the major health messages of the time has been incorporated in everyday discussion and gossip. These messages indicate that informal yet powerful calls for protective action are developing within communities in the face of the spread of HIV/AIDS. In Keesing's terms, these are new cultural blueprints for action.

"Dangerous Women," Culture, and the Gendering of the AIDS Epidemic

Developing HIV/AIDS representations of gender in South Africa may not be as even-handed as Stadler's examples from the Lowveld suggest. In fact, local cultural understandings of health and disease progression in KwaZulu-Natal reflect more accurately the highly gendered and subordinate position of many African women on the continent. Here the specific manner in which blame for driving the epidemic was laid at their door in early years is instructive, and here we begin to appreciate what many regard as the negative side of the current valorization of tradition in parts of Africa. The examples that follow demonstrate the ambiguities in, and controversies around, culture and tradition in contemporary South Africa. They also provide further examples of how culture, in the form of existing local understandings of ill-health and the progression of disease, has adapted to an African alternative to Western medical explanations of HIV/AIDS.

Drawing on the work of Leclerc-Madlala (2001), Reynolds Whyte has investigated ethnomedical theories and disease categorization in KwaZulu-Natal since the beginning of the AIDS epidemic in this region. She was one of the first researchers to note that Zulu-speaking people regard the body as a complex whole, in which the various organs are interconnected by the flow of blood around and between them. Disease—or, as it is conceptualized, "dirt"—in an organ mixes with blood and is moved to other parts of the body, which then become infected. Attempts to understand the new disease built on these accounts, and particularly on the belief that a woman's vagina provides an excellent place for disease to lodge. It was soon even said that HIV was a very strong and persistent disease that could stay hidden for many years. This corresponded with the health information about the long latency period of the disease. Similarly, the spread of HIV largely through sexual relations and transmission by blood fitted well with the notion of disease being spread by blood around the entire bodily system.

Calling again upon the strength of the HIV virus, it was reputed to have the ability to "stick" to the walls of the vagina, where it would later infect women's sexual partners during intercourse. Zulu women were, therefore, conceptualized as the carriers of HIV and responsible for the danger it represented toward men. Following this line of argument, Leclerc-Madlala sought to account for the spate of rapes perpetrated on young girls and even babies in the region in terms of the desire of men to avoid HIV infection by having sex with virgins. Indeed, this was also the interpretation of these events offered by many Africans themselves, who stated that it was widely believed that sex with a virgin would actually cure HIV/AIDS. Thus is the power of rumor and of some of the many myths that have developed around the insecurities and anxieties that surround the epidemic on the continent. Not surprisingly, many lead to drastic action, and in one case a woman, Dudu Dlamini—who disclosed her HIV-positive status—was killed by an enraged and fearful mob in KwaZulu-Natal.

What amounts to demonizing women for carrying and spreading HIV/AIDS, Leclerc-Madlala argues, has contributed to a call from some quarters for steps to be taken to control young unmarried women who are stereotyped as having many sex partners. They are said to have "gotten out of control," and their "promiscuity" now poses a threat not only to the men with whom they have sex but also to the society as a whole. It is in these terms that she interprets the current support for what is popularly known as "virginity testing" in parts of South Africa. In the context of the argument advanced in this chapter, virginity testing might be seen as an active community response to local explanations of the spread of the AIDS epidemic that calls on the idiom of traditional culture and custom as both its vehicle and its major source of appeal.

Virginity Testing and the Control of Women's Sexuality: A Return to Traditional Zulu Culture?

KwaZulu-Natal has for some years seen the revival of what is said to be the traditional custom of examining unmarried young women to ascertain if they are still virgins (Leclerc-Madlala 2001). Coinciding roughly with the advent of HIV/AIDS, the current form of virginity testing may occur informally within families and small local communities, or at more formal and often relatively lengthy ceremonies that draw large numbers of women and girls to engage in them either as spectators or participants. Such occasions are now led by virginity testers. They move around the countryside and a few urban areas putting their expertise into practice. Records are kept, and the girls who pass the test are publicly acclaimed and awarded certificates.

Virginity testing has been welcomed by the South African national and provincial departments of health, which apparently hail the potential of what is beginning to amount to a large social movement, to support their campaigns against high-risk sex. Thus, South African government officials often attend the larger ceremonies and speak publicly in favor of the traditional values of "youthful purity" and chastity before marriage. In some areas, "graduates" of the virginity testing continue to meet for regular social events, which provide occasions for displays of local regalia, singing, dancing, and general socialization. Scorgie (2002) ascribes much of the popularity of virginity testing among girls to these ongoing occasions for socializing, some of which, no doubt, ironically take place away from the watchful gaze of parents.

It would appear that the current popularity of virginity testing appeals to different people for very different reasons. Virginity testing is by no means uncontroversial, however, and public debate on its virtues and detractions rages in both the public and private domains. The controversy is amply reflected in the coverage virginity testing receives in the media and popular press. Scorgie (2002) chronicles and analyzes the major debates that the movement has spawned. These range from objections that—with its focus on chastity and abstinence—there is little room in its agenda for promoting condom use as a protection against HIV infection, to complaints that the procedure of testing for virginity constitutes an infringement of young women's dignity and their right to privacy. In terms of the latter, virginity testing becomes a human rights issue, and, as such, the act of testing for virginity constitutes an infringement of the new South African constitution.

The most vociferous criticism is that virginity testing constitutes a major challenge to gender equality, which is also a key tenet of the constitution, and to the empowerment of African women, which is one of the fundamental objectives of the new government's development policies. The influential South African Gender Commission has criticized the sometimes explicit objective of virginity testing as the revival of traditional controls over women, and particularly the control of men over young women. In response to these attacks, supporters of virginity testing argue that it reinforces "tradition" and serves to support cultural rights that are themselves enshrined in the constitution. The proponents of "cultural rights" and "African tradition" (often expressed strongly in this context as "our tradition" and "our customs") believe that both have a major role to play in the revival of African identity and consciousness.

Such are the ambiguities and paradoxes centered around popular understandings of culture in South Africa today. The very heat of these debates endorses the fact that culture is a continually changing terrain that combines iterative reflection, action, and experimentation in which the roles of human agency, innovation, and adaptability are interwoven in complex and sometimes dramatic ways. The results are not always to the liking or advantage of all, but the controversies that ensue reveal the vibrancy of the terrain and its responsiveness to changing circumstances. The final case study of how HIV/AIDS and culture are intertwined in Africa focuses on changing male identities in relation to accepted sexual behavior.

The Changing Culture of Male Identities in South Africa: Reality versus the Myth of Male Rights to Having Many Partners

The analysis in this chapter has thus far relied heavily on ethnographies of the contemporary social environment. The use of historical sources, including indigenous texts, court records, and interviews with older informants aimed at eliciting their memories and descriptions of past exploits, also serves to underscore the flexibility of culture, and the fact that contemporary perceptions of what is "traditional" may be idealized (and sometimes sanitized) versions of reality. Both have been demonstrated by Hunter (2004), who explored the changing historical nuances of what it once meant, and now means, to be an *isoka*, or a young unmarried man who is much sought after by women in Zulu society. In contrast to young women, having many sexual partners is tacitly approved, and even publicly applauded, for men.

Calling on the traditional practice of polygyny as justification, it is often stated that men "need many partners." Hunter (2004) shows that, in fact, this is a popular misreading of the past. In the late nineteenth century among the Zulu, although certain forms of nonpenetrative sex were lightly policed, full intercourse and particularly impregnating a young woman was a matter for reproach, and a fine was imposed on the perpetrator. More surprisingly, in terms of today's version of traditional Zulu culture, unmarried women were also allowed the license of having a limited number of lovers—once again, providing they did not allow pregnancy to occur. Hunter draws the distinction between sexual relations and fertility, and notes that the latter was protected and both transferred and symbolized when *illibolo* (bridewealth) passed from the family of a man to that of a woman at marriage. The practice of *soma* (sex between thighs) was the mechanism for avoiding pregnancy, and the point at which this limited form of sexual relations was permitted between a couple was publicly marked. This event, furthermore, was seen as merely a stage in the longer process of marriage. A young man celebrated for being an *isoka* (an eligible bachelor) was expected to eventually court and choose one woman, pay *illibolo*, and establish a homestead of his own. When this occurred, his status changed from that of *isoka* to *umnumzana*, a fully mature and respected adult. It was the achievement of this, as much as sexual pleasure itself, that lay behind the well-ordered system of courting and controls on sexuality occurring at this period of history.

Speaking to informants under thirty-five years of age, Hunter (2004) found that none were married or even in the process of getting married. The growing difficulties of achieving marriage were, he notes, a discernable theme in their conversations. He concludes that as marriage and the achievement of the status of *umnumzana* become less and less likely, so the controls on sexuality fall away, leaving the form but not the substance of the traditional conception of the *isoka*. Like other writers, he seeks the roots of this change in the colonial encounter, in the experience of migrant labor, and in the agrarian collapse following the imposition of a money economy in the early years of the twentieth century. However, the AIDS crisis, he argues, may signal the end to the current hegemony of the *isoka* as recognized today by virtue of his many sexual conquests, and by society's acceptance of this state of affairs. According to Hunter (2004: 141–142):

Day by day, funeral by funeral, AIDS bears harder down on the *isoka* masculinity. The symptoms, recognized by even very young children in the townships, couldn't be more emasculating—and de-masculating: some of the most virile, popular and independent bodies are steadily transformed into diseased and dependent skeletons shunned by friends and neighbours . . . and where the contradictions of *isoka* are played out. Consequently, masculinities are under huge scrutiny and critique, even if women are still commonly blamed for "promiscuity" and AIDS.

Hunter (2004) sees in images like the above an intimation that a change in the culture of male sexuality is in the making. His recent interviews with women suggest that in the face of the epidemic, some are also reducing the number of sexual partners they have—or they are relying more frequently on condoms for protection. In this, Hunter substantiates Stadler's belief that new moral scripts are being written in response to the epidemic.

Conclusion

An attempt has been made here to illustrate some of the ways in which what is often loosely referred to as "culture" operates in a number of the African settings where AIDS is common. While important in understanding the behavioral ramifications of the epidemic in particular places and contexts, when looked at from a comparative perspective, a purely "cultural" approach has limitations. Lessons from the global experience of the epidemic suggest, first, that there are important structural and often political regularities that facilitate the spread of HIV and characterize and exacerbate many of its worst local manifestations. In seeking to stem the progression of HIV/AIDS, and to address its repercussions in any particular setting, these regularities have increasingly been shown to outweigh considerations of culture alone.

Among the most important problems facing Africans in controlling the spread of HIV are widespread poverty and deprivation, inequality of access to opportunities for achieving a healthy and adequate lifestyle, and lack of access to public resources for the treatment of ill-health and disease. Increasingly recognized as a universal human right, quality health care is beyond the reach of many Africans, particularly African women, and the millions of children and adolescents who are either infected or more broadly affected by the epidemic on the continent. Other categories of disadvantaged people may also be affected in particular locations, and here local culture may have a role to play in that behavioral factors and cultural stereotypes often set such people apart from the mainstream, and in increasing social stigma (Parker and Aggleton 2003). Indeed, stigmatization is often both the precursor and the effect of the epidemic worldwide.

In concluding this chapter, it may be suggested that the time has come for observers, and also insiders themselves, to dispense with either negative or (in some cases) overly positive and protective attitudes toward culture. While we have seen some of the problems and divisions to which culture, particularly phrased in terms like "our tradition" or "our custom," may lead, we have also seen how, over time, culture changes and adapts to circumstance. The AIDS epidemic presents a crisis and challenge like no other. At the same time, it seems unlikely that the challenge represented by poverty and deprivation will be easily or speedily addressed, so that many of the insecurities and anxieties created by these conditions will continue to plague Africa and other developing regions. This in turn may well mean that reliance on alternative explanations to the Western medical explanations of AIDS continues to offer hope and emotional support to many for some time to come. In such situations, it is not surprising that many individuals consider the resources expended on traditional remedies to be well worth the expense.

References Cited

Ashforth, A. 2002. "An Epidemic of Witchcraft: The Implication of AIDS for the Post-Apartheid State." *African Studies* 61 (1): 121–143.

———. 2005. *Witchcraft, Violence and Democracy in South Africa*. Chicago: University of Chicago Press.

Barnett, T., and A. Whiteside. 2002. *AIDS in the Twenty-first Century: Disease and Globalisation*. London: Palgrave Macmillan.

Beyrer, C., and N. E. Kass. 2002. "Human Rights, Politics and Reviews of Research Ethics." *Lancet* 360 (9328): 246–251.

Boonzaier, E., and J. Sharp, eds. 1988. *South African Keywords: The Uses and Abuses of Political Concepts*. Cape Town, South Africa: David Philip.

Evans-Pritchard, E. E. 1937. *Witchcraft, Oracles and Magic among the Azande*. Oxford: Clarendon Press.

Farmer, P. 1999. *Infections and Inequalities: The Modern Plagues*. Berkeley: University of California Press.

———. 2003. *Pathologies of Power: Health Human Rights and the New War on the Poor*. Berkeley: University of California Press

Geertz, C. 1983. *Local Knowledge*. New York: Basic Books.

Hobsbawm, E., and T. Ranger. 1981. *Invention of Tradition*. Cambridge: Cambridge University Press.

Hunter, M. 2004. "Masculinities and Multiple Sexual Partners, and AIDS: The Making and Unmaking of Isoka in KwaZulu-Natal." *Transformation* 54: 123–153.

Keesing, R. 1981. *Cultural Anthropology: A Contemporary Perspective.* 2nd ed. New York: Rinehart and Winston.

Leclerc-Madlala, S. 2001. "Virginity Testing: Managing Sexuality in a Maturing HIV/AIDS Epidemic." *Medical Anthropology Quarterly* 15 (4): 533–552.

———. 2002a. "On the Virgin Cleansing Myth: Gendered Bodies, AIDS and Ethnomedicine." *Journal of AIDS Research* 1: 87–95.

———. 2002b. "Traditional Healers and the Fight against HIV/AIDS in South Africa." In *Bodies and Politics: Healing Rituals in the Democratic South Africa*, ed. V. Faure, 61–73. Les Noveaux Cahiers de l'IFAS (2). Johannesburg: IFAS.

———. 2002c. "Youth, HIV/AIDS and the Importance of Sexual Culture and Context." *Social Dynamics* 28 (1): 20–41.

Lockhart, C. 2002. "Kunyenga, 'Real Sex,' and Survival: Assessing the Risk of HIV Infection among Urban Street Boys in Tanzania." *Medical Anthropology Quarterly* 16 (3): 294–311.

Makgoba, M. W., ed. 1999. *African Renaissance: The New Struggle.* Cape Town, South Africa: Mafube/Tafelberg

Ngubane, H. 1977. *Body and Mind in Zulu Medicine.* London: London Academic Press.

Niehaus, I. A. 1997. *Witches, Mysteries, Rumours, Dreams and Bones: Tensions in the Subjective Reality of Witchcraft in the Mpumalanga Lowveld, South Africa.* Johannesburg: University of the Witwatersrand, Institute for Advance Social Research.

———. 2002. "Renegotiating Masculinity in the South African Lowveld: Narratives of Male-to-Male Sex in Labour Compounds and Prisons." *African Studies* 61 (1): 77–120.

Parker, R. 2004. *Treatment Access: A Challenge for Public Health and Social Justice.* Seminar presentation for Ethnography in Action, Durban, August.

Parker, R., and P. Aggleton. 2003. "HIV and AIDS-Related Stigma and Discrimination: A Conceptual Framework and Implications for Action." *Social Science and Medicine* 57: 13–24.

Parker, R., and A. Ehrhardt. 2001. "Through an Ethnographic Lens: Ethnographic Methods, Comparative Analysis and HIV/AIDS Research." *AIDS and Behavior* 5 (2): 105–114.

Preston-Whyte, E. M. 2003. "Contexts of Vulnerability: Sex, Secrecy and HIV/AIDS." *African Journal of AIDS Research* 2 (2): 89–94.

Preston-Whyte, E. M., C. Varga, H. Oosthuizen, R. Roberts, and F. Blose. 2000. "Survival Sex and HIV/AIDS in an African City." In *Framing the Sexual Subject: The Politics of Gender, Sexuality and Power*, ed. R. G. Parker, R. M. Barbosa, and P. Aggleton, 165–190. Berkeley: University of California Press.

Ranjani, R., and M. Kudrati. 1996. "The Varieties of Sexual Experience of the Street Children of Mwanza, Tanzania." In *Learning about Sexuality: A Practical Beginning*, ed. S. Zeidenstein and K. Moore. New York: Population Council and International Women's Health Coalition.

Reynolds Whyte, S. 2002. "Subjectivity and Subjunctivity: Hoping for Health in Eastern Uganda." In *Postcolonial Subjectivity in Africa*, ed. R. Werbner, 171–190. London: Zed Books.

Scorgie, F. 2002. "Virginity Testing and the Politics of Sexual Responsibility: Implications for AIDS Intervention." *African Studies* 61 (1): 55–75.

Setel, P. 1999. *A Plague of Paradoxes: AIDS; Culture, and Demography in Northern Tanzania*. Chicago: University of Chicago Press.

Stadler, J. J. 2003a. "Rumor, Gossip and Blame: Implications for HIV/AIDS Prevention in the South African Lowveld." *AIDS Education and Prevention* 15 (4): 357–368.

———. 2003b. "The Young, the Rich, and the Beautiful: Secrecy, Suspicion and Discourses of AIDS in the South African Lowveld." *African Journal of AIDS Research* 2 (2): 127–140.

Susser, I., and Z. Stein. 2004. "Public Health Matters: Culture, Sexuality, and Women's Agency in the Prevention of HIV/AIDS in Southern Africa." In *HIV and AIDS in Africa: Beyond Epidemiology*, ed. E. Kalipen, S. Craddock, J. R. Oppong, and J. Ghosh, 133–143. Malden, Mass.: Blackwell.

UNAIDS. 2004. *2004 Report on the global AIDS epidemic: Executive Summary*. www.unaids.org.

Varga, C. 1997. "Sexual Decision-Making and Negotiation in the Midst of AIDS: Youth in KwaZulu-Natal, South Africa." *Health Transition Review* 7 (Supplement 2): 13–40.

Xaba, T. 2002. "The Transformation of Indigenous Medical Practices in New South Africa 1985 to 2000." In *Bodies and Politics: Healing Rituals in the Democratic South Africa*, ed. V. Faure, 23–40. Les Noveaux Cahiers de l'IFAS (2). Johannesburg: IFAS.

15

Conclusion

It's Not Just About AIDS—The Underlying Agenda to Control HIV in Africa

DOUGLAS A. FELDMAN

The life of man: solitary, poor, nasty, brutish, and short.
—Thomas Hobbes, *Leviathan*, 1651

The world can only be grasped by action, not by contemplation.
The hand is more important than the eye.
—Jacob Bronowski, *The Ascent of Man*, 1973

Clearly, the work of anthropologists on HIV/AIDS in Africa has been enormous and crucial since 1985. It is likely that this trend will continue over the coming decades as well. The role of the applied medical anthropologist is no longer seen as peripheral by those in the public health community, but central to both an understanding of public health and to effectively promoting healthy change.

Africa is a rich, culturally diverse continent with enormous promise. At the same time, however, it is beset with challenging problems. In sub-Saharan Africa alone, 25.4 million adults and children are living with HIV. There are over 3 million newly infected persons with HIV each year. Across the continent south of the Sahara, 7.4 percent of all adults are HIV positive. Indeed, 2.3 million died of AIDS in 2004, while 13.3 million women are living with HIV. Unlike the developed nations of North America and Europe, HIV is transmitted mostly heterosexually—between husband and wife, husband and mistress, husband and multiple wives in polygynous rural areas, and husband and female sex worker.

There is certainly same-sex transmission of HIV among men, but more research is needed to learn the extent of this on the overall HIV epidemiology. There is some transmission of HIV through unclean needles, but it is likely that this plays a relatively small, but not necessarily negligible, role in the transmission of HIV in general. Infants often become HIV infected through the birth process and through breast-feeding.

Unquestionably, the key epidemiologic question concerning HIV transmission is: why is it spreading heterosexually so freely in sub-Saharan Africa, but not in North America and Europe? Quite amazingly, by the second half of the first decade of the twenty-first century, we still do not know. It is possible, however, though not yet proven, that HIV-1 subtype C, which is common in Africa, is more transmissible vaginally than HIV-1 subtype B, which is common in North America and Europe.

Helen Epstein and Daniel Halperin have argued quite persuasively that the prevailing custom throughout much of Africa of men having mistresses functions to significantly augment HIV transmission. While this is undoubtedly true, it is not clear why this not equally true in the West among those white suburban men who also have a mistress.

Other biosocial factors may also play a role in the difference between transmission patterns in the West and in Africa. The combination of lack of male circumcision and poor genital hygiene appears to increase HIV transmission risk, when compared with populations where male circumcision is common and/or genital hygiene is routinely practiced. "Dry sex," the common practice in many parts of Africa where women decrease vaginal secretions prior to sexual activity, is likely to increase genital abrasions, which may lead to increased HIV risk. Ritual "sexual cleansing," where a widow is expected to have sex with her deceased husband's brother, can increase HIV risk. The traditional practice of "curing" sexually transmitted infections by having sex with a young virgin has been extended in some parts of Africa to "curing" AIDS, with tragic results.

Other sociocultural factors also increase HIV transmission. While HIV spread initially among wealthier Africans, poverty today is clearly exacerbating the spread of HIV among the poor. Quite often, female sex workers are paid more by their male clients to have them not use condoms. Teenage girls who are AIDS orphans (born to an HIV positive mother, but HIV negative themselves) are forced to quit school and marry early, putting them at increased risk for HIV. The unequal status of women in most of Africa makes sexual negotiation for safer sex between married couples difficult, if not impossible.

AIDS is only one of many problems, although certainly the most devastating problem, facing Africa today. The population of Africa has grown from 227 million people in 1950 to an astounding 916 million people in

2006, resulting in enormous population pressure. In addition to HIV/AIDS, many other infectious and chronic diseases are common, including cholera, malaria, tuberculosis, childhood diarrhea diseases, and other sexually transmitted infections besides HIV/AIDS. Poverty is pervasive, with most of the population earning less than U.S.$2 a day. Half of the population is under sixteen years of age.

In many African nations, the infrastructure of roads, schools, and health facilities is deteriorating. The limited funds are frequently diverted from health care and education expenditures to the military. Corruption is fairly rampant. Income inequality between the African elite and the poor is alarmingly wide. An image I will never forget on my first day in Dakar, Senegal, was watching a Mercedes-Benz driven by a wealthy African kicking up dust into the faces of the desperately poor in tattered rags living on the sidewalks. Warfare, and at times genocide, has plagued much of the continent in recent years: Rwanda, the Democratic Republic of the Congo, Angola, Liberia, Sierra Leone, Sudan—the list goes on.

Some African nations are mostly dependent upon foreign aid, and are deeply in debt—struggling with the interest on loans that the lenders knew could never be paid off. Most of the workforce is unskilled or poorly skilled. But even skilled and professional workers face high rates of unemployment and underemployment. International trade policies have African countries competing for multinational corporation investment by ensuring an underpaid labor force with no unions and few benefits. This race to the bottom, as is true for much of the rest of the less developed world, drives unregulated capitalism on the African continent.

With the population of Africa quadrupling since 1950, there has been enormous population pressure throughout much of the continent. While AIDS alleviates population growth rates, it actually makes things much worse. For example, it significantly worsens the dependency ratio (the proportion of the young and elderly population who are economically dependent upon gainfully employed adults). AIDS disproportionately kills adults who are in their most economically productive years. As a result, millions of AIDS orphans put a severe strain on the African extended family. While the extended family (aunts, uncles, grandparents, cousins—not just the immediate or nuclear family) has been very resilient throughout Africa in absorbing the problems in the past, AIDS creates a unique burden in which grandparents often are responsible for the many children of several of their children who have died from the disease. Increasingly, many children in Africa are finding that they must fend for themselves. Older children are often made responsible for their younger siblings.

In most African nations, the health infrastructure is not equipped to deal with the AIDS crisis, which diverts funds and attention away from other health concerns. The poor, who comprise the vast majority of the population, are least able to cope.

The epidemic is affecting Africa unevenly. It is most severe in southern Africa, where there are very high adult HIV rates. These include 39 percent in Swaziland, 37 percent in Botswana, 34 percent in Zimbabwe, 29 percent in Lesotho, 22 percent in South Africa, and 21 percent in Namibia. On the other hand, some African nations show very low adult HIV rates. These include 0.8 percent in Senegal, 1.0 percent in Somalia, 1.7 percent in Madagascar, 1.9 percent in Mali, 1.9 percent in Benin, 2.6 percent in Sudan, 3.4 percent in Equatorial Guinea, and 3.9 percent in Angola.

While there have been some successes, in most African nations the epidemic is not controlled by successful HIV interventions. Although condom use has sharply increased, condoms are not used sufficiently to curtail the epidemic. Uganda has shown a sizable drop in HIV seroprevalence since 1986, due to government involvement, initial partner reduction, and, since the early 1990s, condom promotion.

What can be done to prevent the further spread of HIV and to care for and treat persons with HIV, in Africa? What works?

Fear messages promoting abstinence or monogamy do work, but only in the short term. After a few months or years, people tend to ignore fear messages. The evidence we have from two decades of work throughout the world shows that condom promotion, safer sex negotiation skills, peer education intervention programs, involving traditional healers for AIDS prevention, sex work and client education workshops, switching from high-risk (that is, unprotected vaginal and anal sex) to lower-risk (that is, oral sex, interfemoral sex, and mutual masturbation) practices are good medium-term solutions.

The long-term solution for Africa, however, is to change the political economy. Alleviating poverty, reducing income inequality, increasing the status of women, reducing the level of social stigma against persons with HIV/AIDS, eliminating national debt obligations, reducing government corruption, shifting funds from military to social and health needs, and instituting minimum wage regulations, health and other social benefits, and retirement benefits are excellent long-term solutions for not only solving the AIDS crisis in Africa but also solving most of the other social ills currently facing the people of the continent. Medium-term and long-term solutions need to occur simultaneously.

So then, what is being done? The President's Emergency Plan for AIDS

Relief (PEPFAR) is a five-year plan (2004–2008), expected to be renewed again in 2009, to spend $U.S.15 billion (recently increased to $U.S.18.5 billion) for HIV prevention, AIDS treatments, and AIDS care in fifteen countries (twelve of which are in Africa). With PEPFAR, the United States is currently spending half of all the AIDS funding that has been allocated by developed countries for less developed countries. PEPFAR in Africa focuses on Botswana, Côte d'Ivoire, Ethiopia, Kenya, Mozambique, Namibia, Nigeria, Rwanda, South Africa, Tanzania, and Zambia, with only a relatively small allocation to The Global Fund to Fight AIDS, Tuberculosis, and Malaria for the other forty-five African countries and territories.

In reality, PEPFAR actually gives most of the funds to American, not African, organizations—such as the American Red Cross, Catholic Relief Services, Harvard School of Public Health, Columbia University, and others. Indeed, it is possible that the development of PEPFAR and the war in Iraq may have been related. During August 2002, the Bush administration was rapidly moving in the direction of going to war against Iraq at the same time that it was rather cool to the notion of funding HIV/AIDS programs in Africa. Then secretary of state Colin Powell had just returned from Africa, where he all but promised a massive allocation of funds to attack the AIDS crisis in Africa. He was, at that time, reportedly not enthusiastic about the proposed invasion of Iraq. However, in a matter of a few weeks, by early September 2002, the situation had reversed. The Bush administration enthusiastically favored the creation of PEPFAR, while Secretary Powell strongly denied any previous doubts about Iraq.

In any event, the lack of investment by Europe to solve the AIDS crisis in Africa has been baffling. In spite of the numerous speeches by leaders of many European nations about the importance of controlling global AIDS, the pledges for funds have been very meager, and many of those pledges have been later ignored.

The United Nations created The Global Fund to Fight AIDS, Tuberculosis, and Malaria in about 100 countries. The Global Fund formed a "3 by 5 Initiative"—three million people in the less developed world were to receive antiretroviral treatments for AIDS by the end of 2005. But with only 300,000 receiving treatment toward the end of 2005, it was far from reaching its goal. PEPFAR originally planned to have two million people treated for AIDS by 2006. In 2005, the deadline was delayed to the end of 2008.

Why are the Bush administration and the neoconservative members of Congress so generous? What is their agenda? The answer is complex, but it appears that under the guise of "compassionate conservatism," they appear to be trying to use the AIDS crisis as an ideological tool for shaping the values and behaviors of millions of persons in less developed nations.

PEPFAR funding gives precedence to faith-based organizations over other nongovernmental organizations (NGOs). About half of all local organizations being funded through PEPFAR are faith based. During the 1990s, there was a rapid growth of American evangelism and fundamentalist religious thought in much of Africa. PEPFAR will strengthen and fund mostly fundamentalist churches (and perhaps some mosques) that see persons with AIDS as "sinners," further enabling the growth of American evangelical churches in Africa.

Through PEPFAR, abstinence-only programs are given priority funding, and Congress has required that fully one-third of all prevention funds must be used for abstinence-only education. In 2006, this was quietly increased so that two-thirds of all prevention spending went for abstinence-only and fidelity-maintaining education. However, abstinence-only programs have been proven to be the least effective prevention method in several research studies. At best, they do not work; at worst, they lead to more HIV and other sexually transmitted infections by not teaching young people how to use a condom and practice safer sex if and when they do become sexually active.

While abstinence is the Bush administration's answer for how to control premarital sex, monogamy and "partner reduction" are the administration's answers for how to control extramarital sex. When pressed, however, "partner reduction" is simply code for monogamy. As a result, funds for condom promotion are being reduced as a proportion of the total prevention spending, and it is already more difficult for many Africans to find and buy low-cost condoms. Messages about the use of condoms are intentionally stressing inaccurate statements that condoms are ineffective in HIV prevention. In Uganda during 2005, this created an artificial condom shortage, which is likely to reverse the success in lowering the HIV seroprevalence since the early 1990s in that country and lead to an increase in the HIV prevalence rates there. Preliminary data already show an increase in the HIV rate in Uganda.

The first head of PEPFAR, Randall Tobias, was the former CEO of a major pharmaceutical firm. Not surprisingly, PEPFAR required in 2004 that all antiretroviral drugs purchased be American brand-name, rather than generic, drugs. However, the World Health Organization (WHO) has established that the generic drugs work just as well and are substantially less expensive. Fewer persons with AIDS will be helped as a consequence of the

PEPFAR requirements limiting the use of generic medications. By the end of 2005, PEPFAR began allowing the purchase of generic drugs. However, by early 2007 most of the funds for drugs dispensed by PEPFAR were still for brand-name American drugs.

Recipients of PEPFAR funds are now required to sign a statement that they are opposed to sex work and will not use these funds to support sex workers. But sex work is legal in several, mostly Francophone, African nations. As a matter of fact, some NGOs target sex workers for assistance. As a high-risk group, sex workers and their clients need to be a primary focus for HIV prevention, and for assistance if HIV positive.

Some neoconservative members of Congress and the White House director of National Drug Control Policy in 2005 advocated that PEPFAR also prohibit any assistance to recreational injecting drug users (IDUs), and especially to needle exchange programs. While there are relatively few recreational IDUs in most of Africa, this policy would ensure that they would not receive any harm reduction interventions.

Scientists, including some anthropologists, have been appointed to panels based upon their support of the neoconservative agenda on AIDS, or denied promotions based upon their lack of support. Policy in the Bush administration is often based upon political ideology rather than empirical scientific evidence.

The Bush administration policy has substantially cut funding for the Global Fund, while creating a parallel program (PEPFAR) that would promote religious Right/neoconservative values and practices. However, one neoconservative former senator (Pennsylvania senator Rick Santorum) had supported an increase in U.S. funds to the Global Fund—from $U.S.300 million to $U.S.800 million per year. Certainly, this change is unanticipated and perplexing. Though his motives were unclear, it is possible that by "buying out" the Global Fund, one could control it, and thus extend PEPFAR/neoconservative/religious Right policy to the Global Fund as well. The largest donor to the Global Fund would likely have the most say as to how the programs are conducted.

What happens over the next few years at PEPFAR and the Global Fund will shape the direction not only of HIV/AIDS in Africa for many years to come but also politics, values, and human behavior in Africa. Clearly, this massive multibillion dollar intervention into the lives of most Africans needs to be closely watched and carefully evaluated. We need to be wary of the generosity of PEPFAR, while demanding greater generosity from other funding sources.

Anthropologists, then, need to take an activist role in not just understanding the social and biosocial dimensions of HIV/AIDS in Africa, but in working together with the people of Africa to move the continent in the right direction. European nations must be convinced that this is an ideological struggle and that only a huge financial investment at this time can save Africa from the conservative strings attached to PEPFAR funding. Only Europe can bring in the condoms that PEPFAR takes away. Only Europe can ensure that funding is available for high-risk populations, such as sex workers, men who have sex with men, and IDUs. Only Europe can fund antiretroviral medications for all of Africa, not just the PEPFAR-funded nations, and achieve this with generic medications.

Make no mistake: this is an ideological struggle, between secularism and religious fundamentalism, between progressivism and neoconservatism, between empirical science and magical thinking, between socially responsible capitalism and unregulated capitalism, between a people-first policy and the large vested interests—perhaps the most important one of the twenty-first century. Taking a holistic view, a multidimensional cultural understanding, and an empirically based awareness of what works and what does not work, anthropologists, together with the peoples of Africa, can forge an alliance to reduce the scourge of this devastating epidemic, while helping to build a new Africa based in African values, and a promise of a magnificent future for all Africans.

Contributors

Douglas A. Feldman is a professor of anthropology at SUNY Brockport near Rochester, New York. He served as a senior consultant with the Centers for Disease Control and Prevention in Atlanta, and as a consultant with the University of Rochester School of Medicine's AIDS Vaccine Unit. He received the Kimball Award for Public Anthropology in 1996 for his work in the area of AIDS and anthropology. He was on the executive board of the Society for Medical Anthropology (SMA), and has served as treasurer of the National Association for the Practice of Anthropology, as a member of the Nominations Committee of the American Anthropological Association (AAA), as founding chair of the SMA AIDS and Anthropology Research Group, as founding co-chair of the AAA Task Force on AIDS, and as a member of HIV/AIDS advisory committees of the Institute of Medicine, National Academy of Sciences. He has previously served as a professor at Nova Southeastern University, as research associate professor at the University of Miami School of Medicine, and as founding executive director of the AIDS Center of Queens County in New York City.

He was one of the first anthropologists to conduct research on AIDS among gay men in the United States in 1982, and the first anthropologist to do AIDS research in Africa (Rwanda, 1985). He has continued to do funded HIV/AIDS research in Zambia, Senegal, and Uganda, and among gay men in the United States over the years.

Stella Babalola is senior research officer at the Johns Hopkins University Center for Communication Programs. She has conducted research in the areas of positive deviance, adolescent sexual attitudes and behaviors, access to care and support systems among people living with HIV/AIDS, women's empowerment, and the effects of communication programs.

Dr. K. Sridutt Baboo, physician, is an associate professor in the Department of Community Medicine at the University of Zambia School of Medicine in Lusaka, Zambia.

The late Dr. Ganapati Bhat, physician, was a professor and chair of the Department of Paediatrics and Child Health at the University of Zambia

School of Medicine in Lusaka, Zambia. He passed away during the cowriting of his chapter.

Judith E. Brown, anthropologist, has worked in developing nations for the past thirty years, including Liberia, Tunisia, the Democratic Republic of the Congo, Cameroon, Haiti, and Kenya. Her research interests include women's insertion of traditional intravaginal products and male circumcision.

Dr. Ndashi W. Chitalu, physician, is a professor in the Department of Community Medicine at the University of Zambia School of Medicine in Lusaka, and a former member of the Zambian parliament.

Ariela Eshel is a medical anthropologist whose research interests include illness etiology and social support in religious communities, infectious disease, and HIV/AIDS. She is currently employed by the Centers for Disease Control and Prevention in Atlanta.

Orlando Gómez-Marín is a professor and biostatistician in the Department of Epidemiology and Public Health at the University of Miami School of Medicine in Miami, Florida.

Jeffrey Johnson, anthropologist, is a professor at East Carolina State University. He has a strong interest in quantitative research methods in anthropology.

Carl Kendall, anthropologist, is acting chair of the Department of International Health and Development at Tulane University. He is a frequent consultant to HIV/AIDS and child health programs in Latin America, Africa, and Asia.

Ruth Kornfield, anthropologist, is a consultant based in Rwanda. She conducts formative and evaluation research to inform HIV/AIDS prevention and family planning promotion programs throughout Africa and in Asia.

Richard B. Lee is a professor of anthropology at the University of Toronto. Since the 1960s, he has been conducting ethnographic research among the Ju/'hoansi of Botswana and Namibia. He has been actively involved in social research and training on HIV/AIDS in Africa since 1996.

Kim Longfield is a senior researcher for Central and Southeast Asia at Population Services International in Bangkok, Thailand. She conducted her doctoral dissertation research in Africa through Tulane University.

Robert Lorway is a Ph.D. candidate in anthropology at the University of Toronto in Canada. His recent doctoral work in Namibia has explored the intersections among sexuality, gender power relations, national identity, and HIV vulnerability.

Kate Macintyre is an associate professor in the Department of International Health and Development at Tulane University School of Public Health and Tropical Medicine. She has had more than fifteen years of professional international experience in program management, health policy, reproductive health, HIV/AIDS, and behavior change programming for infectious diseases.

Susan McCombie is a medical anthropologist with research interests in international health and infectious disease. She has been involved in health research in Africa, the United States, and Central Asia, and currently teaches at Georgia State University.

Peggy O'Hara Murdock, professor of public health education at Middle Tennessee State University, has wide research and publication experience in HIV/AIDS prevention intervention design and peer education program development in Zambia, South Africa, and the United States.

Dr. Kasonde Mwinga, physician, is the National Professional Officer with the World Health Organization in Zambia.

Elizabeth Onjoro Meassick, anthropologist, works for the Centers for Disease Control and Prevention Global AIDS Program in Zambia, where she is the associate chief of behavioral science. Previously, she was the Global AIDS Coordinator of the U.S. Department of State, and a Fellow at the Presidential Advisory Council on HIV/AIDS in the U.S. Department of Health and Human Services Office of HIV/AIDS Policy.

Eleanor Preston-Whyte, anthropologist, is a research professor in the School of Development Studies and coheads the Centre for HIV/AIDS Networking

(HIVAN) at the University of KwaZulu-Natal in South Africa. Her interests include HIV/AIDS, population studies, the dynamics of family and kinship structures, adolescent sexuality, and reproductive health.

Charles B. Rwabukwali is an associate professor in the Department of Sociology and the deputy dean of the Faculty of Social Sciences at Makerere University in Kampala, Uganda. His research interests are in health resources utilization, socioeconomic impacts of HIV/AIDS, and fertility regulation research.

Anthony Simpson taught English and African history for nearly twenty years at a Zambian boy's boarding school, which became the focus of his doctoral research. Currently lecturing in social anthropology at the University of Manchester, England, he is completing a book on men and masculinities in the time of HIV/AIDS in Zambia.

Ida Susser is a professor of anthropology at the CUNY Graduate Center in New York City. Her current research, funded by the MacArthur Foundation, examines global policies and women's mobilization concerning HIV/AIDS.

Teresa Swezey is a research health sociologist at RTI International. Her area of specialization is gender, health, and development, with an emphasis on the gendered aspects of the HIV/AIDS epidemic in sub-Saharan Africa.

Michele Teitelbaum, anthropologist, is a senior health services specialist at RTI International. Her international work is focused on development of health care systems in lower- and middle-income countries and the integration of HIV/AIDS and reproductive health services into those systems.

Index